Current Concepts in Hernia Surgery

Editor

AJITA S. PRABHU

SURGICAL CLINICS OF NORTH AMERICA

www.surgical.theclinics.com

Consulting Editor
RONALD F. MARTIN

June 2018 • Volume 98 • Number 3

ELSEVIER

1600 John F. Kennedy Boulevard • Suite 1800 • Philadelphia, Pennsylvania, 19103-2899

http://www.surgical.theclinics.com

SURGICAL CLINICS OF NORTH AMERICA Volume 98, Number 3
June 2018 ISSN 0039–6109, ISBN-13: 978-0-323-58422-7

Editor: John Vassallo, j.vassallo@elsevier.com
Developmental Editor: Meredith Madeira

Surgical Clinics of North America (ISSN 0039–6109) is published bimonthly by Elsevier Inc., 360 Park Avenue South, New York, NY 10010-1710. Months of publication are February, April, June, August, October, and December. Business and Editorial Offices: 1600 John F. Kennedy Blvd., Suite 1800, Philadelphia, PA 19103-2899. Periodicals postage paid at New York, NY and additional mailing offices. Subscription prices are $350.00 per year for US individuals, $802.00 per year for US institutions, $100.00 per year for US students and residents, $420.00 per year for Canadian individuals, $1015.00 per year for Canadian institutions, $475.00 for international individuals, $1015.00 per year for international institutions and $225.00 per year for Canadian and foreign students/residents. To receive student/resident rate, orders must be accompanied by name of affiliated institution, date of term, and the *signature* of program/residency coordinator on institution letterhead. Orders will be billed at individual rate until proof of status is received. Foreign air speed delivery is included in all *Clinics* subscription prices. All prices are subject to change without notice. POSTMASTER: Send address changes to *Surgical Clinics*, Elsevier Health Sciences Division, Subscription Customer Service, 3251 Riverport Lane, Maryland Heights, MO 63043. **Customer Service (orders, claims, online, change of address): Telephone: 1-800-654-2452 (U.S. and Canada); 314-447-8871 (outside U.S. and Canada). Fax: 314-447-8029. E-mail: journalscustomerservice-usa@elsevier.com (for print support); journalsonline support-usa@elsevier.com (for online support).**

Reprints. For copies of 100 or more, of articles in this publication, please contact the Commercial Reprints Department, Elsevier Inc., 360 Park Avenue South, New York, New York 10010-1710. Tel. 212-633-3874, Fax: 212-633-3820, E-mail: reprints@elsevier.com.

The Surgical Clinics of North America is also published in Spanish by McGraw-Hill Interamericana Editores S.A., P.O. Box 5-237 06500 Mexico D.F. Mexico; and in Portuguese by Interlivros Edicoes Ltda., Rua Comandante Coelho 1085, CEP 21250, Rio de Janeiro, Brazil; and in Greek by Paschalidis Medical Publications, Athens Greece.

The Surgical Clinics of North America is covered in *MEDLINE/PubMed (Index Medicus)*, *EMBASE/Excerpta Medica, Current Contents/Clinical Medicine, Current Contents/Life Sciences, Science Citation Index*, and *ISI/BIOMED*.

Contributors

CONSULTING EDITOR

RONALD F. MARTIN, MD, FACS
Colonel (ret.), United States Army Reserve, Department of Surgery, York Hospital, York, Maine

EDITOR

AJITA S. PRABHU, MD, FACS
Assistant Professor of Surgery, Comprehensive Hernia Center, Cleveland Clinic, Cleveland, Ohio

AUTHORS

HEMASAT ALKHATIB, MD
Research Fellow, Comprehensive Hernia Center, Digestive Disease and Surgery Institute, Cleveland Clinic, Cleveland, Ohio

PAUL W. APPLEBY, MD
Surgical Resident, Department of Surgery, New Hanover Regional Medical Center, South East Area Health Education Center, Wilmington, North Carolina

LUCAS R. BEFFA, MD
Division of Minimal Access and Bariatric Surgery, Greenville Health System, University of South Carolina School of Medicine – Greenville, Greenville, South Carolina

ALFREDO M. CARBONELL, DO
Vice Chairman of Academic Affairs, Professor of Surgery, Division of Minimal Access and Bariatric Surgery, Greenville Health System, University of South Carolina School of Medicine – Greenville, Greenville, South Carolina

DAVID C. CHEN, MD
Associate Professor of Clinical Surgery, Lichtenstein Amid Hernia Clinic, Department of Surgery, University of California at Los Angeles, Los Angeles, California

DEEPA V. CHERLA, MD
Department of General Surgery, Cleveland Clinic, Cleveland, Ohio

JENNIFER COLVIN, MD
Department of General Surgery, Cleveland Clinic, Cleveland, Ohio

FABIOLA A. ENRIQUEZ, BA
Department of Surgery, Division of Plastic Surgery, University of Pennsylvania, Philadelphia, Pennsylvania

JOHN P. FISCHER, MD, MPH
Assistant Professor, Department of Surgery, Division of Plastic Surgery, University of Pennsylvania, Philadelphia, Pennsylvania

JACOB A. GREENBERG, MD, EdM
Associate Professor of Surgery, University of Wisconsin–Madison, School of Medicine and Public Health, Madison, Wisconsin

WILLIAM W. HOPE, MD, FACS
Director of Surgical Education, Assistant Professor, Department of Surgery, New Hanover Regional Medical Center, South East Area Health Education Center, Wilmington, North Carolina

CHARLOTTE M. HORNE, MD
The Cleveland Clinic, Cleveland, Ohio

Q. LINA HU, MD
Resident Physician, Department of Surgery, University of California at Los Angeles, Los Angeles, California

KYLE L. KLEPPE, MD
Instructor of Surgery, University of Wisconsin–Madison, School of Medicine and Public Health, Madison, Wisconsin

DAVID M. KRPATA, MD
Assistant Professor of Surgery, Comprehensive Hernia Center, Cleveland Clinic, Cleveland, Ohio

MICHAEL LOVE, MD
Department of Surgery, Greenville Health System, Greenville, South Carolina

ALYSSA L. MARGIOTTA, MS
University of South Carolina School of Medicine – Greenville, Greenville, South Carolina

TASHA A. MARTIN, MD
Surgical Resident, Department of Surgery, New Hanover Regional Medical Center, South East Area Health Education Center, Wilmington, North Carolina

BRENT D. MATTHEWS, MD
Professor and Chair, Department of Surgery, Carolinas Medical Center, Charlotte, North Carolina

CHARLES A. MESSA IV, BS
Department of Surgery, Division of Plastic Surgery, University of Pennsylvania, Philadelphia, Pennsylvania

HEIDI J. MILLER, MD, MPH
Assistant Professor, Department of Surgery, University of New Mexico, Sandoval Regional Medical Center, Rio Rancho, New Mexico

LAUREN PATON, MD
Assistant Professor, Department of Surgery, Carolinas Medical Center, Charlotte, North Carolina

CLAYTON C. PETRO, MD
Department of Surgery, Cleveland Clinic, Cleveland, Ohio

BENJAMIN POULOSE, MD, MPH, FACS
Division of General Surgery, Vanderbilt University Medical Center, Nashville, Tennessee

AJITA S. PRABHU, MD, FACS
Assistant Professor of Surgery, Comprehensive Hernia Center, Cleveland Clinic, Cleveland, Ohio

IRFAN A. RHEMTULLA, MD, MS
Department of Surgery, Division of Plastic Surgery, University of Pennsylvania, Philadelphia, Pennsylvania

MICHAEL J. ROSEN, MD, FACS
Professor of Surgery, Cleveland Clinic Lerner College of Medicine, Cleveland Clinic, Cleveland, Ohio

STEVEN ROSENBLATT, MD, FACS
Assistant Professor, Department of General Surgery, Cleveland Clinic Lerner College of Medicine, Cleveland Clinic, Cleveland, Ohio

LUCIANO TASTALDI, MD
Research Fellow, Comprehensive Hernia Center, Digestive Disease and Surgery Institute, Cleveland Clinic, Cleveland, Ohio

SHIRIN TOWFIGH, MD, FACS
President, Beverly Hills Hernia Center, Beverly Hills, California

JEREMY A. WARREN, MD, FACS
Divisions of Minimal Access and Bariatric Surgery, Assistant Professor, Department of Surgery, Greenville Health System, University of South Carolina School of Medicine Greenville, Greenville, South Carolina

Contents

Hernia Repair: Measures of Success and Perioperative Considerations

> More research is needed with regards to gender, race, and socioeconomic status on ventral hernia presentation, management, and outcomes. The role of culture and geography in hernia-related health care remains unknown. Currently existing nationwide registries have thus far yielded at best a modest overview of disparities in hernia care. The significant variation in care relative to gender, race, and socioeconomic status suggests that there is room for improvement in providing consistent care for patients with hernias.

> With growing pressures to formulate easily interpreted quality metrics, potential pitfalls exist that deleteriously affect the ultimate outcome of patients. This article defines what quality means in hernia surgery, how it is measured, who measures it, and how it is reported. Key governmental organizations responsible are highlighted. Although striving for high quality seems relatively straightforward, it is a challenge to account for all variables. Most definitions of quality are based on products and derived from minimum standards. This transition to basing it on health care delivery is ongoing, challenging, and incredibly important for the future of patients.

> Hernia repair is one of the most common operations performed by surgeons; however, there is neither consistency in practice nor broadly accepted guidelines to advise best practices. Hernia programs can help shape guidelines through voluntary participation, inclusion, continuous quality improvement, education, and research by all stakeholders involved in hernia surgery at the institution. Once established, a hernia

program can improve the delivery of care and outcomes of patients with hernia, leading to added value for the institution and health care system.

Prior publications of the *Surgical Clinics of North America* have highlighted the technical challenges of abdominal wall reconstruction. This article provides an update on synthetic, biologic, and biosynthetic mesh research since the 2013 *Surgical Clinics of North America* hernia publication and highlights the future of mesh research. This update features research that has been conducted since the prior publication to guide surgeons to choose the best and most appropriate mesh for their patients.

Incisional and parastomal hernias are a cause of significant morbidity and have a substantial effect on quality of life and economic costs for patients and hospital systems. Although many aspects of abdominal hernias are understood, prevention is a feature that is still being realized. This article reviews the current literature and determines the utility of prophylactic mesh placement in the prevention of incisional and parastomal hernias.

This article reviews the literature that supports routine expectations for smoking cessation; weight loss; diabetic, nutritional, or metabolic optimization; and decolonization techniques before ventral hernia repair. These methods diminish postoperative complications. In an era of value-centric care, an upfront investment in patient optimization can improve the quality of the repair by reducing wound morbidity and hernia recurrence, naturally translating to a reduction in cost. The adoption of these practices and further study aimed at identifying other effective optimization techniques are encouraged.

Enhanced recovery after surgery (ERAS) protocols are spreading throughout various fields in surgery. ERAS protocols involve the implementation of evidence-based elements of care that are applied throughout the entire perioperative period to facilitate optimal recovery for the patient. ERAS protocols have been associated with improvements in quality of care, patient-reported and operative outcomes, and patient safety as well as reductions in cost. Thus, ERAS protocols have led to an overall improvement in health care value for the patient and the health care system.

Incisional and Parastomal Hernias

Flank and lumbar hernias are challenging because of their rarity and anatomic location. Several challenges exist when approaching these specific abdominal wall defects, including location, innervation of the lateral abdominal wall musculature, and their proximity to bony landmarks. These hernias are confined by the costal margin, spine, and pelvic brim, which makes closure of the defect, including mesh placement, difficult. This article discusses the anatomy of lumbar and flank hernias, the various etiologies for these hernias, and the procedural steps for open and robotic preperitoneal approaches. The available clinical evidence regarding outcomes for various repair techniques is also reviewed.

Inguinal Hernias

The success of an inguinal hernia repair is defined by the permanence of the operation while creating the fewest complications at minimal cost and allowing patients an early return to activity. This success relies and depends on the surgeon's knowledge and understanding of groin anatomy and physiology. This article reviews relevant anatomy to inguinal hernia repair and technical steps to open tissue and mesh repairs as well as minimally invasive approaches.

Open inguinal hernia approaches are varied. The best studied approaches are reviewed herein. The common factor among them is the imperative anatomy knowledge of the surgeon. This knowledge is key to improved outcomes. A tailored approach is best to determine which open technique, if any, is most appropriate for the patient. Although the anterior mesh approach is the most commonly applied, there is support in using the posterior approach or a tissue repair for subsets of patients, such as women.

Both the transabdominal preperitoneal approach and the total extraperitoneal approach to inguinal hernias provide an effective means of repairing inguinal hernias. The robotic platform can be used and may help to decrease immediate postoperative pain; however, as this is a fairly new technique, more research will help further determine long-term outcomes. In all methods of fixation, we ensure adequate fixation medially with tacks placed on the Cooper ligament. Awareness of the nerves and vessels helps to guide dissection as well as prevent inadvertent injury during mesh fixation.

Approach to the Patient with Chronic Groin Pain   651

Q. Lina Hu and David C. Chen

Chronic postoperative inguinal pain has become a primary outcome parameter after elective inguinal hernia repair with significant consequences affecting patient productivity, employment, and quality of life. A systematic and thorough preoperative evaluation is important to identify the etiologies and types of pain. Owing to the complex nature of chronic pain, a multimodal and multidisciplinary treatment approach is recommended. Patients with chronic pain refractory to conservative measures may be considered for surgical intervention. Triple neurectomy remains the most definitive and accepted remedial operation performed and provides effective relief in the majority of patients.

SURGICAL CLINICS
OF NORTH AMERICA

ISSUE OF RELATED INTEREST:

Advances in Surgery, 2017 (Vol. 51)
John L. Cameron, *Editor-in-Chief*
Available at: http://www.advancessurgery.com/

THE CLINICS ARE AVAILABLE ONLINE!
Access your subscription at:
www.theclinics.com

Foreword

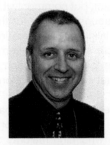

Ronald F. Martin, MD, FACS
Consulting Editor

Some surgical problems are conceptually difficult but technically straightforward. Some problems are conceptually straightforward though technically challenging. There are some surgical problems that have the illusory appearance of being conceptually straightforward and also technically straightforward though they are, in fact, frequently neither. Hernia surgery is a classic example of this illusion.

The technical description of an abdominal hernia, the true variety, not including the sliders, that I was taught in my early days is a defect in the abdominal parieties through which passes a mesothelial-lined sac and its contents. I learned it from a pediatric surgeon who taught me many other surgical life lessons that have formed the very foundation of my career and practice. As with most things he taught me, this definition has been useful because it is simple, direct, and easy to remember when you are tired. Also, it helps one reduce the likelihood of making mistakes by losing situational awareness. At its core, the above-mentioned definition provides us with pretty much everything we need to know about abdominal hernias: there is a defect and there is a sac with stuff in it. What could be simpler? From this, one can ascertain how to fix all such hernias. One simply has to put the stuff and the sac (maybe) back on the right side of the abdominal wall and make the defect such that no stuff will improperly go back through it. Again, what could be simpler? Well, as it turns out, lots of things could be simpler.

In the Army, we have a maxim that no battle plan survives contact with the enemy. We still make plans and prepare and prepare and prepare. Yet, we are always cognizant that we will most likely modify our plans on the fly. This is probably true for hernia surgery as well. One might note that I did actually write "hernia surgery" rather than "hernia operation," since many of the issues that cause hernia repair to become problematic begin long before the operation. Hernia operations can include a range of procedures from relatively straightforward operations to cases that make even the most ardent of surgeons seriously consider instant retirement. Any surgeon who hasn't encountered a hernia repair that has caused her/him to reconsider career choice hasn't done enough of them.

Surg Clin N Am 98 (2018) xiii–xv
https://doi.org/10.1016/j.suc.2018.03.002
0039-6109/18/© 2018 Published by Elsevier Inc.

surgical.theclinics.com

One of the cruel ironies of the really difficult hernia repairs is that they are frequently the "re-do" operations. The ironic bit being the surgeon doing the follow-up repair is rarely the surgeon who did the original repair. Sometimes that is because the patient has moved, the surgeon has retired, or some other such constraint, but commonly it is because the patient lost confidence in the index surgeon and sought another for the re-repair. If you happen to make a substantial portion of your living out of operating on others' complications, you will no doubt feel this irony more acutely than some others. One other thing you may learn over time from being the follow-on surgeon is that the patterns of failure so often lead back to some corner that someone cut along the way that initiates a failure or series of failures.

If one wants to become a good hernia surgeon, one has to treat every hernia repair as if it has to last for life (of the patient, that is). While there are some rare occasions where a staged approach to hernia repair is required, the overwhelming majority of cases will be best served by expertly executing the best repair for definitive success at the correct time. This will invariably involve more than simply being technically capable of performing an operation but will require understanding the patient-substrate one has to work with and how to get a patient optimized for the correct operation under the most ideal circumstances possible. Sometimes the most important aspect of a hernia repair has nothing to do with the procedure itself but requires the patient address issues of inadequate or excess weight, tobacco addiction, or medical fitness. When the clinical situation permits, optimally improving these other patient factors is possibly more likely to contribute to long-term success of the hernia repair more than the operation itself. In addition, improving these other medical factors may do more to benefit the patient's overall quality of life and longevity than any hernia repair may. Parenthetically, when I have been involved with patients who we have worked with to decrease excess body weight in order to improve success with, say, a complex component separation, invariably the patients have been far more verbal in their appreciation with the help with weight loss than the hernia repair itself.

Nothing above should suggest to the reader that the technical component of hernia management should be considered an easy thing. Learning the technical aspects of hernia repair is more challenging than many people give it credit for. For what it is worth, teaching hernia repair is even harder than learning it. Hernia repairs are frequently considered "junior resident cases" though I have seen plenty of chief residents struggle with primary inguinal hernia repairs. As well, I have seen far more junior staff surgeons vexed by hernia repairs, particularly groin hernias, than by more complicated intra-abdominal procedures. Also, for some reason, people seem more reluctant to ask for an extra set of eyes for a difficult hernia repair than they might for a difficult "larger" operation.

Dr Prabhu, our Guest Editor for this issue, and I were both trained in large part by the same surgeons, including the pediatric surgeon mentioned above, Dr Albert W. Dibbins, who taught me how to think about hernia as a process. As with many other things, the real lesson is to understand the problem at its core principles. Once that has happened, testing the possibilities of options and expanding the universe of new treatments become possible. Conversely, developing solutions without understanding the core problem more often than not produces more problems. We must do what we can to assure that our solutions solve our problems rather than try to bend our problems to justify our solutions.

In the hopes that we can all better understand what we need to know about hernia repair, our options, and how to keep from adding more links to the error chain that sometimes occurs, we are fortunate to have this issue by Dr Prabhu and her colleagues. It is a comprehensive look at what we need to know to understand the fullest range of our options and also to understand how the problem of hernia affects patients and society. We are deeply indebted to them for their phenomenal effort. Whether one incorporates hernia repairs as a substantial portion of their practice or whether one simply makes incisions that could be the precursors of a hernia, the material in this issue is of profound importance to you. As always, we welcome your feedback.

Ronald F. Martin, MD, FACS
Colonel (ret.), United States Army Reserve
Department of Surgery
York Hospital
16 Hospital Drive, Suite A
York, ME 03909, USA

E-mail address:
rmartin@yorkhospital.com

Preface

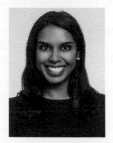

Ajita S. Prabhu, MD, FACS
Editor

Hernia remains one of the most common general surgery diseases in the United States, and yet we still know surprisingly little about the care of these patients. What is the best operation for which patient? Should we use a piece of mesh, and if so, which one? Is there a way to prevent hernias? What about the treatment of recurrences and complications? The list of questions seems unending, while the incidence of hernia continues to increase. In some ways, this has always been the case, ever since Theodor Bilroth said, "If we could artificially produce tissues of the density and toughness of fascia and tendon, the secret of the radical cure of hernia would be discovered." Still, other things are changing. As a society, our health care system has shifted to a value-based priority. If the value equation is defined as outcomes that matter to patients and stakeholders divided by cost, we have to begin to prioritize hernia outcomes, including recurrences, complications, and patient quality of life. In short, we need to be able to evaluate our patients and optimize them for surgery, offer them the best operation we can, and get them through the process with the best possible outcomes. This seems like it should be a simple thing! And yet, here we are.

Since the last Hernia issue of *Surgical Clinics of North America*, there has been a much greater focus on patient experience and health care disparity. There is also a much greater emphasis on evaluating physician performance based upon metrics. This issue of *Surgical Clinics of North America* attempts to get at some of these seismic shifts we are seeing in health care and how they relate to the care of patients with hernias. We delve a little bit into why it's so hard to answer some of the questions I mention above, epidemiology of hernia disease and disparity in hernia care, quality measures, building a hernia program, and getting patients ready for surgery. There is an update on mesh and biomaterials, to inform the reader of exactly what is on the shelf as far as devices go. And then we shift gears into technique and operative approaches to many commonly seen clinical scenarios in hernias of all types. Most of all, I hope that the readers of this issue will benefit as much as I have from the wealth of knowledge contained in these pages, written by some of the most prolific hernia surgeons in America. Each author was chosen for his or her experience and expertise, and I thank them for their generosity with their time and efforts for this endeavor. I am

Surg Clin N Am 98 (2018) xvii–xviii
https://doi.org/10.1016/j.suc.2018.03.001
0039-6109/18/© 2018 Published by Elsevier Inc.

honored to have the opportunity to put this issue together and am hopeful that it will serve as a reference for those in seek of knowledge about hernias for years to come.

Ajita S. Prabhu, MD, FACS
Cleveland Clinic
Cleveland Clinic Comprehensive Hernia Center
9500 Euclid Avenue
Cleveland, OH 44195, USA

E-mail address:
PRABHUA@ccf.org

Epidemiology and Disparities in Care

The Impact of Socioeconomic Status, Gender, and Race on the Presentation, Management, and Outcomes of Patients Undergoing Ventral Hernia Repair

Deepa V. Cherla, MD[a],*, Benjamin Poulose, MD, MPH[b],
Ajita S. Prabhu, MD[a]

KEYWORDS

- Ventral hernia repair • Epidemiology • Disparities in care • Socioeconomic status
- Gender • Race

KEY POINTS

- Moro rocoaroh is needed with regards to gender, race, and socioeconomic status on ventral hernia presentation, management, and outcomes.
- The role of culture and geography in hernia-related health care remains unknown.
- Currently existing nationwide registries have thus far yielded at best a modest overview of disparities in hernia care.
- The significant variation in care relative to gender, race and socioeconomic status suggests that there is room for improvement in providing consistent care for patients with hernias.

The management of hernia disease remains one of the most common surgical problems faced by health care providers across the world. Inguinal hernias are the most common and make up about 3 out of every 4 abdominal wall hernias.[1] Inguinal hernia repair rates range from 10 repairs per 100,000 population in the United Kingdom to 28

Conflicts of Interest: Dr D.V. Cherla has nothing to disclose. Dr A.S. Prabhu receives honoraria from Bard Davol and Medtronic, he serves on the advisory board at Medtronic, and he receives research support from Intuitive Surgical (CRG:09022017). Dr B. Poulose is an employee of the Americas Hernia Society Quality Collaborative, has received consulting fees from Pfizer Medical and Ariste Medical, and has received research grant support from Bard-Davol.
a General Surgery Department, Cleveland Clinic, 9500 Euclid Avenue, Cleveland, OH 44195, USA; b Division of General Surgery, Vanderbilt University Medical Center, 1161 21st Avenue S Medical Center N D-503, Nashville, TN 37232, USA
* Corresponding author.
E-mail address: cherlad@ccf.org

Surg Clin N Am 98 (2018) 431–440
https://doi.org/10.1016/j.suc.2018.02.003
0039-6109/18/© 2018 Elsevier Inc. All rights reserved.

surgical.theclinics.com

repairs per 100,000 population in the United States.[2] The incidence of inguinal repair increases with age in men, who comprise about 95% of primary care encounters.[1]

Ventral hernia represents a heterogeneous subtype of hernia disease that includes primary hernias (epigastric, umbilical, lumbar, Spigelian) and acquired hernias (incisional and parastomal). In 2006, the estimated number of ventral hernia repairs treated in both inpatient and outpatient settings was 348,000 in the United States.[3] Assuming a linear increase with time, it is likely that nearly 500,000 ventral hernia repairs are performed annually in the United States alone. Incisional hernia is unique in that it affects all surgical subspecialties where an incision is made directly into or near the abdomen. In the cancer population alone, 41% of patients developed an incisional hernia up to 2 years after resection.[4] Even laparoscopic or laparoscopic-assisted approaches resulted in hernia formation rates of up to 23%. With an aging population exposed to a higher cumulative risk of developing incisional hernia after both minimally invasive and open surgery, the management of ventral hernia will continue to be a central focus of surgical disease.

Health care disparities are defined as differing rates of health, medical care, morbidity, and mortality among patients of varying demographic groups.[5,6] Specifically, disparities in surgical health care have been identified as a problem because they can lead to poorer functional outcomes, prolonged rehabilitation and recovery times, and lower quality of life, particularly for disadvantaged population groups,[6] and therefore have been targeted by the federal government and the Affordable Care Act for elimination.[7] As such, attention from the American College of Surgeons, the Institute of Medicine, the American Medical Association, and the National Institutes of Health has recently been directed toward developing a national surgical disparities research agenda and appropriate funding priorities.[5,8]

Care for patients with hernias is likely an important area in which to study health care disparity, particularly because more than 350,000 hernias are repaired annually in the United States, at an estimated cost of $3.2 billion.[3] Given the scope of surgical care devoted to this disease process, the elimination of disparity in hernia care could potentially result in better postoperative outcomes (specifically with regard to hernia recurrence) and also a significant savings in health care costs. Still, there is a dearth of literature that can truly determine and/or address the underlying issues associated with hernia care. Indeed, other specialty areas of medical care have identified many systems issues that may conspire to ultimately result in disparate care. Among these are patient-related factors (disproportionate access to care, lack of health literacy, educational status, patient health beliefs, and language barriers), physician factors (unintentional racial biases, poor provider understanding of cultural expectations, physician race, and communication skills/style), and health care system factors (time constraints, lack of education).[9] Surgical and technical specialties may also include additional variables that are less easily quantifiable and yet may affect the ultimate care provided, such as surgeon's technical abilities and number of years in practice. Not surprisingly, the most robust literature surrounding health care disparity seems to be focused on areas in which the disease processes are well-defined, as are treatment algorithms and classification of outcomes.[10–13]

Despite the common nature of hernia disease and the frequent—and increasing— incidence of herniorrhaphy,[3] our collective knowledge regarding best practices is alarmingly rudimentary and largely driven by anecdote. This problem is likely multifactorial; however, the overarching challenge is the fundamental heterogeneity of hernia disease as an entity. In addition, patient-specific characteristics and comorbidities are difficult to capture, yet still must be taken into consideration when designing treatment algorithms. Further compounding this is a lack of commonly accepted and used hernia staging systems, without which it is nearly impossible to meaningfully assess various approaches and techniques for specific hernia disease. Although several ventral hernia staging and grading systems have been proposed and used in various scenarios,[14–16] to date there is not a universally used system with which to guide the conversation regarding best practices in hernia care.

If the disease is heterogeneous, technical operative approaches used for hernia repair are vastly more so,[17] and often largely depend on surgeon preference in absence of high-level data to aid in decision making. The technical approaches offered may also be limited by surgeon education, in that a given surgeon may not be familiar with all technical approaches and may, therefore, simply offer the operation that they know. Even prosthetic mesh devices, which are ubiquitous in the setting of incisional herniorrhaphy, vary greatly in their basic building materials as well as the methods of engineering. Owing to the proprietary nature of the manufacture of these materials as well as the lack of common strength testing methodology and material weight reporting for meshes, the lack of standardized comparisons between devices adds another layer of complexity that ultimately hampers the determination of recommended devices for various types of hernias. Also, although mesh materials are cleared to come to market through the US Food and Drug Administration's 510K process,[18] the lack of long-term patient follow-up and device surveillance substantially limits our ability to meaningfully assess the performance of these often permanent indwelling devices over time. Given the long-term complications inherent to hernia repair with mesh,[19,20] there is a clear imperative for surgeons and industry stakeholders to develop a better understanding of the behavior of these materials as well as the consequences of their placement.

Although defining the disease process and treatment algorithms is needed to pursue best practice recommendations in hernia care, best practices may also only be determined once the outcomes of interest are clearly defined and collected in a consistent manner. Wound morbidity and hernia recurrence are widely regarded to be the most important outcomes of interest with regard to hernia care. Wound morbidity is very relevant because it seems to confer an increased risk of recurrence,[21] and recurrence itself is suspected to beget further recurrence.[22] Still, substantial variability exists with regard to the nomenclature surrounding wound events after ventral hernia repair. Hernia recurrence rates remain difficult to determine, primarily owing to loss of patients to follow-up over time, as well as the lack of robust datasets that may help to better determine the numerator of recurrences over the denominator of repairs.

Because there is a mounting pressure to provide value in health care,[23] there is a need for increased resources to be directed toward research in hernia care to target potential areas for improvement.[24] One potential avenue that may contribute to progress in this regard is a national hernia registry, which would allow the collection of granular hernia-related data and may help to fill some of the knowledge gaps surrounding hernia disease, particularly with regard to choosing the best technical approaches. In more recent years, the design and implementation of this type of platform has occurred through the Americas Hernia Society Quality Collaborative.[24] Although this platform embraces the concept of continuous quality improvement and is similar to the National Surgical Quality Improvement Program[25] in that it collects clinical data as opposed to administrative data, the Americas Hernia Society Quality Collaborative has the added benefit of including granular hernia-specific technical data that may substantially further the field of hernia study in a manner that was previously unprecedented in the United States. However, unlike the National Surgical Quality Improvement Program, where data extractors are made available as a condition of participation,[25] data are entered by the surgeon for the Americas Hernia Society

Quality Collaborative and, therefore, limited in the number of continuous participants. It is likely that further resources will be necessary to continue to grow this invaluable tool.

Although the current status of knowledge surrounding the care of patients with hernias may seem somewhat austere given the considerations mentioned, there is nevertheless some indication in the current body of literature that hints at the presence of disparity in hernia care. After a thorough review of the existing literature currently available that pertains specifically to hernia surgery, we found multiple publications on this topic. Although the body of literature addressing this has thus far relied on small institutional-specific series or larger national databases lacking detailed clinical information, the findings to date suggest that there is indeed a substantial opportunity to improve hernia care given appropriately allocated resources. Indeed, at least 1 publication by Poulose and colleagues[26] demonstrates a disproportionately increased use of resources for certain populations undergoing ventral hernia repair versus others, suggesting what the authors note as "a very real disparity in the distribution of resources used in the inpatient management of ventral hernia repair." We present an overview of our findings from a thorough literature review regarding disparities in hernia care.

GENDER DISPARITIES IN HERNIA CARE

There are several publications pertaining to gender-related disparity in hernia care. The majority of these suggest a gender disparity in terms of presentation, operative management, and outcomes. Although ventral hernias are thought to occur more frequently in males than in females,[27] female patients may be at an increased risk for acute presentation owing to having hernias that are more likely to incarcerate and/or having poor access to health care.[28,29] In terms of operative management, there is some suggestion of a gender disparity in hernia repair approach for at least umbilical hernia repair. Regarding specifically ventral hernia repair, Colavita and colleagues[30] found no significant difference in rates of laparoscopic versus open ventral hernia repair with mesh by gender following a review of 11,804 cases in the 2009 Nationwide Inpatient Sample (NIS). Funk and colleagues,[31] however, found that on both univariate and multivariate analyses using large data also from the NIS, gender remained significantly associated with laparoscopic versus open umbilical hernia repair (female odds ratio [OR], 0.6; 95% confidence interval [CI], 0.4–0.7).

Gender has also been studied in relation to postoperative outcomes of ventral hernia repair (**Table 1**). Female gender been associated with higher rates of surgical site infection,[32] readmission,[33] and chronic pain,[34] and decreased quality-of-life scores in the immediate postoperative period.[35] Conclusions are mixed regarding recurrence rates (higher[30] and lower[36,37]). Surprisingly, however, male gender has been associated with higher total hospital charges.[26]

Table 1
Gender and outcomes in the ventral hernia repair literature

Author, Year	Odds Ratio	95% Confidence Interval	Outcome(s)
Hornby et al,[36] 2015	Female 3.53	1.39–8.97	42-mo recurrence
Helgstrand et al,[33] 2013	Female 1.7	1.1–2.7	Readmission (after laparoscopic repair)
Simon et al,[38] 2015	Female 0.726	0.697–0.757	Complications
	Female 0.654	0.561–0.762	Mortality
Cox et al,[34] 2016	Female 1.7	1.1–2.7	Chronic pain

RACE DISPARITIES IN HERNIA CARE

Individuals of varying races have been shown to have different rates of emergent presentation of their hernias.[38–40] This observation may be due to differences in socioeconomic status (SES),[39] trust and skepticism in the medical community, and communication barriers with physicians.[38] After controlling for SES, Bowman and colleagues[39] found that black individuals were more likely than white individuals to present with acute hernia complications requiring emergent surgery (11% vs 4%; $P<.01$). Wolf and colleagues[41] retrospectively reviewed 453,161 adults from the 2003 to 2011 NIS and also found that race was an independent predictor of emergent repair (black, 1.77 [1.64–1.92]; Hispanic, 1.44 [1.28–1.61]). The clinical impact of emergent repair, more frequent among individuals of black and Hispanic races, is highlighted by the association of acute presentation with greater odds of in-hospital death, higher costs, and greater duration of hospital stay.[40] Black individuals have also been found to be significantly younger than white individuals at the time of operative intervention (48 years vs 56 years; $P<.001$).[39] No significant differences existed among black, Hispanic, and white patients in the rates of presentation of chronically incarcerated hernias.[39]

Regarding operative management, Bowman and colleagues[39] found no significant difference between black and white individuals in terms of intraoperative course, laparoscopic approach, or performance of primary versus mesh repair. Funk and colleagues[31] detected a significantly higher percentage of nonwhite individuals undergoing open repair of incisional hernias (75.9% vs 73.4%; $P = .04$), although significant differences were not detected in umbilical or ventral hernia repair.

Race has also been tied to differences in hernia repair outcomes, with minorities having inferior outcomes with specific regard to hernia recurrence, readmission, and postoperative complications (Table 2). Hispanic patients were found to have higher rates of pulmonary complications and mortality in an analysis of the 2004 to 2008 NIS Database.[42] Caucasian race has been associated independently with decreased probabilities of complications and mortality.[37] Asian race has been associated with greater total hospital charges.[26] These findings within the ventral hernia literature reflect national trends; African American individuals have been found to have higher morbidity and mortality rates for a majority of surgical procedures.[43–54]

SOCIOECONOMIC STATUS DISPARITIES IN HERNIA CARE

Income and insurance coverage (public vs private) have frequently been considered proxies for SES.[39] Bowman and colleagues[39] retrospectively reviewed 321 patients

Table 2			
Race and outcomes in the ventral hernia repair literature			
Author, Year	Odds Ratio	95% Confidence Interval	Outcome(s)
Bowman et al,[39] 2010	~1	—	Recurrence
	Black 2.46	1.07–6.59	Readmission
	~1	—	Postoperative complication
	~1	—	6-mo recurrence
Novitsky & Orenstein,[42] 2013	Hispanic increased (specific data not provided)	—	Pulmonary complications, Mortality
Simon et al,[38] 2015	Caucasian 0.994	0.938–1.054	Complications
	Caucasian 0.994	0.753–1.183	Mortality

who underwent ventral hernia repair from 2005 to 2008 at The Mount Sinai Medical Center in New York. They found that patients with Medicaid were more likely to present with incarcerated or strangulated hernias (39% vs 25%; $P<.001$). Individuals with public insurance (Medicare or Medicaid) were more likely than individuals with private insurance to present with both acutely (9% vs 5%) and chronically incarcerated hernias (30% vs 20%).[42] Individuals of lower SES may more frequently present in a delayed fashion owing to a decreased understanding of disease processes,[9,41,55,56] reduced access to physicians,[57–60] physician mistrust, more formidable physician–patient communication barriers,[55] decreased access to good preventative care and proper health maintenance,[61,62] and process variations in specialty referral.[8]

Regarding operative management, Bowman and colleagues[39] found no difference by patient insurance in terms of intraoperative course, operative approach, or performance of primary versus mesh repair. Funk and colleagues,[31] in an analysis of 112,070 elective ventral hernia repairs from the 2009 to 2010 NIS, however, found that laparoscopic repairs were less likely to be performed in poorer patients presenting with incisional hernias (OR, 0.7 [95% CI, 0.6–0.9] for patients in the lowest income quartile). In larger studies of multiple surgical specialties, process variations in choice of procedure and adherence to guidelines has been observed to vary by SES.[8]

In terms of outcomes, Bowman and colleagues[39] correlated patient's zip codes with the 2000 US Census Bureau data for median household income. After defining low income as a median household income of less than $20,997 per year, these investigators found that patients in this bracket had an increased odds of 30-day readmission compared with average- or high-income patients (**Table 3**). The findings of Novitsky and Orenstein[42] also supported inferior outcomes for individuals of lower SES; they found that individuals in the lowest quartile of median income within the United States had higher rates of postoperative wound disruption and infection (see **Table 3**). They also associated public insurance with increased rates of postoperative fistula, nonroutine discharge, mortality, shock, mortality, infection, pneumonia/atelectasis, and myocardial infarction[42] (see **Table 3**).

Table 3
Socioeconomic status and outcomes in the ventral hernia repair literature

Author, Year	Odds Ratio	95% Confidence Interval	Outcome(s)
Bowman et al,[39] 2010	Public insurance 1.78	0.78–4.08	Readmission
	Low income 2.44	0.94–6.30	Readmission
	~1	NP	Morbidity
	~1	NP	Mortality
	~1	NP	1-y recurrence
Novitsky & Orenstein,[42] 2013	Medicare 1.60[b]		Postoperative fistula
	Medicare 2.52[b]	2.13–2.98	Nonroutine discharge
	Medicare 2.16[b]	1.50–3.13	Mortality
	Medicare 2.90[b]	1.30–6.48	Shock
	Medicaid 2.04[b]	1.15–3.61	Mortality
	Medicaid 1.42[b]	1.13–1.79	Infection
	Medicaid 1.33[b]	1.06–1.67	Pneumonia/atelectasis
	Medicaid 1.44[b]	1.00–2.08	Myocardial infarction
	Median income[a] 0.63	0.47–0.85	Wound disruption
	Median income[a] 0.82	0.68–0.99	Infection
	Median income[a] 1.21	1.01–1.44	Pneumonia/atelectasis

Abbreviation: NP, not provided.
[a] Highest to lowest quartile.
[b] To individuals having private insurance.

FUTURE DIRECTIONS

More research is needed with regard to gender, race, and SES on ventral hernia presentation, management, and outcomes. The role of culture and geography in hernia-related health care also remains unknown. Currently existing nationwide registries have thus far yielded at best a modest overview of disparities in hernia care. The knowledge that a significant variation in care exists relative to gender, race, and SES suggests that there is significant room for improvement in terms of providing consistent care for patients with hernias. Still, the relatively few publications that exist are in general derived from large databases that inherently suffer from lack of disease-specific granular data and could otherwise be used to advise best practices and devise guidelines or algorithms for care.

The Institute of Medicine has already concluded that comprehensive, multilevel strategies are needed to eliminate overall health care disparities.[5] A clear knowledge of hernia-related differences among various populations can be used to most effectively allocate appropriate resources to and develop alternative approaches for patient groups at greater risk for complication.

REFERENCES

1. Jenkins JT, O'Dwyer PJ. Inguinal hernias. BMJ 2008;336(7638):269–72.
2. Devlin HB. Trends in hernia surgery in the land of Astley Cooper. In: Soper NJ, editor. Problems in general surgery, vol 12. Philadelphia: Lippincott-Raven; 1995. p. 85–92.
3. Poulose BK, Shelton J, Phillips S, et al. Epidemiology and cost of ventral hernia repair: making the case for hernia research. Hernia 2012;16(2):179–83.
4. Baucom RB, Ousley J, Beveridge GB, Phillips SE. Cancer survivorship: defining the incidence of incisional hernia after resection for intra-abdominal malignancy. Ann Surg Oncol 2016;23(Suppl 5):764–71.
5. Reducing disparities in health care [AMA website]. Available at: https://www.ama-assn.org/delivering-care/reducing-disparities-health-care. Accessed August 26, 2017.
6. NIH launches research program to reduce health disparities in surgical outcomes [NIH website]. Available at: https://www.nih.gov/news-events/news-releases/nih-launches-research-program-reduce-health-disparities-surgical-outcomes. Accessed August 26, 2017.
7. Adepoju OE, Preston MA, Gonzales G. Health care disparities in the post-affordable care act era. Am J Public Health 2015;105(Suppl 5):S665–7.
8. Haider AH, Danka-Mullan I, Maragh-Bass AC, et al. Setting a national agenda for surgical disparities research: recommendations from the National Institutes of Health and American College of Surgeons summit. JAMA Surg 2016;151(6):554–63.
9. Diette GB, Rand C. The contributing role of health-care communication to health disparities for minority patients with asthma. Chest 2007;132(5 Suppl):802S–9S.
10. Lewis P, Fagnano M, Koehler A, et al. Racial disparities at the point of care for urban children with persistent asthma. J Community Health 2014;39(4):706–11.
11. Grzywacz V 2nd, Hussain N, Ragina N. Racial disparities and factors affecting Michigan colorectal cancer screening. J Racial Ethn Health Disparities 2017. [Epub ahead of print].
12. Easter SR, Rosenthal EW, Morton-Eggleston E, et al. Disparities in care for publicly insured women with pregestational diabetes. Obstet Gynecol 2017; 130(5):946–52.

13. Hess CN, Kaltenbach LA, Doll JA, et al. Race and sex differences in post-myocardial infarction angina frequency and risk of 1-year unplanned rehospitalization. Circulation 2017;135(6):532–43.

14. Kanters AE, Krpata DM, Blatnik JA, et al. Modified hernia grading scale to stratify surgical site occurrence after open ventral hernia repairs. J Am Coll Surg 2012; 215(6):787–93.

15. Petro CC, O'Rourke CP, Posielski NM, Criss CN. Designing a ventral hernia staging system. Hernia 2016;20(1):111–7.

16. Ventral Hernia Working Group, Breuing K, Butler CE, Ferzoco S, et al. Incisional ventral hernias: review of the literature and recommendations regarding the grading and technique of repair. Surgery 2010;148(3):544–58.

17. Kokotovic D, Gogenur I, Helgstrand F. Substantial variation among hernia experts in the decision for treatment of patients with incisional hernia: a descriptive study on agreement. Hernia 2017;21(2):271–8.

18. Premarket notification 510(k) [US Food and Drug Administration website]. Available at: https://www.fda.gov/MedicalDevices/DeviceRegulationandGuidance/HowtoMarketYourDevice/PremarketSubmissions/PremarketNotification510k/default.htm. Accessed October 15, 2017.

19. Kokotovic D, Bisgaard T, Helgstrand F. Long-term recurrence and complications associated with elective incisional hernia repair. JAMA 2016;316(15):1575–82.

20. Kummerow Broman K, Huang LC, Fagih A, et al. Hidden morbidity of ventral hernia repair with mesh: as concerning as common bile duct injury? J Am Coll Surg 2017;224(1):35–42.

21. Sanchez VM, Abi-Haidar YE, Itani KMF. Mesh infection in ventral incisional hernia repair: incidence, contributing factors, and treatment. Surg Infect (Larchmt) 2011;12(3):205–10.

22. Flum DR, Horvath K, Koepsell T. Have outcomes of incisional hernia repair improved with time? A population-based analysis. Ann Surg 2003;237(1):129–35.

23. What are the value-based programs? [CMS.gov website]. Available at: https://www.cms.gov/Medicare/Quality-Initiatives-Patient-Assessment-Instruments/Value-Based-Programs/Value-Based-Programs.html. Accessed October 15, 2017.

24. Poulose BK, Roll S, Murphy JW, et al. Design and implementation of the Americas Hernia Society Quality Collaborative (AHSQC): improving value in hernia care. Hernia 2016;20(2):177–89.

25. About ACS NSQIP [American College of Surgeons website]. Available at: https://www.facs.org/quality-programs/acs-nsqip/about. Accessed October 15, 2017.

26. Poulose BK, Beck WC, Phillips SE, et al. The chosen few: disproportionate resource use in ventral hernia repair. Am Surg 2013;79(8):815–8.

27. Van Ramshorst GH, Nieuwenhuizen J, Hop WC, et al. Abdominal wound dehiscence in adults: development and validation of a risk model. World J Surg 2010;34:20–7.

28. Holihan JL, Alawadi ZM, Harris JW, et al. Ventral hernia: patient selection, treatment, and management. Curr Probl Surg 2016;53(7):307–54.

29. Helgstrand F. National results after ventral hernia repair. Dan Med J 2016;63(7) [pii:B5258].

30. Colavita PD, Tsirline VB, Walters AL, et al. Laparoscopic versus open hernia repair: outcomes and sociodemographic utilization results from the Nationwide Inpatient Sample. Surg Endosc 2013;27(1):109–17.

31. Funk LM, Perry KA, Narula VK, et al. Current national practice patterns for inpatient management of ventral abdominal wall hernia in the United States. Surg Endosc 2013;27(11):4104–12.

32. Craig P, Parikh PP, Markert R, et al. Prevalence and predictors of hernia infection: does gender matter? Am Surg 2016;82(4):E93–5.
33. Helgstrand F, Jorgensen LN, Rosenberg J, et al. Nationwide prospective study on readmission after umbilical or epigastric hernia repair. Hernia 2013;17(4):487–92.
34. Cox TC, Huntington CR, Blair LJ, et al. Predictive modeling for chronic pain after ventral hernia repair. Am J Surg 2016;212(3):501–10.
35. Aho JM, Nourallah A, Samaha MJ, et al. Patient-reported outcomes after laparoscopic ventral hernia repair. Am Surg 2016;82(6):550–6.
36. Hornby ST, McDermott FD, Coleman M, et al. Female gender and diabetes mellitus increase the risk of recurrence after laparoscopic incisional hernia repair. Ann R Coll Surg Engl 2015;97(2):115–9.
37. Memtsoudis SG, Besclides MC, Swamidoss CP. Do race, gender, and source of payment impact on anesthetic technique for inguinal hernia repair? J Clin Anesth 2006;18(5):328–33.
38. Simon KL, Frelich MJ, Gould JC, et al. Inpatient outcomes after elective versus nonelective ventral hernia repair. J Surg Res 2015;198(2):305–10.
39. Bowman K, Telem DA, Hernandez-Rosa J, et al. Impact of race and socioeconomic status on presentation and management of ventral hernias. Arch Surg 2010;145(8):776–80.
40. Mehta A, Hutfless S, Blair AB, et al. Emergency department utilization and predictors of mortality for inpatient inguinal hernia repairs. J Surg Res 2017;212:270–7.
41. Wolf LL, Scott JW, Zogg CK, et al. Predictors of emergency ventral hernia repair: targets to improve patient access and guide patient selection for elective repair. Surgery 2016;160(5):1379–91.
42. Novitsky YW, Orenstein SB. Effect of patient and hospital characteristics on outcomes of elective ventral hernia repair in the United States. Hernia 2013;17(5): 639–45.
43. Lucas FL, Stukel TA, Morris AM, et al. Race and surgical mortality in the United States. Ann Surg 2006;243(2):281–6.
44. Farmer MM, Ferraro KF. Are racial disparities in health conditional on socioeconomic status? Soc Sci Med 2005;60(1):191–204.
45. Rosson GD, Singh NK, Ahuja N, et al. Multilevel analysis of the impact of community vs patient factors on access to immediate breast reconstruction following mastectomy in Maryland. Arch Surg 2008;143(11):1076–81.
46. Dunlop DD, Manheim LM, Song J, et al. Age and racial/ethnic disparities in arthritis-related hip and knee surgeries. Med Care 2008;46(2):200–8.
47. Shugarman LR, Mack K, Sorbero ML, et al. Race and sex differences in the receipt of timely and appropriate lung cancer treatment. Med Care 2009;47(7): 774–81.
48. Osborne NH, Upchurch GR Jr, Mathur AK, et al. Explaining racial disparities in mortality after abdominal aortic aneurysm repair. J Vasc Surg 2009;50(4):709–13.
49. Sosa JA, Mehta PJ, Wang TS, et al. Racial disparities in clinical and economic outcomes from thyroidectomy. Ann Surg 2007;246(6):1083–91.
50. Greenstein AJ, Litle VR, Swanson SJ, et al. Racial disparities in esophageal cancer treatment and outcomes. Ann Surg Oncol 2008;15(3):881–8.
51. Curry WT Jr, Carter BS, Barker FG II. Racial, ethnic, and socioeconomic disparities in patient outcomes after craniotomy for tumor in adult patients in the United States, 1988-2004. Neurosurgery 2010;66(3):427–37.
52. Breslin TM, Morris AM, Gu N, et al. Hospital factors and racial disparities in mortality after surgery for breast and colon cancer. J Clin Oncol 2009;27(24): 3945–50.

53. Kamath AF, Horneff JG, Gaffney V, et al. Ethnic and gender differences in the functional disparities after primary total knee arthroplasty. Clin Orthop Relat Res 2010;468(12):3355–61.

54. Singh TP, Almond C, Givertz MM, et al. Improved survival in heart transplant recipients in the United States: racial differences in era effect. Circ Heart Fail 2011; 4(2):153–60.

55. Alawadi ZM, Leal IM, Flores JR, et al. Underserved patients seeking care for ventral hernias at a safety net hospital: impact on quality of life and expectations of treatment. J Am Coll Surg 2017;224(1):26–34.e2.

56. Levinson W, Hudak PL, Feldman JJ, et al. "It's not what you say…": racial disparities in communication between orthopedic surgeons and patients. Med Care 2008;46(4):410–6.

57. Cunningham PJ. Mounting pressures: physicians serving Medicaid patients and the uninsured, 1997-2001. Track Rep 2002;6:1–4.

58. Schulman KA, Berlin JA, Harless W, et al. The effect of race and sex on physicians' recommendations for cardiac catheterization. N Engl J Med 1999;340(8): 618–26.

59. Andrulis DP. Access to care is the centerpiece in the elimination of socioeconomic disparities in health. Ann Intern Med 1998;129(5):412–6.

60. Groeneved PW, Laufer SB, Garber AM. Technology diffusion, hospital variation, and racial disparities among elderly Medicare beneficiaries: 1989-2000. Med Care 2005;43(4):320–9.

61. Wefer A, Gunnarsson U, Franneby U, et al. Patient-reported adverse events after hernia surgery and socio-economic status: a register-based cohort study. Int J Surg 2016;35:100–3.

62. Weissman JS, Stern F, Fielding SL, et al. Delayed access to health care: risk factors, reasons, and consequences. Ann Intern Med 1991;114(4):325–31.

Quality Measures in Hernia Surgery

Michael J. Rosen, MD

KEYWORDS

• Quality • Measures • Outcomes • AHSQC • Hernia outcomes

KEY POINTS

- With the changing landscape of health care, quality measures are becoming increasingly important.
- Understanding the quality measures that surgeons are being evaluated for is critical to maintain control of the profession and assure optimum patient outcomes.
- Defining and measuring quality in complex hospital systems and surgery is very difficult.

The concept of measuring quality and improving outcomes is ingrained in the surgeon more so than almost any other medical professional. The ability for surgeons to sit with patients, interpret data, make the decision to perform an operation, and put into motion a cascade of events is among the most unique relationships in medicine. It is inherent for the surgeon to do everything within his or her power to achieve the highest quality outcome for the patient. All surgeons have some individual scale that allows them to measure their quality, and likely much of this is happening without conscious recognition. This internal scale allows surgeons to make decisions minute by minute to achieve the best outcomes for patients. Often, in surgery and in particular hernia surgery, high-quality data are not available to help guide these decisions and thus the surgeon relies on judgment, experience, and intuition. Although this is a reasonable approach and has resulted in historically excellent outcomes in many cases, with the introduction of the Affordable Care Act (ACA), many changes have occurred to that process that challenge that way of thinking and have significant implications for the medical and surgical community. Understanding what these changes are, who is making these decisions, who is measuring surgical quality, and how exactly they are measuring quality is critical for surgeons to be fairly assessed in the future and understand the scale.

Dr M.J. Rosen is a salaried employee of the Americas Hernia Society Quality Collaborative, which is a nonprofit 501c3 organization. He has received grant support to his institution for clinical trials by Intuitive and Miromatrix as a Principal Investigator, and he is on the board of Ariste Medical.
Lerner College of Medicine, Cleveland Clinic Foundation, 9500 Euclid Avenue, A-100, Cleveland, OH 44195, USA
E-mail address: rosenm@ccf.org

Surg Clin N Am 98 (2018) 441–455
https://doi.org/10.1016/j.suc.2018.01.007
0039-6109/18/© 2018 Elsevier Inc. All rights reserved.

surgical.theclinics.com

With growing pressures to formulate easily interpreted quality metrics, many potential pitfalls exist that can deleteriously affect the ultimate outcome of patients. This article attempts to define what quality means in surgery, in general, and hernia surgery, specifically; how it is being measured; who is in charge of measuring it; and, when appropriate, how it will be reported. With growing oversight, many organizations have been created to help define and measure quality. The number of governmental acronyms measuring and reporting quality can be overwhelming for the clinician to interpret. This article also attempts to highlight the key governmental organizations that are in charge of defining quality in medicine. This field of health care improvement is evolving and ever-changing based on the practices of politics in Washington, DC. Although the exact layout of this plan likely will continue to evolve, it is certain that surgeons will be measured based on the quality of their outcomes. It is important to be facile in this process for future success in this profession. Although striving for high quality seems relatively straightforward, actually measuring quality is extremely challenging owing to the challenge of accounting for all of the variables that occur in the delivery of health care. Most definitions of quality are primarily based on products and are derived from minimum standards. This transition from product-based quality measurements to health care delivery is ongoing, challenging, and incredibly important for the future of our patients.

When the Institute of Medicine published their seminal paper "To Err is Human: Building a Safer Health System," the call to action of improving quality and safety in the modern health care system was launched.[1] Subsequently, the ACA increased the pace at which this transition was meant to occur. The ACA strives to reduce the fragmentation of the health care system; improve coordination of care; and begin to reward quality, improve outcomes, and lower health care costs. One of the primary goals of the ACA is to transition from a volume-based payment model to a value-based payment model. The definition of value in a health care system originates from economic theory; it is equal to the quality divided by the cost.[2,3] From a payer's perspective, cost is relatively straightforward to measure through reimbursement claims. However, developing judicious quality measures has been the topic of significant research, debate, and ongoing analysis.

One of the initiatives to operationalize the transition to value-based care delivery was the formation of accountable care organizations, within Medicare's Fee for Service program. These organizations are entities that are held accountable for both the cost and the quality of care defined for a population of patients. These are most commonly medical groups and hospital systems but can include skilled nursing facilities and postacute facilities. With the proliferation of these organizations, the Centers for Medicare and Medicaid Services (CMS) has defined specific domains in which quality is measured in health care systems. These quality measures are tools designed to quantify health care processes, outcomes, and patient and caregiver experiences with the overall goal of providing effective, safe, efficient, patient-centered, equitable, and timely care. The 4 most common primary domains used to provide the framework for assessing quality of care are structure, process, outcomes, and patient satisfaction.[4–6]

STRUCTURE MEASURES

Structure measures are defined as a feature of a health care organization or clinician related to the capacity to provide high-quality care.[6,7] These measures are often viewed as less valuable because they are farthest removed from improving patient outcomes.[2,3] Additionally, structural measures indicate the potential for providing high-quality care but do not ensure that the process measures are available to actually provide good outcomes.[3] Structure measures focus on organizational, human, and material resources.[6] In particular, these assess whether providers have the equipment and technology to support health care delivery. The availability of the electronic medical record (EMR) and other health information technology are included in these measures. These structure measures are essentially fixed resources available to the medical staff or organization. Structure measures can often be confused with process measures (see later discussion). For instance, a common quality measure is whether physicians prescribe outpatient medications electronically. The structure measure would be whether the physicians have access to the EMR and the process measure would be the percentage of physicians that actually prescribe these medications electronically.[6] However, the most important measure, which is often not reported, is whether this capability and electronic delivery of medications truly results in a measurable improvement in patient outcomes. It is interesting that there are very few clinical data that EMRs have improved clinical outcomes; however, because they are an easily measured fixed resource they are commonly reported and assessed for structure measures. These structure measures are rarely related to specific surgical entities and are more focused on available institutional global facilities and are likely not attributable to the individual clinician.

PROCESS MEASURES

Process measures assess the efficiency and compliance of health care workers in delivering health care services and procedures. These measures are used to determine the extent to which providers give patients specific services that are aligned with evidence-based guidelines for care.[3] In contrast to outcome measures, these process measures are unable to be influenced by factors outside of the health care system. Inherent to process measures is the goal of reducing variation, thus theoretically improving outcomes. However, process measures should not be confused with measuring quality outcomes. The ease of reporting process measures and the challenges of measuring true outcomes has led to an overwhelming number of process measures serving as surrogates for quality. For instance, of the 78 Healthcare Effectiveness Data and Information Set (HEDIS) measures for 2010, the most widely used quality metrics were process-based delivery with all but 5 being clearly process measures and not true outcomes.[2,4] Likewise, of the 1958 quality indicators in the National Quality Measures Clearinghouse, only 139 (7%) are actual outcomes and only 32 (<2%) are patient-reported outcomes.[8,9]

These measures are supposed to be derived from evidence-based medicine and should be attributed to improved clinical outcomes. Although this is inherent in the definitions, in surgery there are often incomplete data to definitively support some of these measures but guidelines persist nonetheless. In addition, there are cases in which patients may have certain exclusion criteria that are not reflected in the process measures, which can make accurate reporting challenging. An example of a seemingly straightforward process metric is the time that the discharge orders were written and the time the patient was discharged from the hospital. This would demonstrate the discharge process that occurs in a hospital system and would be a measure to evaluate the efficiencies of that system. However, it would not take into consideration the patient that does not have a ride home until the end of the day due to a spouse working, the time it takes for an ambulance to arrive for transportation to a nursing home, or inclement weather that could lead to further delays. All of these examples demonstrate the challenges of easily measuring and reporting even seemingly straightforward process measures in complex hospital systems. In addition to the limitations of process measures being associated with improved outcomes, that organizations become consumed with these measurements and dedicate large resources to their process improvement efforts has led to further skepticism from clinicians about the value of actual quality measurements, which unfortunately include outcome improvements as well.[9]

OUTCOME MEASURES

A clinical outcome is defined as a health state of a patient resulting from health care.[6,7] Clinical outcomes are arguably the most important quality metric measured. However, they are also the most difficult to calculate with administrative data and current methodology. These measures are often controversial and raise significant concerns among clinicians who argue that appropriate illness severity and risk adjustment methods are not accurately represented in these analyses. Although advanced statistical adjustment, data stratification, and analytics are often applied to these data sets, without the appropriate information inherent to the disease process they often cannot account for all of the variability in clinical practice. These measures are additionally criticized for being rudimentary downstream consequences of various different complicated processes.[3] Within hernia surgery there are many features that can affect the clinical outcomes of the patients that cannot be accounted for with administrative data. For example, it has been shown in multiple staging systems that the width of the hernia defect directly relates to the expected surgical outcome and risks.[10,11] It would not seem reasonable to measure the clinical outcome of a 1 cm hernia on the same playing field as a 25 cm defect. However, with administrative data in which the hernia width is not accounted for, this could easily occur. It is paramount that clinicians participate in appropriate data acquisition to allow reasonable risk stratification of their outcomes.

With the shifting focus from provider-measured outcomes to patient-specific outcomes, many quality measures are evolving into patient-reported outcomes. These measures focus on questionnaires to assess symptoms, functional outcomes, and health-related quality of life from pain to social functioning.[6] The National Institutes of Health has responded to this initiative with the development of the Patient-Reported Outcomes Measurement Information System (PROMIS) system.[12] This system contains items that cover the 3 domains of physical, mental, and social health outcomes. There have been several other hernia-specific quality-of-life metrics available for assessing patient-reported hernia outcomes.[13,14] However, among the major limitations of assessing patient-reported outcomes is the process by which these tools are delivered and the long-term data that needs to be assessed, particularly in hernia disease states. The mechanism by which patients will report their outcomes has not been clarified. It is clear with hernia surgery that short-term 30-day to 90-day outcomes will not adequately provide meaningful, complete quality outcomes in these patients. Utilization of social media platforms, texting, email, and telephone calls are all potential means to improve completion of patient-reported outcomes; however, with the current Health Insurance Portability and Accountability Act (HIPPA) laws, there are many challenges in using these avenues to collect data. With the growing need for patient-reported outcomes, it will be important to devise innovative ways to collect these data while protecting patient privacy.

Additionally, it is likely that one will never be able to simply predict the outcomes of all patients undergoing a procedure regardless of location, physician, or patient-determined factors. This inability to limit all variation in health care should be acknowledged and adjusted for as well. An alternative model would be to create a quality improvement process in which all physicians participated to achieve the best possible outcomes within their own practice and capabilities. Possible features of this quality system could include measuring real outcomes, with the principal purpose of enabling innovation and quality improvement, and not comparing provider outcomes; providing periodic feedback real-time; and participating in ongoing quality improvement initiatives.[2] When a physician reaches this participation level, the system would deem them achieving their own individual high-quality outcomes. Perhaps public reporting of the participation of certain physicians in this type of system would allow more accurate delivery of health care information to the consumer to make informed decisions. This would shift the system from measuring a simple binary outcome and instead begin the process of defining the minimum requirements necessary to achieve high-quality outcomes within certain disease states as a system and not as an isolated clinician.

PATIENT AND CAREGIVER EXPERIENCE OF CARE MEASURES

In 2012, the CMS attributed the importance of patient experience to quality metrics. Without a doubt, patient experience in the health care system is important and deserves serious consideration. However, many of these measures are unclear as to whether they should be attributed to the individual physician or the system itself. Some of these measures include the patient's experience with the front office staff, timeliness of care, and impressions of communication by the physician. There are many potential pitfalls in interpreting these data that deserve mention. In large group practices, the individual physicians often do not have any control over or knowledge of who staffs the front. Even more problematic is that physicians often have to have difficult conversations with patients that at times can lead to patient dissatisfaction based on the information that is delivered. As an example in hernia surgery, some patients with chronic groin pain after an operation might see a physician and, after a complete work up and evaluation, the physician determines that the patient cannot be helped with an operation. Although this might be the most appropriate medical treatment, the patient might leave the office dissatisfied (even if the surgeon delivered the information in an empathetic, appropriate manner) and thus report low patient-experience scores. Additionally, a patient's health literacy or lack thereof can contribute to low satisfaction scores based on lack of understanding of the message being delivered. In these cases, it will not be possible for a clinician to achieve a high satisfaction score regardless of their approach.

Currently, patient-experience scores are measured with tools developed by the Agency for Healthcare Research and Quality (AHRQ). These are survey-based and are known as the Consumer Assessment of Healthcare Providers and Systems (CAHPS). The 2 most common versions include the Clinician and Group CAHPS, which measures patients' recent experience with clinicians and staff, and the Hospital CAHPS, which reports on patients who have experienced a recent medical, surgical, or obstetric admission. Inherent to any survey analysis, there is the potential for significant bias in selection of patients with a negative experience or outlook to complete the survey, the minimum number of replies to adequately assess a physician's outcomes, and the lack of validation of the survey tool to adequately report on quality.

Other patient-experience measures are commonly reported on physician-rating Web sites such as Vitals.com and Healthgrades.com. It is concerning that some patients might use these patient-satisfaction scores as a surrogate for the quality of their physician or surgeon. In a recent analysis, patient-reported Web sites were compared with hernia surgeon–reported quality outcome metrics regarding their ability to correlate patient-entered evaluations of surgeons with high-quality surgical outcomes.[15] Although the Web sites did successfully correlate with each other in their ability to discern patient satisfaction, there was no correlation with higher patient-satisfaction reporting for a surgeon and better clinical outcomes for that surgeon. It is thus important for patients to understand that a higher patient-satisfaction score regarding their physician might not directly correlate with a better surgical outcome.

WHO IS MEASURING SURGEONS?

There are several organizations that are tasked with measuring and defining the outcomes of the previously mentioned quality metrics. Although the list is quite long, this article focuses on the high-level organizations that are most important in measuring surgical quality metrics.

The gold standard of health care quality measures is the National Quality Forum (NQF). The NQF is a nonprofit organization that endorses and recommends the use of standardized performance metrics in health care. The NQF is a consensus-based entity that comprises more than 60 public and private organizations, which advises both the federal government and private payers on the best measures to use in quality accountability and payment programs.[7] The NQF evaluates and measures how health care services are delivered and facilitates improvements in safety, equity, transparency, health information technology, provider accountability, and informed consumer decision-making.[6] Almost all surgical quality metrics from the American College of Surgeons' Physician Quality Reporting System (PQRS) and the Quality Clinical Data Registry (QCDR) are vetted and approved by the NQF.

The operational arm of improving the health care of Americans is the National Quality Strategy (NQS). This organization was brought about with the Affordable Care Act to develop and execute a national strategy for quality improvement in health care. It brings together public and private sector stakeholders and is led by the AHRQ. Its overall goal is to ensure Americans receive the right care, at the right time, in the right setting, every time.[16] The NQS also focuses on disseminating best practices to apply to local health care delivery to optimize regional outcomes.

The CMS quality program borrows many of the same principles of the NQS program. There are several unique features to the CMS strategy, including better care at a lower cost, prevention medicine, expanded health care coverage, and enterprise excellence.[6] The CMS program has evolved over the last several years and continues to change based on the ACA and its modifications. The PQRS has been among the more popular quality reporting systems applied to surgeons, although it has recently been overhauled with the new Quality Payment Program introduced by the CMS. The PQRS aimed to assess the quality of care provided throughout the continuum of care from prevention, chronic and acute care, and procedure-related care, to resource utilization and care coordination. Physicians were allowed to select from hundreds of measures to allocate 9 individual measures covering several of the quality domains previously listed. These data are reported on the Medicare Physician Compare Web site. On this Web site, an overall quality rating is given based on a star system and individual performance scores are reported as percentages. Currently, the Web site reports on group practices and accountable care organizations but likely will provide data on individual physicians in the future. Many of these reportable quality metrics involve process measures and very few are easily attributable to surgical outcomes or quality. It is unclear whether these data reported on individual surgeons to the public or payers can be appropriately risk adjusted and understood to truly inform the consumer to make a decision based on achieving the highest quality outcome.

The CMS recently performed a major overhaul of its quality program with the final ruling of the Medicare Access and Children's Health Insurance Program Reauthorization Act (MACRA) of 2015. In this new process, the CMS agreed to end the sustainable growth rate formula in exchange for a new reward system for health care providers. This system would focus on providing better care, not just more care. It combined a multitude of existing quality reporting systems into 1 new program. The goal of the MACRA program is to reduce administrative burden on physicians, allow physicians to focus on care improvements, promote value-based care, and allow for a smooth transition from prior programs. This program in its current form is entitled the Quality Payment Program. It essentially allows for 2 payment models: merit-based incentive payment system (MIPS) and alternative payment models (APMs). The categories for reporting requirements are displayed in **Table 1**.[3]

Table 1
Merit-based incentive payment system performance categories and reporting requirements for the 2017 performance period

MIPS Category	General Reporting Requirements	Available Measure
Quality	Report up to 6 quality measures or specialty measures set for minimum 90 d Report 15 quality measures for 1 full y on Web interface	271 individual measures
Advancing Care Information	Fulfill 5 required measures for a minimum of 90 d Security risk analysis E-prescribing Provide patient access Send summary of care Request or accept summary of care May submit up to 9 measures for additional credit May receive bonus credit for reporting public health and clinical data registry measures	2 available measures set options Option 1: advancing care information objectives and measures[15] Option 2: 2017 advancing care information transition objectives and measures[11]
Improvement Activities	Attest completion of up to 4 improvement activities for minimum 90 d Participants in certified patient-centered medical homes and certain qualifying APMs will automatically earn some points and may receive full credit	92 available measures in 8 subcategories Achieving health equity Behavioral and mental health Beneficiary engagement Care coordination Emergency response and preparedness Expanded practice access Patient safety and practice assessment Population management
Cost or resource use	No data submission required Calculated from claims	

From Squitieri L, Chung KC. Measuring provider performance for physicians participating in the merit-based incentive payment system. Plast Reconstr Surg 2017;140(1):217e–26e; with permission.

The MIPS program encompasses 4 domains: Quality, Improvement Activities, Advancing Care, and Cost. The Quality program replaces the PQRS system, and includes multiple options to choose from, with 6 reported measures. The CMS has recognized that it is difficult to report clear quality metrics, in particular for surgical specialties, and has introduced the QCDR. These are CMS recognized registries or collaboratives that collect patient and treatment information for purposes of improving patient outcomes and quality of care. There are several options for meeting this measure. One of the hernia-specific options is the Americas Hernia Society Quality Collaborative (AHSQC; see later discussion). The improvement activities are based on an attestation statement and include at least 4 measures for 90 days. The advancing care component involves the utilization of an EMR to e-prescribe, report care summaries, and allow patient access. In addition, reporting data in a QCDR can provide bonus points. Currently, cost data will not be analyzed on a per case basis and will be calculated from adjudicated claims. Despite the fluid nature of this quality metric and payment system, it is important for physicians to be aware that they are being measured in 2017 for payment adjustments that will be attributed in 2019.

APMs are another way for the CMS to improve quality outcomes and reduce cost in the system. These incentives involve lump sum payments for caring for CMS beneficiaries to share risk in providing the care for these patients. It is meant to increase transparency of physician-focused payment models. In its current form, APM will receive a lump sum incentive payment equal to 5% of the prior year's estimated aggregate expenditures under the fee schedule. The 5% incentive payment will be available from 2019 to 2024, but in 2026 the fee schedule growth rate will be higher for qualifying APM participants. By 2022, practitioners can expect a potential 9% increase or decrease, depending on their performance.

In summary, the CMS has significantly altered the projected payment models for its beneficiaries and the shift from rewarding volume of care to promoting the value of care delivered has occurred. Because surgeons can provide some of the highest value to patients in a hospital system, it is important for surgeons to be engaged in this process and verify that quality is being measured appropriately. To date, many of the quality metrics that are being measured are not directly related to improving clinical outcomes. It is clear that quality outcomes can be divided into quality metrics and quality improvement. Quality metrics can be defined as improving a number to achieve a higher score on the reporting system without directly improving patient outcomes. Because quality metrics are now being used to rank hospitals and potentially impose payment adjustments, many hospital systems invest in large quality departments to track and optimize these metrics. It is often an unintended consequence of these resources that much of the focus is placed on making the number look better and gaming the system without improving the quality.[17] On the other hand, true quality improvement is the act of improving the quality of care delivered to patients. This is often very expensive, is hard to measure, and can be difficult to obtain from classic data sources; however, it should be the overriding goal of quality improvement programs.

There are multiple examples of quality benchmark adherence failing to be correlated with quality improvement. For instance, timely administration of antibiotics in the emergency department has not been linked to improved outcomes in community-acquired pneumonia, despite its being used as a measurable quality tool.[17] Others have challenged the Surgical Care Improvement Project's quality measure of appropriate timing of antibiotic delivery before surgical incision as not being correlated with any improvement in outcomes.[18] One specific example of a quality metric related to hernia surgery that could be improved without improving patient outcomes is the occurrence of an enterotomy. Although it is well known in reoperative hernia surgery that adhesions can be severe and appropriately risk-adjusting these outcomes can be difficult; patient safety indicators (PSIs) consider enterotomy to be a preventable complication. In brief, PSIs are a set of measures that screen for adverse events as a result of exposure to the health care system. These are reported on a system or provider level. Although these measures were initially intended to provide benchmarks to allow for improved performance and accountability, they have been used to provide a simple count or measure of quality events. This oversimplification of surgical quality often does not result in true quality improvement. For instance, although most surgeons would agree that there are certain technical aspects to reducing bowel injuries during reoperative surgery, the conversation about reducing enterotomies is overshadowed by the attempts to modify the way the complication is being reported. With regard to bowel injury, if the provider appropriately reports that the injury was inherent to the disease process and unavoidable due to the adhesions and nature of the case, the PSI is not reportable. Although this is very appropriate, it shifts the focus away from having a real conversation on why these events are occurring and perhaps developing ways to reduce the complication in the first place. This culture of improving the quality metrics and perhaps not completing true quality improvement is dangerous and could fall short of all of the goals of the quality improvement efforts of the new health care system.

LIMITATIONS OF QUALITY MEASURES

Many authors have begun to question the validity, accuracy, and value of these previously mentioned performance metrics and quality initiatives.[19] One such example is Morgan and colleagues[20] who reported the surgical site infection (SSI) rates in patients undergoing abdominal hysterectomies using the Michigan Surgical Quality Collaborative. This is a particularly important quality metric because it is a CMS-recognized preventable hospital-acquired condition and subject to payment penalties. They reported 2 important flaws in the current system. First, the sites in the bottom quartile of SSI rates were not significantly different from those sites that were not in the bottom quartile. In essence, hospitals could be financially penalized for a difference in infection rates that was entirely based on chance. Second, after risk adjusting the data for evidence-based risk factors associated with SSI, more than 20% of the hospitals changed quartiles. Recently, Haskins and colleagues[15] reported an analysis using the AHSQC that compared hernia surgeon self-reported quality metrics with online patient-reported physician scores. Although they did not find a correlation between physician-reported quality metrics and patient-reported scores, they did report several CMS-approved quality metrics. It is interesting that in many of their analyses the top quartile and the bottom quartile performers differed by only a few percentage points. Although not directly analyzed, it is concerning that potential penalties could be administered to physicians and hospitals with only 1% to 2% differences in outcomes that are likely not statistically significantly different.

Another major limitation of risk adjusting health outcomes is controlling for the severity of illness and social challenges that often cannot be controlled for in models. Investigators have found that safety net hospitals that tend to care for a large volume of ill, lower socioeconomic patients are at the greatest risk of suffering reduced payment penalties and are also more unlikely to receive a bonus payment.[21] This disparity in penalizing hospitals that care for the highest risk patients, while potentially achieving the highest quality outcomes attainable, seems unfair. Any system that adequately measures and rewards quality care, must take into consideration all aspects of the challenges that each of these systems face in delivering health care.

MEASURING QUALITY IN HERNIA SURGERY

Measuring, reporting, and comparing outcomes, according to Michael Porter,[2] a renowned health economist, are the most important steps toward rapidly improving outcomes and making reasonable choices about reducing costs. He also notes that it is important to strive for rigorous outcome measures to assess a patient's comprehensive outcome. In his recommendations for measuring quality, it is also critical to manage the competing outcomes of short-term benefits and long-term functionality when considering the most appropriate option. Within hernia surgery this is paramount. Because a hernia patient often has a medical device implanted for life, there is a major need for the full assessment of quality throughout the lifetime of a patient when measuring outcomes. As an example, if a low-cost implant results in significant cost savings during implantation and the 30-day outcomes are equivalent to a much more expensive implant, it seems logical that that implant will improve value in the system. However, with mesh in particular, the long-term outcomes of these products might result in significant patient harm with reoperations, chronic pain, enterocutaneous fistulae, and other mesh-related complications that must be factored into the equation.[22] The only realistic means of achieving this type of data are through rigorous data collection tools with long-term patient outcomes.

A recent survey analysis of hernia surgeons and hospital administrators suggests a very low rate of tracking hernia patients' outcomes, with only 45% of surgeons and 33% of hospital administrators reporting an active means of tracking short-term and long-term patient outcomes after hernia surgery.[23] Recognizing the importance of measuring clinical outcomes and obtaining the necessary data to fairly risk adjust these outcomes in hernia patients, the AHSQC was founded by the Americas Hernia Society.[24] The mission of the AHSQC is "to maximize quality and value of hernia patient care through collaboration."[24] The AHSQC is a continuous quality improvement organization that measures hernia-related outcomes in patients undergoing ventral, inguinal, and parastomal hernias. Since its inception in 2013, it reports data on more than 200 surgeons from across the United States in various practices, including academic, academic-affiliated, and private practice. The collaborative prospectively collects demographic patient risk factors, perioperative details, and long-term follow-up using validated patient-reported outcome measures, including the PROMIS pain scale, the Ventral Hernia Recurrence Inventory, and the Hernia-Related Quality-of-Life Survey (HERQLES) abdominal wall functional scores.[13,25–27] The data are analyzed and risk adjusted in real time to provide ongoing feedback to surgeons, hospitals, and hernia centers. Core comparisons are performed for surgeon-level and hospital-level outcomes with comparisons available in real time versus the entire collaborative for key hernia-related outcomes. Currently, data from more than 22,000 patients provides the ongoing impetus for improving outcomes in patients undergoing hernia surgery. This group has published multiple manuscripts with evidence-based real world guidelines to improve quality outcomes, including elimination of routine preoperative outpatient chlorhexidine scrubs, elimination of routine bowel preparation before elective hernia repair, the potential downside of epidural utilization in ventral hernia repairs, and methods to reduce readmissions after ventral hernia repair.[28–30] This is an example of surgeons collaborating to take control of quality measurement, collectively report real data in real time, and strive for improving the outcomes of their patients. It will be important for other fields of surgery to collaborate

Table 2
Americas Hernia Society Quality Collaborative Quality Clinical Data Registry metrics

Measure	Type	Description
Unplanned Reoperation within the 30-d Postoperative Period	Outcome	Percentage of patients aged 18 y and older who had any unplanned reoperation within the 30-d postoperative period of the primary procedure
Surgical Site Infection within the 30-d Postoperative Period	Outcome	Percentage of patients aged 18 y and older who had a surgical site infection (superficial, deep, or organ space infection) within the 30-d postoperative period of the primary procedure
Patient-Centered Surgical Risk Assessment and Communication	Process	Percentage of patients aged 18 y or older who underwent elective surgery who had their personalized risks of postoperative complications assessed by their surgical team before surgery using a clinical data-based, patient-specific risk calculator and who received personal discussion of those risks with the surgeon
Ventral Hernia Repair: Surgical Site Occurrence Requiring Procedural Intervention within the 30-d Postoperative Period	Outcome	Percentage of patients aged 18 y and older who have undergone ventral hernia repair who had a surgical site occurrence requiring procedural intervention within the 30-d postoperative period Surgical site occurrences include any surgical site infections (superficial, deep, organ space) or any of the following: wound cellulitis, nonhealing incisional wound, fascial disruption, skin or soft tissue ischemia, skin or soft tissue necrosis, wound serous drainage, wound purulent drainage, chronic sinus drainage, localized stab wound infection, stitch abscess, seroma, infected seroma, hematoma, infected hematoma, exposed biologic mesh, exposed synthetic mesh, contaminated biologic mesh, contaminated synthetic mesh, infected biologic mesh, infected synthetic mesh, mucocutaneous anastomosis disruption, enterocutaneous fistula Procedural interventions include any of the following: wound opening, wound debridement, suture excision, percutaneous drainage, partial mesh removal, complete mesh removal
Unplanned Hospital Readmission or Observation Visit within the 30-Day Postoperative Period	Outcome	Percentage of patients aged 18 y and older who had any unplanned hospital readmission or 23-h observation visit within the 30-d postoperative period

(continued on next page)

Table 2
(continued)

Measure	Type	Description
Abdominal Wall Reconstruction Surgical Site Occurrence Requiring Procedural Intervention within the 30-d Postoperative Period	Outcome	Percentage of patients aged 18 y and older who have undergone abdominal wall reconstruction, defined as ventral hernia repair with myofascial release (abdominal wall fascial layer separated from muscular layer), who had a surgical site occurrence requiring procedural intervention within the 30-d postoperative period. Surgical site occurrences include any surgical site infections (superficial, deep, organ space) or any of the following: wound cellulitis, nonhealing incisional wound, fascial disruption, skin or soft tissue ischemia, skin or soft tissue necrosis, wound serous drainage, wound purulent drainage, chronic sinus drainage, localized stab wound infection, stitch abscess, seroma, infected seroma, hematoma, infected hematoma, exposed biologic mesh, exposed synthetic mesh, contaminated biologic mesh, contaminated synthetic mesh, infected biologic mesh, infected synthetic mesh, mucocutaneous anastomosis disruption, enterocutaneous fistula Procedural interventions include any of the following: wound opening, wound debridement, suture excision, percutaneous drainage, partial mesh removal, complete mesh removal This measure is reported as 3 performance rates stratified by hernia width: 1. Abdominal wall reconstruction surgical site occurrence requiring procedural intervention within the 30-d postoperative period; any hernia width (overall rate) 2. Abdominal wall reconstruction surgical site occurrence requiring procedural intervention within the 30-d postoperative period-hernia width of ≤10 cm 3. Abdominal wall reconstruction surgical site occurrence requiring procedural intervention within the 30-d postoperative period-hernia width of >10 cm
Abdominal Wall Reconstruction Preoperative Diabetes Assessment	Process	Percentage of diabetic patients aged 18 y and older who have undergone abdominal wall reconstruction defined as ventral hernia repair with myofascial release (abdominal wall fascial layer separated from muscular layer) with hemoglobin A1c assessment within 6 mo before operation
Ventral Hernia Repair: Biologic Mesh Prosthesis Use in Low-Risk Patients	Efficiency	Percentage of patients aged 18 y and older who have undergone low risk (elective, class I wound, no active skin infection, no stoma present) ventral hernia repair using biologic mesh placement

(continued on next page)

Table 2 (continued)		
Measure	Type	Description
Ventral Hernia Repair: Pain and Functional Status Assessment	Patient-reported outcome	Percentage of patients aged 18 y and older who have undergone ventral hernia repair with completed preoperative (baseline) and at least 1 follow-up patient-reported pain and functional status assessment (patient-reported outcome) These patient-reported outcomes can be completed with an in-person clinical visit, telephone call, smartphone, or email This measure is reported as 2 performance rates: 1. Ventral hernia repair: pain and functional status assessment; overall completion rate 2. Ventral hernia repair: pain and functional status assessment; email engagement completion rate

and devise similar quality initiatives and collaboratives to ensure adequate and fair reporting of quality outcomes in the future.

Recently, the AHSQC was recognized as a QCDR. As previously mentioned, this distinction allows surgeons to use the data reported within the collaborative to satisfy the MIPS requirement for quality reporting. These quality metrics have been designed by the AHSQC, recognizing the importance of risk adjustment and the complexity of hernia surgery. As noted in **Table 2**, the AHSQC has elected to focus on clinical outcome measures to improve quality with 6 of the 9 reported measures falling into the outcomes or patient-reported outcomes category. Equally important, the AHSQC has recognized the importance of risk adjustment and has elected to measure wound morbidity and surgical outcomes based on hernia width when stratifying physicians. This is an example of surgeons with clinical expertise in their field developing, measuring, and reporting their outcomes, and is an ideal model for other surgical fields to follow. Moving forward, the next phase of this model will be the development of public reporting mechanisms to allow the consumers (patients) to appropriately evaluate their surgeons. It is the overwhelming opinion of the AHSQC that simple binary reporting of individual outcomes will not provide a reasonable means for patients to accurately assess their surgeon's quality. Instead, the AHSQC suggests that the process of surgeons being involved in continuous quality improvement, tracking and analyzing their data, participating in improvement activities, and reassessing their outcomes will produce high-quality hernia surgeons. Thus, it would seem most appropriate that the surgeons who are in good standing within the AHSQC could be publicly reported as hernia surgeons of excellence based on the process of continuous quality improvement and not based on a single individual outcome.

SUMMARY

The outcomes that occur after surgical procedures are complex, highly variable, and difficult to measure. However, the importance of quality improvement and quality metrics are here to stay. All stakeholders in medicine must find ways to measure, report, and improve the quality of care that they deliver to patients. The process of defining and measuring quality is an extremely challenging proposition and yet is critically important for the future of the health care system. It is paramount that clinically active physicians who care for patients are at the table when these complex decisions are being made, and that it is not simply delegated to politicians and administrators. Although it is out of our comfort zone, and often was not our primary objective in going into medicine, if these changes are not being selected, validated, and implemented in a thoughtful, reasonable manner, our patients and our ability to care for our patients will be compromised.

REFERENCES

1. Kohn LT, Corrigan JM, Institute of Medicine, editors. To err is human: building a safer health system. Washington, DC: National Academic Press; 2000.
2. Porter ME. What is value in health care? N Engl J Med 2010;363(26):2477–81.
3. Squitieri L, Chung KC. Measuring provider performance for physicians participating in the merit-based incentive payment system. Plast Reconstr Surg 2017; 140(1):217e–26e.
4. NCQA (National Committee for Quality Assurance). NCQA HEDIS measures: summary table of measures, product lines and changes. Washington, DC: NCQA; 2014. Available at: http://www.ncqa.org//Portals/0/Hedisqm/hedis2014/List_of _HEDIS_Measures.pdf.
5. Donabedian A. The quality of care. How can it be assessed? JAMA 1988;260(12): 1743–8.
6. Kessell E, Pegany V, Keolanui B, et al. Review of medicare, medicaid, and commercial quality of care measures: considerations for assessing accountable care organizations. J Health Polit Policy Law 2015;40(4):761–96.
7. AHRQ (Agency for Healthcare Research and Quality). Principles for the National Quality Strategy (NQS). 2014. Available at: www.ahrq.gov/workingforquality/nqs/principles.htm. Accessed January 15, 2017.
8. National Quality Measures Clearinghouse (NQMC) home page: Available at: http://wwww.qualitymeasures.ahrq.gov/faq.aspx. Accessed January 15, 2017.
9. Porter ME, Larsson S, Lee TH. Standardizing patient outcomes measurement. N Engl J Med 2016;374(6):504–6.
10. Petro CC, O'Rourke CP, Posielski NM, et al. Designing a ventral hernia staging system. Hernia 2016;20(1):111–7.
11. Muysoms F, Campanelli G, Champault GG, et al. EuraHS: the development of an international online platform for registration and outcome measurement of ventral abdominal wall hernia repair. Hernia 2012;16(3):239–50.
12. Broderick JE, DeWitt EM, Rothrock N, et al. Advances in patient-reported outcomes: the NIH PROMIS((R)) measures. EGEMS (Wash DC) 2013;1(1):1015.
13. Krpata DM, Schmotzer BJ, Flocke S, et al. Design and initial implementation of HerQLes: a hernia-related quality-of-life survey to assess abdominal wall function. J Am Coll Surg 2012;215(5):635–42.
14. Heniford BT, Lincourt AE, Walters AL, et al. Carolinas comfort scale as a measure of hernia repair quality of life: a reappraisal utilizing 3788 international patients. Ann Surg 2018;267(1):171–6.
15. Haskins IN, Krpata DM, Rosen MJ, et al. Online surgeon ratings and outcomes in hernia surgery: an Americas Hernia Society Quality Collaborative analysis. J Am Coll Surg 2017;225(5):582–9.

16. 2013 Annual Progress Report to Congress: National Strategy for Quality Improvement in Health Care. Washington, DC: US Department of Health and Human Services; 2013.
17. Esposito ML, Selker HP, Salem DN. Quantity over quality: how the rise in quality measures is not producing quality results. J Gen Intern Med 2015;30(8):1204–7.
18. Hawn MT, Richman JS, Vick CC, et al. Timing of surgical antibiotic prophylaxis and the risk of surgical site infection. JAMA Surg 2013;148(7):649–57.
19. Jenkins TR. The use of quality metrics in health care: primum non nocere and the law of unintended consequences. Am J Obstet Gynecol 2016;214(2):143–4.
20. Morgan DM, Swenson CW, Streifel KM, et al. Surgical site infection following hysterectomy: adjusted rankings in a regional collaborative. Am J Obstet Gynecol 2016;214(2):259.e1–8.
21. Gilman M, Adams EK, Hockenberry JM, et al. Safety-net hospitals more likely than other hospitals to fare poorly under Medicare's value-based purchasing. Health Aff (Millwood) 2015;34(3):398–405.
22. Kokotovic D, Bisgaard T, Helgstrand F. Long-term recurrence and complications associated with elective incisional hernia repair. JAMA 2016;316(15):1575–82.
23. Park AE, Zahiri HR, Pugh CM, et al. Raising the quality of hernia care: is there a need? Surg Endosc 2015;29(8):2061–71.
24. Poulose BK, Roll S, Murphy JW, et al. Design and implementation of the Americas Hernia Society Quality Collaborative (AHSQC): improving value in hernia care. Hernia 2016;20(2):177–89.
25. Muysoms FE, Deerenberg EB, Peeters E, et al. Recommendations for reporting outcome results in abdominal wall repair: results of a Consensus meeting in Palermo, Italy, 28-30 June 2012. Hernia 2013;17(4):423–33.
26. Revicki DA, Chen WH, Harnam N, et al. Development and psychometric analysis of the PROMIS pain behavior item bank. Pain 2009;146(1–2):158–69.
27. Baucom RB, Ousley J, Feurer ID, et al. Patient reported outcomes after incisional hernia repair-establishing the ventral hernia recurrence inventory. Am J Surg 2016;212(1):81–8.
28. Krpata DM, Haskins IN, Phillips S, et al. Does preoperative bowel preparation reduce surgical site infections during elective ventral hernia repair? J Am Coll Surg 2017;224(2):204–11.
29. Prabhu AS, Krpata DM, Perez A, et al. Is it time to reconsider postoperative epidural analgesia in patients undergoing elective ventral hernia repair?: an AHSQC analysis. Ann Surg 2017. [Epub ahead of print].
30. Prabhu AS, Krpata DM, Phillips S, et al. Preoperative chlorhexidine gluconate use can increase risk for surgical site infections after ventral hernia repair. J Am Coll Surg 2017;224(3):334–40.

Establishing a Hernia Program

David M. Krpata, MD

KEYWORDS

- Hernia program • Hernia repair • Hernia outcomes • Hernia value

KEY POINTS

- Hernia Programs should be inclusive, center around teamwork, and be voluntary.
- Continuous quality improvement through collaboration is a principal concept of a Hernia Program.
- The mission should center on improving the quality and value of care delivered to hernia patients.

INTRODUCTION

Despite the fact that hernia surgery comprises one the most common operations performed by general surgeons, the field remains one with little consistency or guidelines for best practices and operative approaches. One major reason for this is that hernia surgery tends to have less interest from academics, resulting in limited resources for research funding, inadequate long-term follow-up, and an underappreciation for patient-centered outcomes. One potential method of countering these challenges is to establish an institutional Hernia Program. Hernia Programs are gaining in popularity; however, there will always be room for more programs and growth within each program.

DEFINING A HERNIA PROGRAM

The blueprint for establishing a Hernia Program is one more of internal direction than architectural. More is gained with motivation than with a brick-and-mortar building. More is achieved with desire than with an extensive network of administrative assistants or physician extenders. In essence, a Hernia Program only requires commitment and an interest in improving patient outcomes.

Six key concepts define a Hernia Program. The single most important concept that establishes the foundation for a Hernia Program is that a Hernia Program is distinct from a "Center of Excellence." Centers of Excellence have traditionally been designed to drive the care of a disease to a single area with higher volumes, more resources,

Disclosure Statement: The author has nothing to disclose.
Comprehensive Hernia Center, Cleveland Clinic, 9500 Euclid Avenue, A-100, Cleveland, OH 44195, USA
E-mail address: krpatad@ccf.org

and a theoretic improvement in outcomes.[1] The "Center of Excellence" model of providing care is exclusive and can be punitive toward centers without a designation. This model is not realistic for hernia surgery because of the sheer volume of hernia operations performed as well as the variability in the complexity of hernias. Any general surgeon should perform most hernias. Thus, a Hernia Program is the opposite of a "Center of Excellence"; it is meant to be inclusive, with the goal of all participants in the program working collaboratively to identify strengths and improve on each other's weaknesses. This model ultimately improves the performance of those in the program, reduces cost, and delivers the most value to patients.

The second concept builds on the inclusive nature of a Hernia Program, and it is teamwork. Hernia Programs are meant to encourage all participants to work together to improve the delivery of care to hernia patients. If you are looking to start a Hernia Program to make yourself better than your partner or to put the neighboring hospital out of business, you have completely missed the point. Members of a program should work as a team to achieve the common goal of betterment of the end product for the consumer, not betterment of self.

The next concept gets at one of the main roots of a Hernia Program. It is the idea of continuous quality improvement. Continuous quality improvement is the process of reflection for a system. Within every system, we should be asking ourselves questions that drive improvement: "Is this the most efficient way to complete this process?" and "What happens when we change our approach?" It requires engagement and belief in the process so that strengths and weaknesses are not only identified but also acted upon. Identified strengths should be implemented system-wide, and weakness should be abandoned. After changes are made, the cycle repeats, asking again, "How can we improve?"

The fourth concept defining a Hernia Program is that it should be voluntary. All those who have the desire to participate in a Hernia Program should be allowed to; however, the key words here are desire and participation. Forcible participation leads to insincerity, which clouds opportunities for continuous quality improvement. Providing members of your hospital with a Hernia Program gives them the opportunity to improve the delivery of hernia care in your system; however, if individuals do not participate, they should then be excluded from the program because success is so heavily dependent upon active participation by all members.

Hernia Programs should serve as stewards of information to both patients and other providers who are looking to improve the delivery of hernia care. As such, education is the fifth component of a Hernia Program. The door should always be open to accepting and providing feedback. Staying current with the literature allows a program to implement new techniques and perioperative management strategies to improve the hernia care provided.

The final concept that defines a Hernia Program is research. It is important to recognize that research does not necessarily mean publishing outcomes in the highest-level journals. The Merriam-Webster's Dictionary defines research as "the investigation or experimentation aimed at the discovery and interpretation of facts, revision of accepted theories or laws in the light of new facts, or practical application of such new or revised theories or laws". As such, being a Hernia Program means pushing ourselves to test and review current hernia practices to establish new standards for the field. Importantly, this should be conducted in a controlled and organized fashion rather than haphazardly experimenting within the field. Sharing results with others completes the process and can be achieved through conversation, presentations, or publication.

Collectively, these 6 concepts provide the foundation for a Hernia Program and its mission. As with all businesses and corporations, institutional Hernia Programs should have a mission statement. Our program's mission statement is as follows:

The institutional drive, through the work of all its individuals, to improve the care of hernia patients through quality improvement, cost reduction, research and education of all who care for patients with hernias.

ASSEMBLING THE TEAM AND PROTOCOLS

After defining your Hernia Program and its mission, the next step in establishing a Hernia Program is to understand and identify the stakeholders involved. A Hernia Program goes beyond a few surgeons. Hospital administrators are also considered stakeholders based on the potential for a Hernia Program to standardize approaches and reduce costs associated with the care of hernia patients.

Hernia Program stakeholders include any and all surgeons who are involved with abdominal wall disease at an institution. Surgical stakeholders include not only general surgeons but also plastic surgeons, colorectal surgeons, and trauma surgeons. Bringing all of these surgeons to the table provides an opportunity to approach decisions in a multidisciplinary fashion. In addition to the surgical teams, hospital administrators should be included as well. Including division chiefs and surgical chairs in the discussion not only legitimizes the establishment of the program, but provides additional oversight and input. The addition of quality officers to the Hernia Program can aid with monitoring outcomes and identifying opportunities for improvement. Surgical Operations, including the operating room purchasing team, should also be included so that the program can get involved in mesh and device contract negotiations. This is important for 2 reasons: first, it gives participants in the program an understanding of the costs associated with their intraoperative choices for devices or meshes, and second, it provides the end user, the surgeon, a voice during contract negotiations for devices. A director is named once all stakeholders are brought to the table. The director of the Hernia Program should have the most vested interest in the program and is typically one of the surgical members.

After identifying key players, all stakeholders should be brought to the table to begin establishing institutional protocols and guidelines for hernia repair. This step is one of the most critical steps in the process. The essential part of this step is that all members must agree on the protocol and guidelines based on their comfort level and style of practice. Importantly, there is no correct protocol here. Indeed, it is meant to be an agreement between all involved; in absence of this, members may feel alienated and subsequently lose their interest and belief in the program.

The agreed-upon protocol is now the starting point for the program. As the program moves forward, outcomes are monitored, and changes are made to the initial protocols based on those outcomes. **Fig. 1** demonstrates our institutional protocol for ventral hernia repairs. The protocol includes recommendations for the surgical approach, mesh selection based on Centers for Disease Control and Prevention (CDC) wound class, and techniques. Noticeably, our group tends to be more aggressive with synthetic mesh in potentially contaminated cases. This protocol is based on our comfort, and we fully recognize that others may not have the same comfort or agreement with synthetic mesh or even our preferred techniques, and this is okay. Again, the most important part is to establish a protocol for your institution based on everyone's comfort and then follow your outcomes.

MAINTENANCE PHASE

At this point, the Hernia Program is established, and it is time to move on to the maintenance phase. Think of the maintenance period as an opportunity to give back to the members of the Hernia Program and keep participants engaged. For example, our

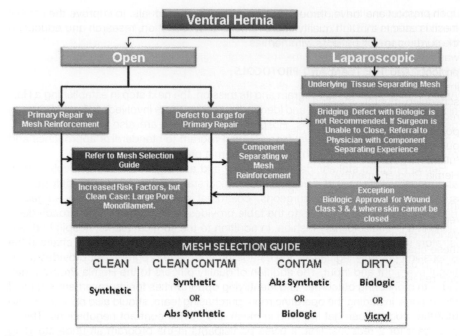

Fig. 1. Protocol-based use for ventral hernia.

program provides educational opportunities through multiple avenues. Our monthly conference allows members of the program an opportunity to present challenging cases and discuss patient selection for various techniques, mesh selection, and post-operative management strategies. In addition, we have quarterly journal clubs to re-view recent additions to the hernia literature which provides an opportunity to critically evaluate studies and learn from others as we consider methods to assess our program.

A critical part of the maintenance phase is the feedback that is provided to the mem-bers. To understand how feedback is provided, first, the group must know how the data are acquired. To record outcomes, surgeons can either establish a prospective data-base at their institution or use a database that is already created. Our program uses the Americas Hernia Society Quality Collaborative (AHSQC; AHSQC.org), which is an online, surgeon-entered database that allows surgeons to review their outcomes as well as compare themselves to other surgeons from across the nation.[2] There are several benefits to using this resource, including the following: (1) it allows surgeons to sort their surgeon-specific data as well as their institutional data; (2) it includes patient as well as operative details, allowing a more granular review of approaches and out-comes; and (3) it is free for members of the Americas Hernia Society (for more details, please see Michael J. Rosen's article, "Quality Measures in Hernia Surgery," in this issue). Importantly, the data entered into the AHSQC can be cross-referenced against administrative data, which informs the director of the Hernia Program of how many pa-tients are being entered by each surgeon of the program. Our program requires that 90% of cases are entered for a surgeon to be considered a participating member of the Hernia Program. Using the AHSQC and administrative data, surgeons are provided feedback on participation, outcomes such as readmissions, wound morbidity, and protocol compliance. This feedback comes in multiple forms, including direct feedback from the director of the Hernia Program when there is a discrepancy between the agreed upon protocol and the implemented practice. For example, at our institution, if a biologic mesh is used in a CDC 1, clean, ventral hernia repair, the director of the program will call the surgeon to better understand the indications for biologic mesh in that case. If there was no acceptable indication, then the director will review the institutional agreed-upon protocol. Additional feedback is provided in monthly Hernia Program meetings reviewing institutional data. For example, all Hernia Program readmissions are reviewed at a scheduled monthly meeting, and the members of the program discuss readmission reduction strategies based on the cases. At these meetings, additional topics, including postoperative analgesia strategies such as epidurals versus patient-controlled analgesia pumps versus transversus abdominis plane blocks have been changed. At our own institution, we have also changed our deep vein thrombosis prophylaxis strategies based on Hernia Program member feedback and review of the program data.

The third component of the maintenance phase is active continuous quality improvement. The program's outcomes and the feedback provided to surgeons are regularly reviewed for quality improvement opportunities. As problems are identified, various changes are made and implemented in an organized fashion. The impact of these changes is then assessed, and changes are again made. The quality improvement process becomes a cycle of assessment, problem identification, modification, and reassessment.

GETTING BUY-IN

One of the most frequent questions asked about establishing a Hernia Program is, how do you get buy-in to the program? Getting busy surgeons to buy into the concept of a Hernia Program is not an easy task; however, using basic business principles may create the most favorable position to succeed. Most importantly, the vision must be clearly laid out which means you must understand and believe in the reason for starting a Hernia Program and be able to articulate it in a clear, concise manner. The vision should be rooted in improved patient outcomes and optimizing the value of the care delivered. Second, members in the program should be engaged with personalized tasks. Giving members tasks allows them to provide personal input and to help shape the Hernia Program. Expect that this will lead to fruitful discussions and even debates about the program. The director should be open to all opinions and give everyone an opportunity to voice theirs.

The third principle to get buy-in is to follow up with members and participants. A Hernia Program cannot be left on autopilot; otherwise, participants may begin drifting away from the program. Staying engaged with all of the members demonstrates 2 things: (1) your own investment in the program and (2) attention is given to those participating in the group and what they are doing. Fourth, manage resistance early. Disgruntled members can spread negative energy throughout the program and influence others' opinions. Begin by addressing the concerns of any members who are resistant and try to find common ground for resolution of their concerns. Persistent resistance to the Hernia Program should be viewed as involuntary participation, and those members should be removed from the program immediately.

The fifth and most crucial principle to getting buy-in is to accept feedback. As a director, you must be willing to openly listen to criticism about the program and make changes based on this feedback. Failure to accept feedback from members of the program may alienate the participants because of the perception of inflexibility, lack of compassion, or poor leadership. There will be many challenges along the way as the Hernia Program is grown and maintained, but keeping a clear vision, engaging members with personalized tasks, following up with members, addressing resistance early, and accepting feedback give the best chance for success.

IMPACT OF THE HERNIA PROGRAM

The impact of a fully established Hernia Program can be tremendous. As an example, we reviewed our own Hernia Program's experience and the compliance to our ventral hernia protocol, as seen in **Fig. 1**. It is important to note that in our protocol, one area of focus was the elimination of biologic mesh use in CDC wound class 1 cases.

Using mesh utilization practices as a surrogate for Hernia Program protocol compliance, we compared the 19 months before initiation of the Hernia Program with the first 16 months of the Hernia Program.[3] After reviewing 13,937 ventral hernia repairs within the institution, we found that members of the Hernia Program reduced biologic mesh use in CDC wound class 1 cases after the Hernia Program was initiated. In fact, members were 100% compliant and eliminated biologic mesh used in these clean cases. In addition, there was a statistically significant reduction in biologic mesh in all wound classes.

This significant decrease in biologic mesh utilization practices ultimately led to cost savings for the institution of more than $527,000 in 16 months. This example shows that the simple act of getting all stakeholders on the same page concerning the management of ventral hernias can significantly influence the value of care delivered at an institution.

SUMMARY

In summary, a Hernia Program should be inclusive, center around teamwork, strive for continuous quality improvement, be voluntary, provide education for its members and patients, and in some manner contribute to the field through research. Before establishing your Hernia Program, the mission should be clear and center on improving the quality and value of care delivered to hernia patients. While maintaining the program, stick to the mission, get others involved, and be receptive to their opinions. In the end, this will maximize buy-in from the people around you, continuously improve outcomes for patients, and add value to the health care system.

REFERENCES

1. Mehrotra A, Dimick JB. Ensuring excellence in centers of excellence programs. Ann Surg 2015;261(2):237–9.
2. Poulose BK, Roll S, Murphy JW, et al. Design and implementation of the Americas Hernia Society Quality Collaborative (AHSQC): improving value in hernia care. Hernia 2016;20(2):177–89.
3. Krpata DM, Haskins IN, Rosenblatt S, et al. Development of a disease-based Hernia Program and the impact of cost for a hospital system. Ann Surg 2018;267(2):370–4.

Updates in Mesh and Biomaterials

Brent D. Matthews, MD[a], Lauren Paton, MD[b],*

KEYWORDS

- Hernia • Abdominal wall • Biological mesh • Synthetic mesh • Biosynthetic mesh

KEY POINTS

- Additional evidence highlighting the low morbidity associated with synthetic mesh and biosynthetic mesh in clean-contaminated and contaminated fields is provided.
- Additional evidence discussing the limitations of using biologic mesh is provided.
- The future of mesh research may involve trialing novel polymers, alternative ways to deliver antibiotics to surgical sites, and involve data registries including patient-centered outcomes and direct surgeon feedback.

INTRODUCTION

Prior publications of the *Surgical Clinics of North America* have highlighted the technical challenges of abdominal wall reconstruction. In 2008, the issue dedicated to abdominal wall reconstruction discussed the biology of hernia formation, the history of hernia repair, open and laparoscopic ventral hernia repair, and the benefits of the use of prosthetic mesh on patient outcomes. Despite the vast selection of mesh brands available, nearly all mesh continues to use 1 of 3 basic materials—polypropylene, polyester, or polytetrafluoroethylene in various combinations with or without barrier coating. The mesh types differ in many characteristics, including their tensile strength, elasticity, and weight, which depends on pore size and the weight of the polymer. Heavy weight mesh uses thick polymers, small pore size, and high tensile strength, whereas light weight mesh uses thinner polymers and larger pores.

In the 2008 *Surgical Clinics of North America* publication, Bachman and Ramshaw[1] discussed the wide variety of mesh products available for abdominal wall reconstruction and the challenge facing surgeons to choose the most appropriate mesh for ventral hernia repair. Interestingly, they concluded that there was no "best" mesh. Still

Disclosures: The authors have nothing to disclose.
[a] Department of Surgery, Carolinas Medical Center, 1000 Blythe Boulevard, 2nd Floor Administrative Suites, Charlotte, NC 28203, USA; [b] Department of Surgery, Carolinas Medical Center, 1000 Blythe Boulevard, Medical Education Building 6A, Charlotte, NC 28203, USA
* Corresponding author.
E-mail addresses: Lauren.paton@carolinashealthcare.org; Lauren.paton@carolinas.org

Surg Clin N Am 98 (2018) 463–470
https://doi.org/10.1016/j.suc.2018.02.007
0039-6109/18/© 2018 Elsevier Inc. All rights reserved.

a decade later, the decision of which mesh to use is based on several factors: the type of procedure being performed, the clinical situation (elective vs emergent, Centers for Diseased Control and Prevention [CDC] wound classification, etc), the desired handling characteristics to optimize mesh placement, material costs, and the products available to the surgeon based on hospital material contracts.[1] In the same publication, Jin and Rosen[2] described the limited data available specifically when comparing the long-term outcomes of for synthetic to biologic mesh. It seemed that most mesh selections were based on surgeon's anecdotal experience. Clearly, prospective studies comparing clinical outcomes for the variety of meshes available is needed.[2] In that same issue, Earle and Mark[3] discussed the many variables of mesh designs, including the polymer used, fiber size, fiber strength, elasticity, pore size, density, and bioreactivity. These multiple variables do not allow for direct comparisons. Earle and Mark also stressed that, as more mesh types are being developed, surgeons must balance the uncertainty of long-term outcomes when introducing a new prosthetic against the more certain outcomes of existing products.[3] This challenge remains true a decade later.

The 2013 publication of the *Surgical Clinics of North America* on abdominal wall reconstruction further addressed the clinical outcomes of biologic mesh and the safety of prosthetic mesh repair in contaminated settings. The literature exploring the use of biologic grafts in infected and contaminated fields was disappointing. Preclinical animal studies failed to demonstrate consistent evidence of biological mesh remodeling and long-term clinical outcomes using biologics revealed higher than expected recurrence rates.[4] Alternatively, Carbonell and Cobb[5] cited a relatively low morbidity rate associated with the use of light weight and even heavy weight polypropylene mesh in clean-contaminated and contaminated fields. At that time, however, many surgeons remained reluctant to change their practice based on this literature owing to fears of complications, specifically wound and mesh infections, and using prosthetic mesh off-label in CDC class II and III wounds.

The *Surgical Clinics of North America* is dedicating another publication to abdominal wall reconstruction in 2018, and this article provides an update on biomaterial research. This article specifically reviews synthetic, biologic, and biosynthetic mesh research and concludes with thoughts about the future of mesh research. This update highlights research that has been conducted since the prior publication to guide surgeons to make evidence-based choices about biomaterial for ventral hernia repair that are most appropriate for their patients.

UPDATE ON SYNTHETIC MESH RESEARCH

Since Usher and associates[6] first introduced polypropylene prosthetics for incisional hernia in the late 1950s, synthetic mesh has been the predominate material used for hernia repair. Permanent synthetic meshes provide long-term mechanical support to the hernia defect and have been shown to reduce recurrence rates compared with sutured or primary repair. As the use of synthetic mesh became more commonplace, clinical outcomes studies have been conducted that directly impact the surgeon's decision making with regard to mesh selection. Although permanent synthetic meshes have been engineered for strength and durability, short- and long-term complications have been attributed to their use. As such, additional modification in fiber diameter and pore size to decrease the density of the material were implemented. These meshes are categorized into heavy weight, midweight, and light weight depending on the grams per square meter.[7] Studies before 2013 demonstrated an improved quality of life (QOL) with light weight mesh. However, Groene and colleagues[8] published a study in 2016 from the International Hernia Mesh Registry database that analyzed both surgical and QOL outcomes after open ventral hernia repair with heavy weight, midweight, and light weight mesh. This multinational, multi-institutional, prospective registry captured QOL surveys at 1, 6, 12, 24, and 36 months. Of the 549 open ventral hernia repairs, patients with midweight meshes had fewer surgical site infections and shorter durations of stay. Recurrence rates were equal (6.1%) among the 3 types of mesh. Nevertheless, light weight mesh was associated with an overall worse QOL at 6 months and more pain at 1 year. Other studies have reported unfavorable consequences of using light weight mesh, specifically mesh fracturing.[9] Whether this finding is a consequence of technique or related to patient comorbidities is not known. However, the benefits of a reduced foreign body reaction owing to the decreased density of material do not seem to be offset by the physicomechanical properties of the mesh.

In the majority of clean-contaminated and contaminated ventral incisional hernia repairs over the past decade, biologic and more recently bioabsorbable synthetic mesh have been used to reduce the incidence of mesh infection and unplanned reoperation. Prospective, longitudinal trials have demonstrated a 2-year recurrence rate of 20% to 30% and 5-year recurrence rates more than 50%.[10] Owing to the disappointingly high recurrence rate and cost of the biomaterials ($2500-$25,000), surgeons began to use permanent synthetic mesh in CDC class II and III wounds. With this off-label use of synthetic mesh, there is now mounting evidence that certain synthetic meshes, particularly wide pore or light weight mesh, may serve as a viable option in contaminated settings.[11] In 2017, Majumder and colleagues[12] published a multicenter, retrospective review of patients undergoing open ventral hernia repair in clean-contaminated/contaminated fields using biologic and synthetic mesh. A total of 126 patients were analyzed with surgical site infections found to be less frequent in the synthetic group (12.3% vs 31.9%) and a lower rate of hernia recurrence in the synthetic group (8.9% vs 26.3%). The synthetic mesh used was most commonly polypropylene (91%), mostly midweight with a microporous design (92%), and placed in a sublay position. Despite recent studies like this, additional evidence will likely be needed to convince surgeons to use synthetic mesh selectively in clean-contaminated and contaminated fields. If one is to consider the total cost of care to manage wound infections, reoperations for ventral hernia recurrence, and so on, synthetic mesh may eventually prove to be superior to biologic reinforcement in select patient populations.

UPDATES IN BIOLOGIC MESH RESEARCH

Biologic mesh was introduced in hopes that the patient's immune cells would infiltrate the material to defend against the bacterial load in a contaminated case and eventually replace the biologic mesh with the host tissue (tissue remodeling). Preclinical evidence that some biologic meshes enabled revascularization of soft tissue repair sites and improved pathogen clearance in contaminated and infected surgical sites.[13,14] The molecular composition of biologic mesh impacts the biocompatibility and biodegradability.[15,16] One aspect of the manufacturing process of biologic mesh is the cross-linking process that results in the creation of bonds between collagen, which is believed to enhance the strength and durability of the mesh.[17,18] The histologic remodeling profile and biomechanical properties of biologic mesh in particular had not been examined until Cavallo and colleagues[19] compared cross-linked (Permacol) or non–cross-linked (Strattice) porcine dermis over a 1-year period in a porcine model of ventral hernia repair. They found that cross-linked mesh demonstrated significant improvement over time in every remodeling category except for scaffold degradation.

Remodeling characteristics of non–cross-linked mesh remained relatively unchanged over time except for fibrous encapsulation and neovascularization. Remodeling scores for non–cross-linked mesh were significantly higher after 1 month compared with non–cross-linked biologic mesh. The tensile strength and stiffness of both cross-linked and non–cross-linked graft tissue composites were greater than the tensile strength and stiffness of the native porcine abdominal wall in the very early postoperative period, but there was no difference in tensile strength or stiffness by the end of the study period (12 months). Researchers concluded that cross-linked biologic mesh reduces the early histologic remodeling profile but does not significantly impact the tensile strength or stiffness of the graft–tissue composites in the long term. Although limitations of biologic mesh exist, they still are being used. Basic science, translational, and clinical research should still be helpful in aiding the decision of which biologic mesh to use, and what technique to apply to optimize mesh integration and overall tissue remodeling to decrease hernia recurrence.

Since the last *Surgical Clinics of North America* update, additional clinical trials have been reported in patients undergoing ventral incisional hernia repair with biologic mesh. Huntington and colleagues[20] prospectively examined the cost and comparative effectiveness of different biologic meshes used for abdominal wall reconstruction at a tertiary hernia center over a 10-year study period. In their study, 223 patients underwent open ventral hernia repair with either Alloderm Regenerative Tissue Matrix (Allergan, Dublin, Ireland), AlloMax Surgical Graft (Bard Davol, Warwick, RI), Flex HD Acellular Dermis (MTF/Ethicon, Inc., Somerville, NJ), Strattice Reconstructive Tissue Matrix (Allergan) or Xenmatrix Surgical Graft (Bard Davol). Their hernia defects were on average 257 ± 245 cm^2 with a mesh size of 384 cm^2. Of the patients studied, 31% had an infection at the time of operation and 28% had a mesh infection at the time of the operation. Hernia recurrence rates varied significantly by mesh type: 35% Alloderm, 34.5% AlloMax, 37% Flex HDTM, 14.7% Strattice, and 59.1% Xenmatrix over a mean follow-up of 18.2 months. Although 36.6% had postoperative wound infections, the rate of mesh infections requiring explantation was less than 1%.[19] Clearly, the choice of biologic mesh affects the long-term postoperative outcomes in ventral hernia repair and clinical outcome studies such as this can also aid a surgeon in which biologic mesh to choose. Abdelfatah and colleagues[21] published their results regarding long term outcomes with the use of porcine acellular dermal matrix for patients at high risk of infection. After a mean follow-up more than 5 years in 59 of 65 patients, they reported the need to explant mesh owing to infection and hernia recurrence of 25% and 66%, respectively. Patients who had grossly infected wounds had a 100% hernia recurrence rate. Owing to the unreliability of short- and long-term outcomes in patients with infected wounds, biologic mesh should not be used routinely with the expectations of a successful outcome. Several clinical studies have demonstrated that biologic meshes do not necessarily need to be removed when infected and can be managed with serial washout and negative pressure and/or passive dressings. The issue of high-risk patients has also altered mesh selection in patient with class I wounds through multiple grading scales evaluating the risk of surgical site occurrence related to patient comorbidities.

Preclinical and clinical trials, risk stratification, hernia grading, and aggressive marketing have contributed to an increase in demand for biologic mesh over the past decade.[14,22] This push has contributed to an increasing cost of care for the complex ventral incisional hernia patient. There is a lack of level 1 evidence that biologic mesh provides superior outcomes. This controversy continues more than 15 years after their introduction into hernia care.

UPDATE IN BIOSYNTHETIC AND SYNTHETIC ABSORBABLE MESH RESEARCH

The long-term absorbable synthetic materials, termed biosynthetic mesh, are relatively new to surgeons performing abdominal wall reconstruction and were not a focus in the *Surgical Clinics of North America* publication in 2013. Because of its breakdown via hydrolysis, biosynthetic mesh is believed to offer a unique advantage when challenged with bacterial colonization during complex abdominal wall reconstruction.[21] Using biodegradable polymers instead of xenogeneic or allogeneic tissue, biosynthetics provide a temporary scaffold for the deposition of the proteins and cells necessary for tissue ingrowth, neovascularization, and host integration. A variety of absorbable synthetic/biosynthetic meshes are now available and have emerged as a less costly and potentially effective alternative to biologic meshes. One type, GORE BIO-A Tissue Reinforcement (W. L. Gore & Associates, Newark, DE), is a biosynthetic mesh composed of a bioabsorbable polyglycolide-trimethylene carbonate copolymer. This polymer is gradually absorbed by the body within 6 to 7 months.[21] The COBRA (Complex Open Bioabsorbable Reconstruction of the Abdominal Wall) study published by Jin and Rosen[2] in 2017 was a multicenter prospective longitudinal study evaluating the performance of GORE BIO-A for reinforcement of the midline fascial closure in the single staged repair of contaminated ventral incisional hernias. Patients included had a clean-contaminated or contaminated wounds, a hernia defect at least 9 cm, and GORE BIO-A in a sublay, retrorectus, or intraperitoneal position (with at least a 4-cm overlap) with primary fascial closure (n = 104). Concomitant procedures in this cohort typically included enterocutaneous fistula takedown or infected mesh removal. Over a 24-month follow-up period (with 84% completing the study), hernia recurrence rate was 17% by physical examination. Although 29 patients (28%) experienced wound-related complications, no patients required mesh explantation. QOL and return to function significantly improved from baseline for these patients, illustrating that biosynthetic absorbable mesh showed efficacy in several patient-centered metrics. In similar groups of patients, this particular biosynthetic should provide an alternative to biologic and permanent meshes in complex hernia repairs.[10]

A different biosynthetic mesh, Phasix (Bard Davol) and its counterpart Phasix ST (Bard Davol), were evaluated by Scott and colleagues[23] assessing its mechanical and histologic properties. Phasix is composed of poly-4-hydroxybutyrate and Phasix ST composed of poly-4-hydroxybutyrate and an absorbable separate coating made of hydrogel to reduce adhesions. These novel biosynthetic meshes were compared with a partially absorbable permanent synthetic mesh, Ventralight ST (Bard Davol), and a biologic derived dermal mesh, Strattice. In this porcine model, mesh was placed as a sublay repair. Mechanical testing revealed Phasix ST and Phasix demonstrated comparable mechanical and histologic properties to Ventralight ST at 12 and 24 weeks. In addition, the results suggested that fully absorbable meshes with longer term resorption profiles may provide improved mechanical and histologic properties compared with biologically derived scaffolds and serve as a cost-effective alternative for complicated abdominal wall reconstruction cases. There are no prospective comparative studies regarding these devices at the time of this publication to suggest which clinical scenario is suited for their use. Further study is necessary to determine this.

TIGR Matrix (Novus Scientific, Singapore) is an alternative long-term absorbable synthetic mesh. Consisting of a slow-absorbing fiber made of lactide and trimethylene carbonate and a fast-absorbing fiber made of glycolide, lactide, and trimethylene carbonate, this device is designed to fully resorb in 3 years as per the manufacturer description. There are some limited animal models comparing the use of TIGR Matrix with biologic meshes, Gore BIO-A, and polypropylene, which showed no clear benefit to the use of absorbable meshes in large abdominal wall hernias in rabbits.[24] There is also a single-arm clinical trial in which 40 primary inguinal hernias were repaired with TIGR Matrix with favorable short-term and long-term outcomes.[25] As is likely true with all resorbable meshes, further study in terms of comparative trials are needed to further elucidate their potential context for use.

UPDATE IN HYBRID MESH RESEARCH

More recent iterations of innovative devices include hybrid meshes, which consist of a class of meshes best described by the hybrid use of both biologic components and synthetic components. In theory, the biological components of the meshes are meant to protect the synthetic mesh devices from their surrounding environments. An example of such a device is Zenapro Hybrid Hernia Repair Device (Cook Medical, Bloomington, IN), a combination of extracellular matrix and large pore polypropylene mesh. Similarly to other innovative mesh devices, there are very few human studies—1 to date—that describe its use, and none are comparative head-to-head trials with other devices. The aforementioned study is a 12-month single arm study in 63 patients with Ventral Hernia Working Group Grade 1 and 2 hernias.[26] Likely, the follow-up time frame is too short to make any true conclusion regarding hernia recurrence rates. Further study is needed to determine any potential use for these types of devices, because their biologic component certainly will increase the cost of production, which begs further proof of concept in the opinion of these authors.

FUTURE OF MESH RESEARCH

The best mesh for patients still depends on multiple factors, including wound contamination, patient comorbidities, and surgical technique. Although uncertainty about clinical decision making related to mesh selection remains, the development of additional synthetic, biologic, and biosynthetic meshes continues including novel technologies. For instance, Grafmiller and colleagues[27] investigated a polymer that provides controlled release of an antibiotic in a linear fashion over a 45-day period and found that vancomycin drug-releasing polymers in the form of microspheres adequately cleared a bacterial burden of Staphylococcus aureus and prevented mesh infection in a rat model. Poppas and colleagues[28] developed a novel nonbiodegradable hydrogel coated polypropylene mesh and found that it led to a significant decrease in foreign body reaction, oxidative stress, and apoptosis compared with uncoated polypropylene in a rat model. Last, Klinger and colleagues[29] created a model for a "living mesh" with decellularized porcine small intestinal submucosa as a scaffold for human adipose-derived stem cells and analyzed the neovascularization and tensile strength in a rat ventral hernia model. The clinical gap these novel technologies could ultimately cover is to be determined. Nonetheless, innovation in biomaterial development will likely lead to improved patient outcomes. As these clinical studies are completed to evaluate novel technologies, data registries such as the American Hernia Society Quality Collaborative will have a significant role. The American Hernia Society Quality Collaborative was formed in 2013 by hernia surgeons in private practice and academic medical centers using the concepts of continuous quality improvement to improve clinical outcomes, to improve efficiencies of care, and to optimize costs. The patient-centered data collection platform provides ongoing, real-time performance feedback to clinicians in a setting of collaborative learning.[30] The American Hernia Society Quality Collaborative will hopefully provide a mechanism for long-term outcomes research and postmarket surveillance of new products to aid surgeons who perform ventral incisional hernia repair or abdominal wall reconstruction to select the mesh most appropriate and effective for their patients.

SUMMARY

Since the *Surgical Clinics of North America* publication in 2013, clinical research focusing on the use of biologic and synthetic mesh has brought more, but still limited, clarity to the efficacy of these materials as well as their limitations in particular clinical scenarios. Evidence to support the use of biosynthetic meshes, as an alternative to biologic mesh, in CDC class II and III wounds is intriguing. The use of synthetic mesh in these patients is even more disruptive as the accountability to increasing cost of care increases. It will be important that over the next 5 to 10 years of biomaterial research focuses on patient-centered outcomes and value-based metrics. Surgeon-led initiatives such as the American Hernia Society Quality Collaborative should transform the surgeons' capacity to make evidence-based decision regarding biomaterial selection for abdominal wall reconstruction.

REFERENCES

1. Bachman S, Ramshaw B. Prosthetic material in ventral hernia repair: how do I choose? Surg Clin North Am 2008;88(1):101–12.
2. Jin J, Rosen MJ. Laparoscopic versus open ventral hernia repair. Surg Clin North Am 2008;148:1083–100.
3. Earle DB, Mark LA. Prosthetic material in inguinal hernia repair: how do I choose? Surg Clin North Am 2008;88(1):179–201.
4. Novitsky YW. Biology of biological meshes used in hernia repair. Surg Clin North Am 2013;93(5):1211–6.
5. Carbonell AM, Cobb WS. Safety of prosthetic mesh hernia repair in contaminated fields. Surg Clin North Am 2013;93(5):127–39.
6. Usher FC, Oshsner J, Tuttle LL Jr. Use of Marlex mesh in the repair of incisional hernias. Am Surg 1958;24(12):967–74.
7. Cobb WS, Kercher KW, Heniford BT. The argument for lightweight polypropylene mesh in hernia repair. Surg Innov 2005;12:63–9.
8. Groene SA, Prasad T, Lincourt AE, et al. Prospective, multi-institutional surgical and quality-of-life outcomes comparison for heavyweight, midweight, and light-weight mesh in open ventral hernia repair. Am J Surg 2016;212:1054–62.
9. Zuvela M, Galun D, Djuric-Stefanovic A. Central rupture and bulging of low-weight polypropylene mesh following recurrent incisional sublay hernioplasty. Hernia 2014;18:135–40.
10. Rosen MJ, Bauer JJ, Harmaty M, et al. Multicenter, prospective, longitudinal study of the recurrence, surgical site infection, and quality of life after contaminated ventral hernia repair using biosynthetic absorbable mesh- the COBRA study. Ann Surg 2016;265:205–11.
11. Beale EW, Hoxworth RE, Livingston EH. The role of biologic mesh in abdominal wall reconstruction: a systematic review of the current literature. Am J Surg 2012;204(4):510–7.
12. Majumder A, Winder JS, Wen Y, et al. Comparative analysis of biologic versus synthetic mesh outcomes in contaminated hernia repairs. Surgery 2017;160(4): 828–38.
13. Millennium Research Group 2010 US markets for soft tissue repair devices. Millennium Research Group Incorporated, Toronto; 2010.

14. Hartha KC, Broome AM, Jacobs MR, et al. Bacterial clearance of biologic grafts used in hernia repair: an experimental study. Surg Endosc 2011;25(7):2224–9.
15. Le D, Deveney CW, Reaven NL, et al. Mesh choice in ventral hernia repair: so many choices so little time. Am J Surg 2013;205:602–7.
16. Cevasco M, Itani KM. Ventral hernia repair with synthetic composite and biologic mesh: characteristics, indications and infection profile. Surg Infections (Larchmt) 2012;13:209–15.
17. Liang HC, Chang Y, Hsu CK, et al. Effects of crosslinking degree on an acellular biologic tissue on its tissue regeneration pattern. Biomaterials 2004;25(17):3541–52.
18. Badylak SF, Freytes DO, Gilbert TW. Extracellular matrix as a biological scaffold material: structure and function. Acta Biomater 2009;5(1):1–13.
19. Cavallo JA, Greco SC, Liu J, et al. Remodeling characteristics and biomechanical properties of crosslinked versus non-crosslinked porcine dermis scaffolds in a porcine model of ventral hernia repair. Hernia 2015;19:207–18.
20. Huntington CR, Cox TC, Blair LJ, et al. Biologic mesh in ventral hernia repair: outcomes, recurrence, and charge analysis. Surgery 2016;160(6):1517–27.
21. Adelfatah MM, Rostambeigi N, Podgaetz E, et al. Long-term outcomes (>5 year follow-up with porcine acellular dermal matric (Permacol) in incisional hernias at risk for infection. Hernia 2015;19:135–40.
22. Kim H, Bruen K, Vargo D. Acelluluar dermal matrix in the management of high-risk abdominal wall defects. Am J Surg 2006;192(6):705–9.
23. Scott JR, Deeken CR, Martindale RG, et al. Evaluation of a full absorbable poly-4-hydroxybuterate/absorbable barrier composite mesh in a porcine model of hernia repair. Surg Endosc 2016;20:3691–701.
24. Peeters E, van Barneveld KW, Schreinemacher MH, et al. One-year outcome of biological and synthetic bioabsorbable meshes for augmentation of large abdominal wall defects in a rabbit model. J Surg Res 2013;180(2):274–83.
25. Ruiz-Jasbon F, Norrby J, Ivarsson ML, et al. Inguinal hernia repair using a synthetic long-term resorbable mesh: results from a 3-year prospective safety and performance study. Hernia 2014;18(5):723–30.
26. Bittner JG 4th, El-Hayek K, Strong AT, et al. First human use of hybrid synthetic/biologic mesh in ventral hernia repair: a multicenter trial. Surg Endosc 2018;32(3):1123–30.
27. Grafmiller KR, Zuckerman ST, Petro C, et al. Antibiotic releasing microspheres prevent mesh infection in vivo. J Surg Res 2016;206(1):41–7.
28. Poppas DP, Sung JJ, Magro CM, et al. Hydrogel coated mesh decreases tissue reaction resulting from polypropylene mesh implant: implication in hernia repair. Hernia 2016;20:623–32.
29. Klinger A, Kawata M, Villalobos M, et al. Living scaffolds: surgical repair using scaffolds seeded with human adipose-derived stem cells. Hernia 2016;20:161–70.
30. American Hernia Society Quality Collaborative. Available at: https://www.ahsqc.org/faqs. Accessed August 1, 2017.

Role of Prophylactic Mesh Placement for Laparotomy and Stoma Creation

Irfan A. Rhemtulla, MD, MS[a], Charles A. Messa IV, BS[a],
Fabiola A. Enriquez, BA[a], William W. Hope, MD[b],
John P. Fischer, MD, MPH[a],*

KEYWORDS

- Incisional • Hernia • Prevention • Mesh • Augmentation • Parastomal
- Prophylactic

KEY POINTS

- Incisional and parastomal hernias remain a challenge to treat, morphing into a cycle of complications and reoperations with increased cost and decreased quality of life.
- Prevention of abdominal hernias with mesh may have a higher upfront cost, but could lead to a larger benefit by halting the progression of complications and reoperations.
- Use of an onlay mesh with minimal fixation can easily be taught and implemented to prevent incisional hernias in high-risk populations among many surgical subspecialties.
- Use of a retrorectus mesh may be more favorable in parastomal hernia prevention.
- The ideal type of mesh to be used in these surgeries is a topic of debate that will become clearer when more data on bioabsorbable meshes become available.

INTRODUCTION

A cornerstone of modern medical practice is in the institution of preventative, risk-reductive measures to improve outcomes. This is a concept that has been implemented across many specialties with great success, but only sparingly in surgery, a field uniquely equipped to impact patient outcomes by performing prophylactic operations. A few examples include mastectomies and colectomies to prevent cancer in

Disclosure Statement: Dr J.P. Fischer is a consultant for Bard-Davol, Gore, Integra, LifeSciences, and Misonix. He also has research support from Integra LifeSciences and Misonix. Dr W. Hope is a consultant for Intuitive and Lifecell. He has research support from CR Bard and WL Gore. He is a speaker for CR Bard, WL Gore, and Intuitive. He is an honorarium for CR Bard. Drs I.A. Rhemtulla, C.A. Messa, and F.A. Enriquez have nothing to disclose.
[a] Department of Surgery, Division of Plastic Surgery, University of Pennsylvania, South Pavilion – 14th Floor, 3400 Civic Center Boulevard, Philadelphia, PA 19104, USA; [b] Department of Surgery, New Hanover Regional Medical Center, 1725 New Hanover Medical Park Drive, Wilmington, NC 28403, USA
* Corresponding author.
E-mail address: John.Fischer2@uphs.upenn.edu

high-risk patients, insertion of ureteral stents during colorectal surgery to identify ureteral injury, and creation of muscle flaps in vascular procedures to prevent groin infections.[1-4] Similarly, there may be an opportunity to prevent incisional hernias (IH) and parastomal hernias (PH) through surgery with prophylactic mesh placement (PMP).

Considering morbidity, cost, and quality of life, effective primary prevention of IH and PH could improve the lives of patients and reduce the strain of IH and PH on the health care system. Hernias are a cyclical chronic disease with a high recurrence rate, substantial complications, and increased expenses linked to treatment. Flum and colleagues[5] described the high cumulative rates of reoperative repairs for ventral hernias and concluded that adverse outcomes were not decreasing despite efforts at improving repair techniques. Holihan and colleagues[6] took this further and showed that a recurrent hernia has increased complications leading to reoperation, more complications, and an ongoing "vicious cycle" that does not stop. This cycle can be thought of as a conceptual framework, outlined in **Fig. 1**, where roughly one-third of the 350,000 IH repairs in the United States will fail, perpetuating this ongoing cycle and leading to more than \$3 billion in cost.[7-9]

Hernias continue to remain an issue with solutions that are only partially effective. There are emerging data on techniques for PMP to prevent IH and PH. To improve and enhance knowledge, this article summarizes and critically examines the literature evaluating the prevention of abdominal hernias (AH) through the placement of prophylactic mesh.

BACKGROUND

There are estimates that up to 4 to 5 million abdominal surgeries are performed annually in the United States.[10] Midline laparotomies are associated with significant morbidity in the perioperative and postoperative period. One of the most common and challenging postoperative consequences of a laparotomy is an IH, which occurs in roughly 5% to 20% of the general population but is seen in approximately 30% and as high as 73.1% of high-risk patients.[11,12] A study by Bosanquet and colleagues[13] showed through metaregression that the incidence of IH was 12.8% among 83 different patient groups. The authors of that study were also able to identify specific patient groups at high risk for IH, which included increasing age, patients with a history

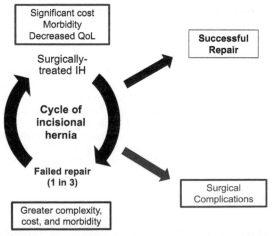

Fig. 1. Conceptual framework for cycle of incisional hernia. QoL, quality of life.

of or operation for abdominal aortic aneurysm (AAA), patients undergoing bariatric surgery, and patients with previous laparotomies or IHs.[13]

In a similar fashion, PH has been shown time and again in the literature as being the most common complication following creation of a colostomy, with incidence rates of 56%.[14–17] Approximately 120,000 PH are repaired in the United States annually with recurrence rates of 80.6% after suture repair, 41.7% after laparoscopic repair, and 28.6% after open mesh repair.[18] Risk factors particular to PH include surgery-specific issues, such as ostomy defect diameter, intraperitoneal compared with extraperitoneal technique, small bowel compared with large bowel stoma, and end ostomy compared with loop ostomy.[19]

When considering AH surgery as an ecosystem, there are multiple interventions that can help to reduce the incidence of AH. These are illustrated in **Fig. 2** and include PMP at the time of initial operation, optimizing treatment at the time of hernia repair, and managing surgical morbidity after hernia repair. The focus of this article is on prevention with prophylactic mesh, because it is the earliest in the cycle and one in which surgeons are able to initially impact.

TECHNIQUE OF MESH PLACEMENT

The technique of fascial closure during abdominal surgery is crucial to the discussion of preventing AH. Before the advent of mesh, the only way fascia was reapproximated was primarily with the use of suture material in a running fashion or with interrupted bites.[20] Studies later found that continuous, slowly absorbing suture was in fact better than interrupted bites at reducing IH.[21] Israelsson and Millbourn[22] described through several studies that the ideal suture to wound length should be at least 4:1, which was again reiterated by the European Hernia Society in their recent published guidelines on the closure of abdominal wall incisions.[23] To our knowledge, this method has not been studied in patients with hernias.

Although the ideal technique to primarily close fascia has been refined over the years, it is not the only method of reapproximating fascia. Hernia surgery was significantly

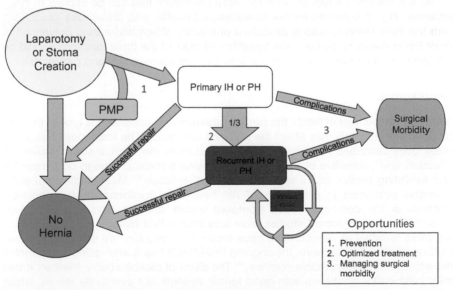

Fig. 2. Opportunities to intervene within the hernia ecosystem.

advanced by data demonstrating that a mesh-reinforced closure reduced the risk of hernia recurrence, regardless of size.[24–26] The concept of using mesh to reapproximate and reinforce fascia during hernia repair can be generalized to hernia prevention through similar techniques.

In the context of prophylactic augmentation, mesh placement can broadly be grouped into three categories: (1) onlay, (2) sublay, and (3) underlay. An onlay mesh is fixed above the muscle to the anterior rectus sheath and is accomplished without entering the abdominal cavity.[27] Theoretically, it is simple, fast, and poses little visceral risk. A systematic review conducted by Borab and colleagues[28] showed that onlay placement of mesh reduced IH despite a high seroma and infection rate. A more recent randomized control trial looking at the prevention of IH with onlay and sublay mesh compared with primary suture closure (PSC), the PRImary Mesh closure of Abdominal midline wound (PRIMA) trial, showed a lower IH rate in the onlay arm compared with the sublay and PSC arms.[11] It should be noted that although it was suggested that the PSC arm use a 4:1 suture to wound ratio, the investigators state that they were unable to confirm that all surgeons participating in the study followed this suggestion.

A sublay mesh, which is typically placed in the retrorectus plane between the posterior sheath and the undersurface of the rectus muscle, allows the mesh to be separated from intraperitoneal structures.[29] Additionally, it is not adjacent to the skin, which could lead to decreased wound complications. The authors believe a retrorectus repair may better resist fascial disruption from Valsalva pressure and has a better tension distribution. This type of mesh placement has been shown to reduce IH, but the technical skill and increased time required may not be ideal for surgeons from different backgrounds in the prophylactic setting.[28]

Another variant is placement of an underlay mesh in the intraperitoneal plane. The mesh in this approach is also below the abdominal musculature, which again may help prevent fascial disruption from Valsalva pressure while also distributing tension like retrorectus placement. However, there is a risk of complications from close adherence to the viscera and it is also less effective at reducing IH when compared with the onlay and retrorectus techniques.[28]

There is not one perfect location for mesh placement that can be applied to every situation. **Fig. 3** summarizes the hypothetical benefits and drawbacks associated with the three mesh locations described previously. When addressing prevention of IH or PH at the initial surgery, the benefits and risks of the three locations should be weighed on an individual basis, taking into account surgeon skill and patient risk.

MESH MATERIAL

Along with placement of mesh, the surgeon also needs to consider the type of mesh to be used and how this may affect the patient's outcomes. The ideal mesh has previously been described to be inert, flexible, resistant to mechanical strain, resilient to infection, and protective of viscera, while causing a minimal foreign body reaction and exhibiting similar tensile strength to the native tissue.[28] Most studies that show favorable outcomes in prevention of AH have used synthetic meshes, possibly because of the decreased cost, increased tensile strength, and composite barriers.[30–34] However, recent studies have also shown that biologic meshes,[35] which are more resistant to infection and have strong incorporation, are successful at preventing hernias. Furthermore, the ongoing PREBIOUS trial is attempting to determine the efficacy of bioabsorbable meshes.[36] The allure of bioabsorbable meshes is that they behave like synthetics with good tensile strength but eventually resorb, which could lead to less chronic pain and a possible decreased infection risk as seen with

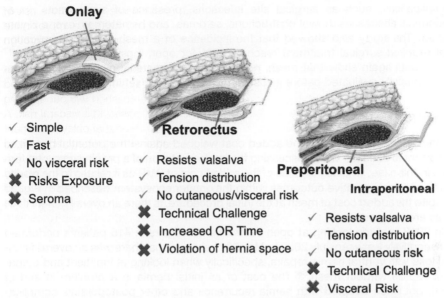

Onlay

✓ Simple
✓ Fast
✓ No visceral risk
✗ Risks Exposure
✗ Seroma

Retrorectus

✓ Resists valsalva
✓ Tension distribution
✓ No cutaneous/visceral risk
✗ Technical Challenge
✗ Increased OR Time
✗ Violation of hernia space

Preperitoneal

Intraperitoneal

✓ Resists valsalva
✓ Tension distribution
✓ No cutaneous risk
✗ Technical Challenge
✗ Visceral Risk

Fig. 3. Mesh placement characteristics. OR, operating room. (*Adapted from* Lanni MA, Tecce MG, Shubinets V, et al. The state of prophylactic mesh augmentation. Am Surg 2018;84(1):99–108; with permission.)

biologics. Along with the aforementioned theoretic benefits, all three mesh types have potential drawbacks, such as increased infection risk and chronic pain for synthetics, increased cost for biologics, and lack of long-term data for bioabsorbables, which are listed in **Table 1**.

Long-term complications associated with mesh placement should be considered. A recent study by Kokotovic and colleagues[37] showed a progressive increase in mesh

Table 1
Potential advantages and drawbacks of synthetic, biologic, and bioabsorbable meshes

Mesh Type	Advantages	Drawbacks
Synthetic	• Cheaper • Long-term tensile strength • Composite barriers • Most data	• Visceral damage • Poor infection resistance • Complicates future procedures • Increased mesh pain/long-term foreign body reaction
Biologic	• More infection resistant • Strong incorporation	• Bulging • Cost • Complications • Efficacy?
Bioabsorbable	• Handles like synthetics • More infection resistant • Short-term tensile strength • Resorbs after wound heals • Less risk for chronic mesh pain/short-term foreign body reaction	• Lack of long-term data • Cost

Adapted from Lanni MA, Tecce MG, Shubinets V, et al. The state of prophylactic mesh augmentation. Am Surg 2018;84(1):99–108; with permission.

complications, such as surgical site infections, presence of sinus tracts, intra-abdominal abscesses, bowel obstructions, seromas, and hematomas, over a 5-year period. The study also showed that the incidence of a mesh-related complication that required surgical treatment reached 5.6% for open mesh cases at 5 years.[37] These data again show that mesh, regardless of the material or placement, needs to be carefully evaluated before its use in the prophylactic setting.

ECONOMIC VALUE

Economic value, defined as the added cost weighed against the potential benefit, is important to consider when discussing the implementation of a prophylactic intervention. In this case, what is the value of the added cost of PMP as it relates to the quality of life and postoperative outcomes within the greater ecosystem described in **Fig. 2**? Despite the added cost of mesh at the initial procedure, is there an overall benefit if AH rates are reduced?

In 2013, a study looking at open ventral hernia repairs in 415 patients performed consecutively between July 2008 to May 2011 showed that there was an overall financial loss with ventral hernia repairs, specifically when looking at inpatient and outpatient repairs without mesh.[38] The cost of an initial hernia is a problem in and of itself, but when coupled with hernia recurrence and other postoperative complications, cost increases and quality of life suffers. Prevention of hernias could improve not only the health of patients, but also the health of society.

Looking at this from another perspective, if the recurrence rate of IH could be decreased by just 1%, this would result in a cost savings of $32 million.[9] Referring back to the "vicious cycle" of hernias, patients undergoing multiple hernia repairs have higher numbers of reoperations, longer operative times, higher incidences of surgical site infections, and higher rates of recurrence.[6] In the context of the hernia framework, the ineffectiveness and high cost associated with treatment and surgical morbidity of AH highlights the need for an intervention at the time of the initial surgery.

Furthermore, a cost-utility analysis assessing health state utilities, modern costs, and published probabilities for PMP showed that mesh cost could be as high as $3700 and still be cost-effective with an absolute IH rate reduction of 15%.[39] Despite the higher upfront cost of mesh, there is value in reducing IH and stopping the "vicious cycle" from being initiated. A primary investment in PMP could lead to a large potential benefit by decreasing overall cost and improving the inefficiency of treatment.

Although not as prevalent as IH, PH still has a noteworthy burden. With greater frequency and higher recurrence rates, there may be an even larger economic value with prevention compared with IH. Beyond the similar postoperative costs associated with IH, patients with PH often have to use more supplies and have more office and emergency room visits because of their ostomy appliances not functioning properly or causing leakage and skin irritation.[40] Something as simple as frequent leakage, which is common with PH, can cost the patient several hundred dollars more per month.[40] A study in 2014 looking at costs for PH in patients undergoing an abdominoperineal resection showed that the average cost to repair a PH is roughly $4683,[41] which when compounded with the previous costs mentioned add up to a substantial financial load for patients and hospital systems.

Another cost-utility analysis looked at the use of prophylactic mesh to prevent PH in patients with stage I-IV rectal cancer undergoing abdominoperineal resection.[41] The study showed that a mesh could cost up to $4556 in stage I and up to $601 in stage IV cancer and still be cost-effective despite the higher incidence of infection.[41] Again, like IH, the value of prevention for PH by spending more up front is of large benefit to mitigate further complications and costs.

SUCCESS OF PROPHYLACTIC MESH PLACEMENT

The idea of using prophylactic mesh to decrease IH is not a new concept. In 2002, Strzelczyk and colleagues[42] showed that after a year follow-up, 0% of patients that had PMP compared with 20% of patients that had PSC after open Roux-en-Y gastric bypass surgery developed IH. More recently, Abo-Ryia and colleauges[30] in 2013 expanded on these results with a randomized controlled trial to include patients with open gastric sleeve procedures and open Roux-en-Y gastric bypass with an average follow-up of 49 months, showing an IH rate of 11% in PMP and 28% in PSC. Two more recent studies in 2015 and 2016 by Bali and colleagues[43] and Muysoms and colleagues,[33] respectively, performed randomized control trials assessing PMP and PSC in another cohort at risk of IH, patients undergoing open AAA repairs. With follow-up between 24 and 36 months, both studies showed an IH incidence of 0% in PMP and 28% to 30% in PSC.[33,43]

These results are not just limited to obese patients and those suffering from an AAA. Randomized controlled trials have focused on other patient populations at high risk including open colorectal cases,[44] where IH incidence was reduced from 31.5% to 11.3% and other elective laparotomies,[31] where the IH incidence was reduced from 37.5% to 2.5% with implementation of PMP. It should be noted that no randomized controlled trial to this point has been able to compare PMP with a confirmed 4:1 suture to wound ratio in the PSC arm. Although there is a need for such a study, the evidence for prevention of IH with PMP is still present, despite the heterogeneity regarding mesh placement throughout these studies.

The PRIMA group attempted to address this heterogeneity and released 2-year follow-up data in 2017 that showed again the rate of IH with PSC (30%) is high, but there was also a difference between onlay (13%) and sublay (18%) placement of mesh.[11] This is an interesting finding in the context of multispecialty use of PMP. A retrorectus repair has the lowest incidence of IH when performed by experienced abdominal wall surgeons, but it is technically challenging and time consuming.[45] This type of repair may not be advisable in a prophylactic setting because of the increased operative time and potential for distorting tissue planes for future surgeries. As a result, the placement of an onlay mesh as described in the PRIMA study with a 3-cm overlap of the fascia and fibrin sealant instead of tacking sutures is effective and easily implemented by surgeons from different specialties.[11]

A recent systematic review by Wang and colleagues[46] looked not only at IH rates in PMP, but other postoperative complications to assess if there were any major adverse outcomes with mesh placement in high-risk laparotomies. They demonstrated that when compared with PSC, although PMP had a higher rate of seromas, they had an improved quality of life and decreased incidence of IH across 12 randomized control trials.[46] Another systematic review expanded on this and showed that the increased seroma rate is more often seen with the onlay technique, but these patients rarely need reoperation and it was viewed as an insignificant postoperative complication by the general population based on a survey of health states.[28,39] In both studies, no other differences in postoperative outcomes were found.[28,46]

Data in support of PMP to prevent PH are also compelling. The early results of a randomized controlled trial for colostomy creation released this year showed the rate of PH at 2 years is 4.5% with retrorectus PMP and 24.2% with PSC.[47] A systematic review by Chapman and colleagues[48] in 2017 showed a decrease in PH from 32.4% to 10.8% with PMP across seven randomized control trials with no difference seen in stoma-related complications. Another systematic review by Cross and colleagues[49] in the same year showed a similar decrease of PH with PMP from 36.6% to 16.4%, but was able to conclude more specifically that there was no difference in parastomal infection, stomal stenosis, or stomal necrosis. Another concern in patients receiving mesh is if there is any increase in wound infection, which was not the case in a study by Lopez-Cano and colleagues.[50]

As with laparotomies, a significant debate exists about mesh type and location during ostomy creation. In a systematic review by Patel and colleagues,[51] a subgroup analysis showed that synthetic mesh was associated with a lower incidence of IH, but this was not appreciated with biologic mesh. This was corroborated by Pianka and colleagues[18] but they were also able to show that mesh placement is ideal in patients with a sublay placement compared with intraperitoneal placement. Most randomized control trials focus on end colostomies compared with loop colostomies, perhaps because they are less likely to be reversed and therefore have more time to form a PH.[18,48–51] As compared with laparotomies, placement of a mesh in the retrorectus plane during the formation of an ostomy may be more feasible because general and colorectal surgeons would likely be performing the index operation. Additionally, placement of the mesh around the ostomy site does not distort tissue planes in the rest of the abdominal wall, specifically the midline.

SUMMARY

IH and PH represent a common, costly, and morbid complication of abdominal surgery; however the selective, targeted use of risk-reductive mesh techniques has shown early promise in positively impacting the hernia ecosystem. Mesh placed as an onlay, retrorectus, or underlay can reduce IH. The other important consideration is that although hernia repairs are performed by general and plastic surgeons (hernia specialists) hernia prevention is in the hands of all surgeons who operate on the abdomen. The method that needs to be implemented by surgeons who do not perform hernia repairs regularly should ideally be easy to perform without addition of time or complexity to the original case. Use of an onlay mesh with minimal fixation can easily be taught and implemented to prevent IH in high-risk populations to a broad variety of surgical subspecialties. Thus, in the context of prevention, onlay mesh has promise to be the simplest, most generalizable option.[11] A bioabsorbable mesh has potential to be the ideal mesh for PMP because it handles like a synthetic and resorbs once the wound heals, but further studies need to be conducted to determine short- and long-term outcomes.

PH has data to support PMP, but placement in a retrorectus plane seems to be more favorable, especially in patients receiving end colostomies. This procedure is not as generalizable across specialties because specialized colorectal or general surgeons are typically creating ostomies. More evidence exists in favor of synthetic meshes for this use, but again long-term studies using bioabsorbable mesh need to be conducted to determine if infection rates can be reduced while having similar tensile strength.

There are no randomized controlled trials in the United States regarding the use of mesh in the primary prevention of AH. This is shocking because the United States is among world leaders in the number of laparotomies, stoma creations, and IH repairs performed. However, the reimbursement structure may explain why hernia prevention has not been embraced up to this point. With the health care crisis in this country, this perspective has to change. Economic value needs to be addressed and the emphasis should shift to prevention instead of repair to remedy the situation.

In conclusion, fewer complications, fewer surgeries, and less time in the hospital can improve patients' quality of life. The data are becoming clearer on the benefits of PMP to accomplish this, but how this relates to the American population needs to be described further. PMP is not the ideal solution for every high-risk person receiving abdominal surgery. One must consider patient selection, surgeon experience, reapproximation of the midline fascia, the effect of reinforcement on postoperative outcomes, type of mesh to use, and placement of the mesh. Taking this all into account, if PMP can help patients and improve the health care system, should it deserve more attention?

REFERENCES

1. Ludwig KK, Neuner J, Butler A, et al. Risk reduction and survival benefit of prophylactic surgery in BRCA mutation carriers, a systematic review. Am J Surg 2016;212(4):660–9.
2. Kalady MF, Church JM. Prophylactic colectomy: rationale, indications, and approach. J Surg Oncol 2015;111(1):112–7.
3. da Silva G, Boutros M, Wexner SD. Role of prophylactic ureteric stents in colorectal surgery. Asian J Endosc Surg 2012;5(3):105–10.
4. Fischer JP, Nelson JA, Mirzabeigi MN, et al. Prophylactic muscle flaps in vascular surgery. J Vasc Surg 2012;55(4):1081–6.
5. Flum DR, Horvath K, Koepsell T. Have outcomes of incisional hernia repair improved with time? Ann Surg 2003;237(1):129–35.
6. Holihan JL, Alawadi Z, Martindale RG, et al. Adverse events after ventral hernia repair: the vicious cycle of complications. J Am Coll Surg 2015;221(2):478–85.
7. Bower C, Roth JS. Economics of abdominal wall reconstruction. Surg Clin North Am 2013;93(5):1241–53.
8. Criss CN, Petro CC, Krpata DM, et al. Functional abdominal wall reconstruction improves core physiology and quality-of-life. Surgery 2014;156(1):176–82.
9. Poulose BK, Shelton J, Phillips S, et al. Epidemiology and cost of ventral hernia repair: making the case for hernia research. Hernia 2012;16(2):179–83.
10. Deerenberg EB, Harlaar JJ, Steyerberg EW, et al. Small bites versus large bites for closure of abdominal midline incisions (STITCH): a double-blind, multicentre, randomised controlled trial. Lancet 2015;386(10000):1254–60.
11. Jairam AP, Timmermans L, Eker HH, et al. Prevention of incisional hernia with prophylactic onlay and sublay mesh reinforcement versus primary suture only in midline laparotomies (PRIMA): 2-year follow-up of a multicentre, double-blind, randomised controlled trial. Lancet 2017;390(10094):567–76.
12. Veljkovic R, Protic M, Gluhovic A, et al. Prospective clinical trial of factors predicting the early development of incisional hernia after midline laparotomy. J Am Coll Surg 2010;210(2):210–9.
13. Bosanquet DC, Ansell J, Abdelrahman T, et al. Systematic review and meta-regression of factors affecting midline incisional hernia rates: analysis of 14,618 patients. PLoS One 2015;10(9):e0138745.
14. Robertson I, Leung E, Hughes D, et al. Prospective analysis of stoma-related complications. Colorectal Dis 2005;7(3):279–85.
15. Pilgrim CH, McIntyre R, Bailey M. Prospective audit of parastomal hernia: prevalence and associated comorbidities. Dis Colon Rectum 2010;53(1):71–6.
16. Carne PW, Robertson GM, Frizelle FA. Parastomal hernia. Br J Surg 2003;90(7):784–93.
17. Helgstrand F, Gogenur I, Rosenberg J. Prevention of parastomal hernia by the placement of a mesh at the primary operation. Hernia 2008;12(6):577–82.

18. Pianka F, Probst P, Keller AV, et al. Prophylactic mesh placement for the PREvention of paraSTOmal hernias: the PRESTO systematic review and meta-analysis. PLoS One 2017;12(2):e0171548.

19. Hotouras A, Murphy J, Thaha M, et al. The persistent challenge of parastomal herniation: a review of the literature and future developments. Colorectal Dis 2013; 15(5):e202–14.

20. Clark JL. Ventral incisional hernia recurrence. J Surg Res 2001;99(1):33–9.

21. Diener MK, Voss S, Jensen K, et al. Elective midline laparotomy closure: the INLINE systematic review and meta-analysis. Ann Surg 2010;251(5):843–56.

22. Israelsson LA, Millbourn D. Prevention of incisional hernias: how to close a midline incision. Surg Clin North Am 2013;93(5):1027–40.

23. Muysoms F, Antoniou S, Bury K, et al. European Hernia Society guidelines on the closure of abdominal wall incisions. Hernia 2015;19:1–24.

24. Luijendijk RW, Hop WCJ, Van Den Tol MP, et al. A comparison of suture repair with mesh repair for incisional hernia. N Engl J Med 2000;342(6):392–8.

25. Christoffersen MW, Helgstrand F, Rosenberg J, et al. Lower reoperation rate for recurrence after mesh versus sutured elective repair in small umbilical and epigastric hernias. A nationwide register study. World J Surg 2013;37(11): 2548–52.

26. Nguyen MT, Berger RL, Hicks SC, et al. Comparison of outcomes of synthetic mesh vs suture repair of elective primary ventral herniorrhaphy: a systematic review and meta-analysis. JAMA Surg 2014;149(5):415–21.

27. Holihan JL, Alawadi ZM, Harris JW, et al. Ventral hernia: patient selection, treatment, and management. Curr Probl Surg 2016;53(7):307–54.

28. Borab ZM, Shakir S, Lanni MA, et al. Does prophylactic mesh placement in elective, midline laparotomy reduce the incidence of incisional hernia? A systematic review and meta-analysis. Surgery 2017;161(4):1149–63.

29. Bauer JJ, Harris MT, Gorfine SR, et al. Rives-Stoppa procedure for repair of large incisional hernias: experience with 57 patients. Hernia 2002;6(3):120–3.

30. Abo-Ryia MH, El-Khadrawy OH, Abd-Allah HS. Prophylactic preperitoneal mesh placement in open bariatric surgery: a guard against incisional hernia development. Obes Surg 2013;23(10):1571–4.

31. Caro-Tarrago A, Olona Casas C, Jimenez Salido A, et al. Prevention of incisional hernia in midline laparotomy with an onlay mesh: a randomized clinical trial. World J Surg 2014;38(9):2223–30.

32. Bevis PM, Windhaber RA, Lear PA, et al. Randomized clinical trial of mesh versus sutured wound closure after open abdominal aortic aneurysm surgery. Br J Surg 2010;97(10):1497–502.

33. Muysoms FE, Detry O, Vierendeels T, et al. Prevention of incisional hernias by prophylactic mesh-augmented reinforcement of midline laparotomies for abdominal aortic aneurysm treatment: a randomized controlled trial. Ann Surg 2016; 263(4):638–45.

34. Strzelczyk JM, Szymanski D, Nowicki ME, et al. Randomized clinical trial of postoperative hernia prophylaxis in open bariatric surgery. Br J Surg 2006;93(11): 1347–50.

35. Llaguna OH, Avgerinos DV, Nagda P, et al. Does prophylactic biologic mesh placement protect against the development of incisional hernia in high-risk patients? World J Surg 2011;35(7):1651–5.

36. Lopez-Cano M, Pereira JA, Lozoya R, et al. PREBIOUS trial: a multicenter randomized controlled trial of PREventive midline laparotomy closure with a

BIOabsorbable mesh for the prevention of incisional hernia: rationale and design. Contemp Clin Trials 2014;39(2):335–41.

37. Kokotovic D, Bisgaard T, Helgstrand F. Long-term recurrence and complications associated with elective incisional hernia repair. JAMA 2016;316(15):1575–82.

38. Reynolds D, Davenport DL, Korosec RL, et al. Financial implications of ventral hernia repair: a hospital cost analysis. J Gastrointest Surg 2013;17(1):159–66 [discussion: 66–7].

39. Fischer JP, Basta MN, Wink JD, et al. Cost-utility analysis of the use of prophylactic mesh augmentation compared with primary fascial suture repair in patients at high risk for incisional hernia. Surgery 2015;158(3):700–11.

40. Aquina CT, Iannuzzi JC, Probst CP, et al. Parastomal hernia: a growing problem with new solutions. Dig Surg 2014;31(4–5):366–76.

41. Lee L, Saleem A, Landry T, et al. Cost effectiveness of mesh prophylaxis to prevent parastomal hernia in patients undergoing permanent colostomy for rectal cancer. J Am Coll Surg 2014;218(1):82–91.

42. Strzelczyk J, Czupryniak L, Loba J, et al. The use of polypropylene mesh in midline incision closure following gastric by-pass surgery reduces the risk of postoperative hernia. Langenbecks Arch Surg 2002;387(7–8):294–7.

43. Bali C, Papakostas J, Georgiou G, et al. A comparative study of sutured versus bovine pericardium mesh abdominal closure after open abdominal aortic aneurysm repair. Hernia 2015;19(2):267–71.

44. Garcia-Urena MA, Lopez-Monclus J, Hernando LA, et al. Randomized controlled trial of the use of a large-pore polypropylene mesh to prevent incisional hernia in colorectal surgery. Ann Surg 2015;261(5):876–81.

45. Albino FP, Patel KM, Nahabedian MY, et al. Does mesh location matter in abdominal wall reconstruction? A systematic review of the literature and a summary of recommendations. Plast Reconstr Surg 2013;132(5):1295–304.

46. Wang XC, Zhang D, Yang ZX, et al. Mesh reinforcement for the prevention of incisional hernia formation: a systematic review and meta-analysis of randomized controlled trials. J Surg Res 2017;209:17–29.

47. Brandsma HT, Hansson BM, Aufenacker TJ, et al. Prophylactic mesh placement during formation of an end-colostomy reduces the rate of parastomal hernia: short-term results of the Dutch PREVENT-trial. Ann Surg 2017;265(4):663–9.

48. Chapman SJ, Wood B, Drake TM, et al. Systematic review and meta-analysis of prophylactic mesh during primary stoma formation to prevent parastomal hernia. Dis Colon Rectum 2017;60(1):107–15.

49. Cross AJ, Buchwald PL, Frizelle FA, et al. Meta-analysis of prophylactic mesh to prevent parastomal hernia. Br J Surg 2017;104(3):179–86.

50. Lopez-Cano M, Brandsma HT, Bury K, et al. Prophylactic mesh to prevent parastomal hernia after end colostomy: a meta-analysis and trial sequential analysis. Hernia 2017;21(2):177–89.

51. Patel SV, Zhang L, Chadi SA, et al. Prophylactic mesh to prevent parastomal hernia: a meta-analysis of randomized controlled studies. Tech Coloproctol 2017; 21(1):5–13.

Preoperative Planning and Patient Optimization

Clayton C. Petro, MD, Ajita S. Prabhu, MD*

KEYWORDS

- Ventral hernia repair • Preoperative patient optimization • Modifiable risk factors

KEY POINTS

- Ventral hernia repair is becoming an increasingly complex field of surgery.
- Hernia dimensions, operative history, and wound class are just a few of the variables that create an infinite number of patient permutations for which there is no standardized classification scheme.
- The variety of repair techniques and prosthetic reinforcement types in the context of such an amorphous group of patients makes controlled study of surgical morbidity and outcomes an extreme challenge.
- In a field in which consensus can be rare, preoperative patient optimization can be something that all surgeons champion.

Ventral hernia repairs (VHRs) comprise a wide degree of complexity. Hernia size, location, number and type of previous repairs, loss of domain, use of prior component separation techniques, previous mesh use, wound class, and abdominal wall compliance all affect decision-making regarding the operative approach. These variables encompass the 1 cm primary umbilical defect, as well as the concurrent midline and lateral defects, commonly associated with a permanent ostomy. If the patient is fortunate enough not to have an emergent presentation related to bowel obstruction or strangulation, the surgeon can plan for definitive repair of the hernia in an elective setting. Although surgeons have little control over the complexity of the patient's hernia and operative history, there are certain patient variables that can be optimized before elective abdominal wall reconstruction. This article reviews the literature that supports routine expectations for smoking cessation; weight loss; diabetic, nutritional, or metabolic optimization; and decolonization techniques. These methods aim to diminish postoperative complications such as wound infections and recurrence. The authors advocate routine adherence to these requirements before elective surgery not just to optimize the most complex cases but also to prevent smaller hernias from becoming complex.

The authors have nothing to disclose.
Department of Surgery, Cleveland Clinic, 9500 Euclid Avenue, Cleveland, OH 44195, USA
* Corresponding author.
E-mail address: prabhua@ccf.org

Surg Clin N Am 98 (2018) 483–497
https://doi.org/10.1016/j.suc.2018.01.005
0039-6109/18/© 2018 Elsevier Inc. All rights reserved.
surgical.theclinics.com

SMOKING CESSATION

Perhaps the most well-studied modifiable patient risk factor is smoking. The deleterious effect of smoking on wound healing has several mechanisms. Fundamentally, smoking leads to elevated blood levels of carbon monoxide, which binds hemoglobin, shifts the oxygen-hemoglobin dissociation curve to the left, and decreases oxygen tissue delivery by as much as 15%.[1,2] Also, although blood levels of neutrophils are increased by 20% in smokers, both neutrophil and monocyte chemotactic–mediated migration into wounds is impaired, blunting the inflammatory response.[3,4] For those neutrophils and monocyte-macrophages that do arrive in the wound bed, in vivo studies have indicated that their oxidative burst–mediated phagocytosis (responsible for the effective destructive of pathogens such as *Staphylococcus aureus* and *Escherichia coli*) is reduced by more than half in smokers.[5,6] Finally, fibroblast dysfunction, coupled with imbalanced protease and antiprotease levels in smokers' tissue, impairs collagen deposition, granulation tissue formation, and remodeling.[7–9] Nonetheless, smokers are at a severe disadvantage in regard to wound healing and their ability to overcome wound morbidity, particularly surgical site infection (SSI).

The evidence to support the negative effect of smoking on postoperative wound morbidity in all surgical patients has consequently accrued. A meta-analysis of cohort studies and randomized controlled trials encompassing nearly 480,000 subjects across surgical subspecialties associated smoking with increased rates of wound necrosis (odds ratio [OR] 3.8), dehiscence (OR 2.1), SSI (OR 1.8), all wound complications (OR 2.3), and subsequent hernia formation (OR 2.1).[10] Specifically in the context of VHR, smoking has been routinely associated with wound morbidity. In a large cohort of 1505 subjects undergoing VHRs from 13 veterans' hospitals using all techniques, logistic regression identified smoking as the only modifiable risk factor associated with a 5% wound infection rate.[11] Furthermore, multivariate analysis from data extracted from the American College of Surgeons' National Surgical Quality Improvement Program (NSQIP) database for more than 72,000 open and laparoscopic repairs associated smoking within 12 months of surgery with deep wound infection (OR 1.6). Interestingly, any history of smoking was also associated with superficial (OR 1.1), deep (OR 1.6), and organ space (OR 1.3) infection, as well as a host of other postoperative complications (eg, pneumonia, reintubation, sepsis, reoperation).[12] A separate NSQIP study specifically looking at all VHRs in 2011 (n = 12,673) found that, in addition to its association with all complications, smoking was independently associated with 30-day readmission.[13] Although administrative databases such as NSQIP are often limited by 30-day follow-up, retrospective analyses with longer follow-up have found a 4-fold increase of incisional hernia after a primary laparotomy in smokers.[14]

Fortunately, the harmful effects of smoking in regard to wound morbidity and hernia occurrence seem to be mitigated by smoking cessation before elective surgery. In a Cochrane review of 13 randomized controlled trials recruiting smokers before elective surgery, 7 trials looked at the association of preoperative abstinence with postoperative complications. For the 2 trials (n = 210) that initiated intensive interventions (defined as multisession face-to-face counseling at least 4 weeks before surgery) a reduction in all complications (relative risk [RR] 0.42) and wound morbidity (RR 0.31) was found. Brief interventions or those less than 4 weeks from surgery were not able to demonstrate a significant impact on morbidity, and were less likely to lead to long-term smoking cessation.[15] Based on these available data, the authors counsel patients on smoking cessation during at least 2 preoperative visits, and require abstinence for a minimum of 4 weeks before elective operations.

Regarding tools to aid smoking abstinence, randomized controlled data specifically looking at nicotine replacement therapy showed no association between nicotine use and postoperative wound morbidity. Therefore, we allow the use of nicotine patches, gum, and lozenges.[16] Alternatively, we do not allow patients to use electronic cigarettes (e-cigarettes). Although the US Food and Drug Administration adopted regulation of e-cigarettes as of August, 2016, their cultivation, marketing, and dissemination in a regulation-free environment allowed for the creation of a wide array of products of which little is known, let alone their consequences relative to surgery.[17,18] It is worth noting that chromatographic and spectroscopy methods have identified trace amounts of carcinogens varying anywhere from 9 to 450 times less than cigarette smoke.[19] This wide variability in available products elucidates the difficulty in making a uniform assessment regarding the safety of their usage.

For patients who report smoking abstinence, the authenticity of their claim can sometimes be difficult to discern. Cessation even after counseling has been reported as low as 19%; therefore, the authors think that it is important to have some tool to help confirm abstinence.[20] Because we allow for nicotine replacement therapy, we test urine for the tobacco plant alkaloid anabasine, an insecticide found in cigarettes. Anabasine can help identify smokers who use nicotine replacement therapy.[21] Admittedly, urine anabasine is an imperfect test. Although nonsmokers will almost always test negative (100% specificity), smokers can still test negative (sensitivity 41%).[22] Most importantly, patients know there is some objective measure by which they are being held accountable. We typically counsel patients that they will be tested when they return to clinic. Although the details regarding the test's sensitivity are left ambiguous, the nature of the test ultimately gives the patient the benefit of the doubt. Patients who sincerely report complete cessation and test negative for urine anabasine are considered abstinent.

How the Authors Do It

- Conduct at least 2 counseling sessions before scheduling of elective surgery, or until 100% abstinence is reported.
- When patients report 100% abstinence, urine is tested for anabasine to corroborate their cessation.
- If urine anabasine is negative, surgery is scheduled for at least 4 weeks after the reported quit date.

WEIGHT LOSS

Obesity also has a well-documented impact on complications following VHR, including wound necrosis, SSI, reoperation, and hernia recurrence.[23–25] Important historical randomized controlled data comparing open to laparoscopic gastric bypass in subjects with a mean body mass index (BMI) of 48 kg/m^2 identified an incisional hernia rate of 39% in the open group compared with 5% in the laparoscopic group ($P<.01$), emphasizing the dramatic impact of obesity on subsequent hernia formation. Specifically, after hernia repair, Sauerland and colleagues[24] found an increase in recurrence with a rate ratio of 1.10 per unit of BMI. Regarding wound morbidity in hernia repair subjects, Fischer and colleagues[26] reported a graded relationship with obesity: OR 1.25, 1.42, and 1.66 for a BMI of 30 to 35, 35 to 40, and greater than 40, respectively.

Consequently, most surgeons agree on the extreme boundaries of offering elective surgery to those with a BMI of less than 30 kg/m^2 and considering a BMI greater than 50 kg/m^2 as prohibitive.[20] However, although most would agree that weight loss is beneficial in regard to minimizing perioperative morbidity, the effect of weight loss on improving outcomes has not been well studied. Medical and surgical weight loss are certainly options but, again, evidence that these interventions have an impact on outcomes of a subsequent VHR is currently unavailable. Therefore, there is currently no consensus on the best approach to achieve weight loss goals or what BMI goal is optimal. There is an ongoing trial assessing the effectiveness of preoperative exercise and weight loss on outcomes after VHR that will provide valuable insight and guidance on the matter (clinicaltrials.gov identifier NCT02365194).

In the absence of good prospective data, the authors provide a detailed description of our approach.[27] Obese patients seeking a VHR are counseled on the importance of weight loss (along with other modifiable risk factors such as smoking cessation and diabetes optimization) before their elective repair. The attending surgeon emphasizes that outcomes are a result of successful operation as well as what the patient brings to the table. The goal of the discussion is to empower patients, allowing them to realize they can have a positive impact on their surgical outcome. Part of empowering patients involves them setting a realistic weight loss goal; most patients will set a goal of 7 to 14 kg (~15–30lbs). The importance of the patients setting the goal themselves cannot be underscored enough. The patients are then seen every 3 months and positive reinforcement is given when they are successful until they reach their goal. Nutritional and exercise counseling is provided when necessary. Although there is no ideal finish line, typically the aim is a BMI of approximately 35 kg/m^2 before scheduling an operation, with the expectation that patients will continue to lose weight until their operation date in weeks to months. The surgeon should recognize that the sincerity of patients' efforts and appreciation of their own role in their outcome is as important as the amount of weight lost.

Patients who are not successful when they return at 3-month intervals are asked to grade their effort from A through F with a plus or minus scale. When they admit that their performance was poor, they are then asked to acknowledge that they would not accept a C-minus effort from their surgeon. This conversation tends to highlight that the operation and expectations after surgery are a team effort, and this reality is meant to cultivate the patient–doctor relationship.

When patients are not successful or their weight plateaus at a prohibitive BMI, the authors tend to refer patients to a medical weight loss specialist to institute a protein-sparing modified fast (PSMF) to achieve the targeted weight loss goal. The PSMF provides 800 calories per day, including 1.2 to 1.5 g/protein/kg of ideal body weight (BMI 25 kg/m^2). Because this is not nutritionally complete, supplements are added and a dietician or physician monitors their progress closely (**Box 1**).[28] In the authors' early experience using a PSMF, patients lost an average of 24 kg, correlating with a drop in BMI of 9 kg/m^2 before surgery. Importantly, 88% of patients successfully maintained their weight loss for an average of 18 months after surgery.[27]

For selective patients who have associated medical comorbidities, appropriate insurance coverage, and whose abdominal wall is not so complex to prohibit laparoscopic access, bariatric surgery is also an option. The authors have no reluctance about bariatric surgical consultation when appropriate; however, we would not advocate definitive hernia repair at the time of their bariatric procedure.

Finally, and importantly, routine surgeon involvement is critical. Asking patients to return after they have lost 100 kg or referring them back to their primary care provider to lose weight before surgery, in the authors' experience, tends not to be successful. Seeing patient at 3-month intervals to monitor success increases compliance, demonstrates the surgeon's commitment to the patient, and is meant to improve the patient–doctor relationship. Working from a tertiary referral center for complex hernia patients, the authors understand that patients often view our referral as a last chance, granting us a degree of leverage when counseling the patient on weight loss and other

Box 1
The protein-sparing modified fast program at Cleveland Clinic

At baseline and ongoing
  Baseline assessment (history, physical examination, electrocardiography) by physician or
  nurse practitioner and dietitian, with continued follow-up
  Dietitian visits every 2 weeks for first month and monthly thereafter; physician or nurse
  practitioner visits every 6 to 8 weeks
  Laboratory tests at baseline, every 2 weeks for first month, and monthly thereafter
  Comprehensive metabolic panel: uric acid
  Behavior modification
  Exercise

Intensive phase (up to 6 months) per day
  1.5 g protein/kg ideal body weight (typically a total of 12–17 oz in the form of lean meat,
  poultry, fish, seafood, eggs, low-fat cheese, tofu)
  Less than 20 g carbohydrate (2 servings of low-starch vegetables, unlimited lettuce salad)
  Trace carbohydrates from other foods and shakes
  Restriction of fats not found in protein sources (no butter, margarine, oils, nuts, seeds, or
  dips; protein sources should contain <3 g fat per ounce)
  Required supplements: multivitamin or mineral tablet; potassium 16 to 20 mEq; calcium 1000
  to 1200 mg; magnesium 400 to 500 mg; sodium 1500 to 2000 mg
  At least 64 oz of fluid

Refeeding phase (6–8 weeks)
  Slowly reintroduce complex carbohydrates and fats; reduce protein
  Month 1: up to 45 g carbohydrate
  Month 2: up to 90 g carbohydrate
  Low-glycemic, high-fiber cereals, fruits, vegetables
  Low-fat foods
  Daily protein reduced by 1 to 2 oz each month
  Stop potassium and magnesium supplements after week 2

From Bakhach M, Shah V, Harwood T, et al. The protein-sparing modified fast diet: an effective and safe approach to induce rapid weight loss in severely obese adolescents. Glob Pediatr Health 2016;3:2333794X15623245; with permission.

modifiable risk factors. However, the authors think most surgeons have nothing to lose and much to gain by adopting this approach.

How the Authors Do It

- Counsel patients on the importance of accountability regarding their modifiable risk factors in regard to their outcomes.
- Ask that patient set a realistic weight loss goal and measure progress at 3-month intervals, lauding success and making unsuccessful attempts unacceptable.
- Implement a medically supervised PSMF or bariatric surgical consultation when appropriate.
- Aim for a BMI of approximately 35 kg/m^2 before scheduling an operation.

DIABETES OPTIMIZATION

Although not studied in a dedicated fashion relative to VHR, considerable data exist regarding the negative impact of poorly controlled diabetes in the basic science realm, as well as clinically in regard to wound morbidity after general, orthopedic, and cardiothoracic surgery. Mechanistically, chronic hyperglycemia diminishes cellular and growth factor response, which leads to less peripheral blood flow and blunted angiogenesis.[29] In vivo studies have also found that artificially glycosylated collagen matrices result in impaired fibroblast function; subsequent collagen remodeling;

and, ultimately, collagen strength.[30] Finally, akin to smoking, leukocyte function, including chemotaxis, oxidative burst, and effective phagocytosis, is dulled.[31]

These basic science findings have a significant clinical consequence. A large-scale review of 5199 coronary artery bypass graft operations found that each unit increase in hemoglobin A_{1c} (HbA_{1c}) corresponded with a 31% increase in deep sternal wound infection (DSWI), and those with an HbA_{1c} value greater than 7 had a 2.88-fold increase in DSWI when compared with those with a value less than 7.[32] In a separate context, a review of 1702 total joint replacements identified an HbA_{1c} greater than 6.7 as a risk factor for developing a wound complication (OR 9.0).[33] Similarly, review of 345 spinal operations revealed no wound infections in those with an HbA_{1c} less than 7, versus a 35% wound infection rate in those greater than 7.[34] Furthermore, in a retrospective review of 647 noncardiac operations extracted from the Veterans Affairs' NSQIP, an HbA_{1c} greater than 7 was associated with a postoperative rate of any infection of 20%, versus an infection rate of 12% in those with an HbA_{1c} level less than 7 ($P = .007$). Unfortunately, the granularity of the data does not specify which infections were from wounds or how many of the operations were hernia repairs.[35]

Given the dramatic association with wound morbidity and poorly controlled diabetes, the authors typically require patients to have an HbA_{1c} less than 8. Those with poorly controlled diabetes are managed similarly to obese patients in that they are not scheduled for surgery, are instructed to set a goal for their HbA_{1c}, and are scheduled to return to the clinic in 3 months. However, the surgeon must be sure the patients are being offered adequate medical management and attempt to distinguish poor compliance from an absence of medical attention all together. Patients are often frank about their poor compliance if they see a doctor regularly who is trying to control their diabetes, whereas others may have been naïve to their poor control. For those who express sincerity in their medical compliance, referral to an endocrinologist is preferred. It is not uncommon for diabetes and obesity to come as a pair, and addressing either will correspondingly address the other. Referral to a nutritionist can also be helpful if indicated. Finally, particularly for poorly controlled diabetics, bariatric surgery should be considered for a select group of patients (see previous discussion).

How the Authors Do It

- Require an HbA_{1c} less than 8 before scheduling an operation
- Endocrinology referral for poorly controlled diabetics
- Monitor weight loss at 3-month intervals with when appropriate.

NUTRITIONAL OPTIMIZATION

The consequences of perioperative malnourishment have been well supported by the National Veterans Affairs surgical risk study. Sixty-seven variables in 87,078 noncardiac operative patients collected prospectively identified a preoperative albumin of less than 3.0 as the single largest predictor of postoperative morbidity.[36] Additional retrospective review of gastrointestinal foregut surgery has identified an inverse relationships between preoperative serum albumin and complications, length of stay, intensive care unit stay, mortality, and resumption of oral intake.[37] Though serum albumin may be an imperfect surrogate for nutrition, it does seem to correlate consistently with poor postoperative events.

Although most hernia patients are not severely malnourished, the most relevant group of abdominal wall reconstruction patients are those in a chronic inflammatory state secondary to an enterocutaneous fistula or enteroprosthetic fistula. These patients can be relatively catabolic or nutritionally depleted when adequate enteral nutrition cannot be provided due to a high-output fistula. In this context, Fazio and colleagues[38] showed that a preoperative serum albumin less than 2.5 g/dL carried a 42% mortality rate versus a 0% mortality rate for those with a level greater than 3.5 g/dL, corroborating the importance of preoperative nutritional optimization. Importantly, for patients identified as severely malnourished[a], prospective randomized data have shown that perioperative total parenteral nutrition demonstrates a reduction in noninfectious postoperative complications (5% vs 43%, P = .03, RR 0.12) without increasing the perioperative infection risk. However, one must appreciate that this is a relatively small patient population and that even most moderately malnourished patients did not appreciate any benefit.[39]

For these select enterocutaneous fistula patients who may benefit, the timing of the reoperation can pose a challenging dilemma. At a minimum, the patient must be sufficiently remote from their index procedure, 6 to 8 weeks before resolution of obliterative peritonitis.[38] In reality, most surgeons will wait 6 months to optimize the patient but nutritional optimization can be difficult to measure.[40] Compared with the 18-day to 20-day half-life of serum albumin, prealbumin (transthyretin) is a short-term nutrition parameter with a 2-day to 3-day half-life that responds rapidly to both malnutrition and adequate protein intake.[41] However, prealbumin is also an acute phase reactant, and preoperative elevation in acute phase response proteins can correspond with negative postoperative outcomes, including mortality.[42] As a consequence, the authors typically trend prealbumin levels concurrently with C-reactive protein (CRP) levels. Ideally, the combination of an increasing prealbumin level and downtrending or normal CRP level gives assurance that the patient's nutritional status is improving. Although this strategy seems to be intuitive, data to support it are admittedly absent.

More recently, malnutrition in the elderly has been identified as an area for improvement because it has traditionally been underrecognized. Because weight and serum protein levels can be influenced by so many factors in the elderly, there has been a growing advocacy for the use of objective nutritional assessment tools. Indices such as the Mini Nutritional Assessment (MNA) take 15 minutes for the patient to complete and give information on the patient's overall health, mobility, diet, and anthropometrics.[43] For hospital inpatients, low MNA scores are associated with mortality, prolonged length of stay, and greater likelihood of discharge to nursing homes. Use of the MNA can identify malnutrition before weight loss or serum protein changes, and can be used to monitor improvement after timely interventions have been made. Effective interventions include increasing the protein and energy density of meals, adapting meals to oral health, additional help during meals, and adding supplements between meals.[44] Although these can stabilize nutrition and improve weight, translation into effective clinical outcomes (eg, reduced mortality, length of stay, resource utilization) is the subject of ongoing study.[45]

How the Authors Do It

- Identify severely malnourished patients as indicated by albumin, prealbumin, and CRP trends.
- Await uptrending prealbumin and downtrending CRP.

METABOLIC OPTIMIZATION

Distinct from addressing malnourishment is the concept of metabolic optimization through immune-enhancing diets (IED) for the nutritionally sound patient. Decades

---

[a] Nutritional Risk Index score (1.519 × serum albumin, g/L + 0.417 × present weight/usual weight × 100). Severely malnourished is indicated by a value less than 83.5.

of basic science work have found that in an acute traumatic or elective surgical setting, arginine levels drop dramatically owing to myeloid cells expressing arginase I, making it a conditionally essential amino acid, even if preoperative levels are normal. The relatively depleted arginine levels blunt the inflammatory and immune responses because the amino acid supports T-cell proliferation; formation of collagen; and formation of the nitric oxide, a critical inflammatory signaling molecule.[46] Further work has found that the administration of omega-3 alters the body's prostaglandin profile, and diminishes the activation of myeloid cells and arginase I, thereby inhibiting the mechanism of arginine breakdown. Therefore, IEDs are arginine and omega-3 rich substances meant to be given preoperatively to overcome this relative deficiency during the acute stress response of a traumatic or surgical event.[47]

The direct translation of these basic science findings into meaningful clinical outcomes is staggering. A meta-analysis of 35 randomized controlled trials of subjects undergoing elective surgery found that subjects receiving perioperative arginine and omega-3 supplementation had fewer infectious complications (RR 0.59) and shorter hospital length of stay (−2.4 days), with no difference in mortality.[48] A criticism of this study (and several other similar meta-analyses with similar findings) was that the control group included both standard unsupplemented diets and diets with standard oral nutritional supplements (ONSs). A subsequent meta-analysis found that IEDs were actually no different than standard ONSs, which still contained varying levels of arginine and omega-3, as well as protein, vitamins, and minerals.[49] These data support the notion that standard ONSs that are inexpensive, widely distributed, and commonly used by subjects (ie, Boost, Nestle, Inc; Ensure, Abbott Laboratories) can be used for the same desired effect as that touted by traditional IEDs (ie, IMPACT Advanced Recovery, Nestle, Inc). To be clear, there is no defined amount of arginine and omega-3 necessary to gain the touted postoperative benefits.

Of note, the benefits of arginine and omega-3 supplementation are unique to the trauma and surgical populations that become transiently arginine deficient.[46] Early investigators abandoned arginine-supplemented diets due to increased rates of mortality in septic critically ill subjects. Further elucidation has found that septic patients are not arginine deficient, and that additional arginine administration increased nitric oxide synthesis that potentiated the hypotension in septic shock.

How the Authors Do It

- Highly motivated patients are encouraged to use any IED or ONS for 5 days before their operation.

METHICILLIN-RESISTANT *STAPHYLOCOCCUS AUREUS* DECOLONIZATION

Two major studies published in the *New England Journal of Medicine* (NEJM) support the effectiveness of *S aureus* decolonization in regard to a reduction in nosocomial infections. The first was a randomized, double-blind, placebo-controlled, multicenter trial in which 1270 of 6771 (19%) *S aureus* carriers identified by nasal swab polymerase chain reaction (PCR) assay were randomized to decolonization versus placebo. Decolonization consisted of mupirocin nasal ointment twice a day and daily chlorhexidine soap for 5 days total. This resulted in a reduction in *S aureus* infection (RR 0.42), most significantly deep SSI (RR 0.21), compared with placebo. Time to onset of infection was also decreased in the placebo group (P = .005).[50] Although decolonization is no doubt effective, its implementation is work-intensive. Screening must be collected, results reviewed, and decolonization techniques administered. The second NEJM article addresses the effectiveness of universal decolonization of methicillin-resistant

S aureus (MRSA). Patients who were universally decolonized without screening had the most dramatic decrease in MRSA infections compared with historical controls (hazard ratio [HR] 0.63), whereas those who underwent targeted decolonization after positive screening showed a more tempered response (HR 0.75), and subjects who underwent MRSA screening and isolation alone had the most modest response (HR 0.92). Interestingly, universal decolonization (using the same aforementioned technique of mupirocin and chlorhexidine) led to a decrease in all bloodstream pathogens, preventing 1 episode of bacteremia for every 99 subjects decolonized (HR 0.56, 3.6 vs 6.1).[51]

More recently, a retrospective review of 632 hernia repair subjects found that MRSA colonization was not independently associated with SSO (surgical site occurrence) or SSOPI (surgical site occurence requiring procedural intervention) after multivariate analysis. Obesity, mesh repair, immunosuppression, and operative time were found to be more significantly associated with wound morbidity.[52] Although these findings are noteworthy, the value of well-designed prospective studies should offset the interpretation of retrospective data subject to selection bias.

Unexpectedly, the authors' retrospective review of 3924 subjects extracted from the AHSQC (Americas Hernia Society Quality Collaborative) found that preoperative chlorhexidine scrub was actually associated with an increase in SSO and SSI using both multivariate logistic regression (SSO, OR 1.34; SSI, OR 1.46) and propensity score modeling (SSO, OR 1.39; SSI, OR 1.45). Although some studies have found a benefit of preoperative chlorhexidine scrubbing, a 2015 Cochrane Review found no benefit in rates of SSI.[53,54] The authors' study was the first to find a statistical disadvantage to this practice. A potential mechanism to explain this finding is that a disruption in the skin's local microbiome of a healthy individual can actually allow for overgrowth of pathogenic bacteria (dysbiosis), increasing susceptibility to nosocomial infections.[55] For example, *S epidermidis* has been shown to produce modulins that inhibit skin pathogens and enhance host antimicrobial peptides against bacteria such as *S aureus* and Group A *Streptococcus*.[56,57] These findings suggest that the innate immune system is well equipped to defend the host from bacteria that the chlorhexidine intends to eliminate, and that these efforts are in fact counterproductive. Due to this finding, the authors have eliminated the preoperative chlorhexidine scrub from the universal decolonization protocol, and have proceeded with only using the mupirocin ointment.

How the Authors Do It

- The authors perform universal decolonization with nasal mupirocin (without chlorhexidine) for 5 days perioperatively, regardless of the day of the operation.
- All patients receive 24 hours of perioperative antibiotic prophylaxis.
- Patients who are known carriers of MRSA or have a chronic or active infection with MRSA are given 24 hours of a perioperative antibiotic prophylaxis that covers MRSA.

PREHABILITATION

One of the newer areas of interest is the concept of prehabilitation, which takes measures to improve a patient's functional status in preparation for surgery. In a systematic review of pooled abdominal and cardiothoracic studies, subjects receiving preoperative inspiratory muscle training for 2 to 10 weeks had fewer pulmonary complications, and some studies showed a reduced length of stay.[58] Although promising, most of these data were influenced by cardiothoracic patients. A more recent meta-analysis of randomized controlled trials that included subjects undergoing abdominal surgery and who were randomized to prehabilitation techniques or not, found that inspiratory muscle training, aerobic exercise, and/or resistance training can decrease postoperative complications (OR 0.59, $P = .03$). Most dramatic was the reduction in pulmonary complications (OR 0.27). The data were insufficient to show a reduction in length of stay.[59] Currently, there are 48 ongoing trials registered on clinicaltrials.gov designed to elucidate the effectiveness of prehabilitation techniques in regard to abdominal surgery. These efforts will help to standardize and support their implementation.

MISCELLANEOUS EFFORTS

Given the degree of bowel manipulation inherent to many recurrent hernia repairs, a preoperative bowel preparation could be considered beneficial for a reduction in postoperative wound morbidity. Using the AHSQC, 12.6% of extracted ventral hernia cases received a preoperative bowel preparation. These 313 subjects were matched to a similar cohort and, after logistic regression, a bowel preparation was associated with an increased incidence of postoperative SSO (OR 1.76) for clean cases but had no statistical effect on SSI or SSOPI. Contaminated cases receiving a bowel preparation were associated with an increased incidence of SSOPI (70% vs 33%, $P = .02$) and length of stay (7 days vs 6 days, $P<.01$).[60] Notably, the touted benefits of a bowel preparation in the colorectal literature in regard to decreased SSI and anastomotic leak rates are in reference to concurrent mechanical and oral antimicrobial bowel preparations.[61] In the authors' aforementioned analysis, 1% of the clean cases and less than 25% of the contaminated cases received both a mechanical and oral antimicrobial bowel preparation. Given these findings, the authors do not routinely administer a bowel preparation unless there is a planned bowel resection (ie, Hartmann reversal), in which case we would administer both a mechanical and oral antimicrobial preparation.

Another early AHSQC analysis investigated the potential benefits of using an iodine-impregnated surgical drape. There was no statistical difference between the group using the iodine impregnated drape (7%) and the group not using the drape (2%).[62] These findings are consistent with a Cochrane review of 1113 subjects that compared iodine-impregnated adhesive drapes with no adhesive drapes, finding no difference in postoperative SSI (RR 1.03). Interestingly, the same review found that noniodinated adhesive drapes actually increased rates of SSI when compared with no drapes (RR 1.23).[63] Currently, to minimize the exposure of incision to the colonized wound, we only use such drapes to isolate stomas, or open or unhealed wounds.

Most recently, the authors set out to evaluate the effectiveness of epidural anesthesia for subjects undergoing VHR. The AHSQC identified 763 subjects receiving postoperative epidural anesthesia and matched them to a similar cohort of 763 subjects not using epidural anesthesia. Subjects with epidurals had an increased length of stay (5.49 vs 4.90 days, $P<.05$), more complications (26% vs 21%, $P<.05$), and worse pain as measured by pain intensity-scaled scores (47.6 vs 44.0, $P = .04$). A limitation was that the matched cohort was 13% less likely to have a case last greater than 2 hours and 6% more likely to have drains placed, indicating this may be a more complex group of subjects. In a subgroup analysis of high-risk pulmonary subjects carrying a history of chronic obstructive pulmonary disease, recent smoking, or dyspnea, subjects with an epidural still had an increased length of stay (6.09 vs 5.26 days, $P<.001$).[64] The authors have speculated that epidurals increase fluid boluses for hypotension and delay transition to enteral pain medication and Foley catheter removal, all of which are counterproductive to enhanced-recovery paradigms. Supporting this suspicion are similar retrospective reviews of pancreaticoduodenectomy patients that found significant rates of hypotension (6%–18%) and catheter dysfunction (9%–14%) associated with epidural use.[65,66]

How the Authors Do It

- For VHR, the authors do not routinely use
  o Bowel preparation
  o Iodine-impregnated adhesive surgical drapes
  o Epidural anesthesia.

SUMMARY

VHR is becoming an increasingly complex field of surgery. Hernia dimensions, operative history, and wound class are just a few of the variables that create an infinite number of patient permutations for which there is no standardized classification scheme. The variety of repair techniques and prosthetic reinforcement types in the context of such an amorphous group of patients makes controlled study of surgical morbidity and outcomes an extreme challenge. However, in a field in which consensus can be rare, preoperative patient optimization can be something that all surgeons champion.

Decades of data accrued for topics such as smoking, weight loss, and diabetes optimization provide valuable insight into their clinical benefit. Furthermore, the financial impact of these optimization techniques has been the subject of more recent study. Subjects undergoing open VHR with 1, 2, or 3 of the aforementioned comorbidities (smoking, diabetes mellitus, obesity) were subject to increasing complication rates (28% vs 35.4% vs 62%, $P<.05$). Subjects with modifiable comorbidities were charged more than $25,000 higher than those without comorbidities ($P = .04$). Even when no complications occurred, subjects with modifiable risk factors generated significantly more total hospital charges than subjects without those risk factors ($65,453 vs $31,788, $P \leq .001$). Furthermore, there was a statistical difference in charges between subjects with 1 modifiable risk factor compared with 2 or 3, suggesting that eliminating 1 risk factor preoperatively can have a greater than $20,000 effect on that patient's medical bill.[67] In an era of value-centric care, an upfront investment in patient optimization can improve the quality of the repair by reducing wound morbidity and hernia recurrence, naturally translating to a reduction in cost. The authors strongly advocate the adoption of these practices and encourage further study aimed at identifying other effective optimization techniques.

REFERENCES

1. Pearce AC, Jones RM. Smoking and anesthesia: preoperative abstinence and perioperative morbidity. Anesthesiology 1984;61(5):576–84.
2. Sheps DS, Herbst MC, Hinderliter AL, et al. Production of arrhythmias by elevated carboxyhemoglobin in patients with coronary artery disease. Ann Intern Med 1990;113(5):343–51.
3. Noble RC, Penny BB. Comparison of leukocyte count and function in smoking and nonsmoking young men. Infect Immun 1975;12(3):550–5.
4. Michaud SE, Dussault S, Groleau J, et al. Cigarette smoke exposure impairs VEGF-induced endothelial cell migration: role of NO and reactive oxygen species. J Mol Cell Cardiol 2006;41(2):275–84.
5. Chambers AC, Leaper DJ. Role of oxygen in wound healing: a review of evidence. J Wound Care 2011;20(4):160–4.
6. Debbia EA, Schito GC, Gualco L, et al. Microbial epidemiology patterns of surgical infection pathogens. J Chemother 2001;13 Spec No 1(1):84–8.

7. Agren MS, Jorgensen LN, Andersen M, et al. Matrix metalloproteinase 9 level predicts optimal collagen deposition during early wound repair in humans. Br J Surg 1998;85(1):68–71.
8. Janoff A. Elastases and emphysema. Current assessment of the protease-antiprotease hypothesis. Am Rev Respir Dis 1985;132(2):417–33.
9. Nakamura Y, Romberger DJ, Tate L, et al. Cigarette smoke inhibits lung fibroblast proliferation and chemotaxis. Am J Respir Crit Care Med 1995;151(5):1497–503.
10. Sorensen LT. Wound healing and infection in surgery. The clinical impact of smoking and smoking cessation: a systematic review and meta-analysis. Arch Surg 2012;147(4):373–83.
11. Finan KR, Vick CC, Kiefe CI, et al. Predictors of wound infection in ventral hernia repair. Am J Surg 2005;190(5):676–81.
12. Kubasiak JC, Landin M, Schimpke S, et al. The effect of tobacco use on outcomes of laparoscopic and open ventral hernia repairs: a review of the NSQIP dataset. Surg Endosc 2017;31(6):2661–6.
13. Lovecchio F, Farmer R, Souza J, et al. Risk factors for 30-day readmission in patients undergoing ventral hernia repair. Surgery 2014;155(4):702–10.
14. Sorensen LT, Hemmingsen UB, Kirkeby LT, et al. Smoking is a risk factor for incisional hernia. Arch Surg 2005;140(2):119–23.
15. Thomsen T, Villebro N, Moller AM. Interventions for preoperative smoking cessation. Cochrane Database Syst Rev 2014;(3):CD002294.
16. Sorensen LT, Karlsmark T, Gottrup F. Abstinence from smoking reduces incisional wound infection: a randomized controlled trial. Ann Surg 2003;238(1):1–5.
17. Farsalinos KE, Polosa R. Safety evaluation and risk assessment of electronic cigarettes as tobacco cigarette substitutes: a systematic review. Ther Adv Drug Saf 2014;5(2):67–86.
18. Breland A, Soule E, Lopez A, et al. Electronic cigarettes: what are they and what do they do? Ann N Y Acad Sci 2017;1394(1):5–30.
19. Goniewicz ML, Knysak J, Gawron M, et al. Levels of selected carcinogens and toxicants in vapour from electronic cigarettes. Tob Control 2014;23(2):133–9.
20. Liang MK, Holihan JL, Itani K, et al. Ventral hernia management: expert consensus guided by systematic review. Ann Surg 2017;265(1):80–9.
21. Moyer TP, Charlson JR, Enger RJ, et al. Simultaneous analysis of nicotine, nicotine metabolites, and tobacco alkaloids in serum or urine by tandem mass spectrometry, with clinically relevant metabolic profiles. Clin Chem 2002;48(9):1460–71.
22. Feldhammer M, Ritchie JC. Anabasine is a poor marker for determining smoking status of transplant patients. Clin Chem 2017;63(2):604–6.
23. Kaoutzanis C, Leichtle SW, Mouawad NJ, et al. Risk factors for postoperative wound infections and prolonged hospitalization after ventral/incisional hernia repair. Hernia 2015;19(1):113–23.
24. Sauerland S, Korenkov M, Kleinen T, et al. Obesity is a risk factor for recurrence after incisional hernia repair. Hernia 2004;8(1):42–6.
25. Desai KA, Razavi SA, Hart AM, et al. The effect of BMI on outcomes following complex abdominal wall reconstructions. Ann Plast Surg 2016;76(Suppl 4): S295–7.
26. Fischer JP, Wink JD, Tuggle CT, et al. Wound risk assessment in ventral hernia repair: generation and internal validation of a risk stratification system using the ACS-NSQIP. Hernia 2015;19(1):103–11.
27. Rosen MJ, Aydogdu K, Grafmiller K, et al. A multidisciplinary approach to medical weight loss prior to complex abdominal wall reconstruction: is it feasible? J Gastrointest Surg 2015;19(8):1399–406.

28. Bakhach M, Shah V, Harwood T, et al. The protein-sparing modified fast diet: an effective and safe approach to induce rapid weight loss in severely obese adolescents. Glob Pediatr Health 2016;3. 2333794X15623245.
29. Brem H, Tomic-Canic M. Cellular and molecular basis of wound healing in diabetes. J Clin Invest 2007;117(5):1219–22.
30. Liao H, Zakhaleva J, Chen W. Cells and tissue interactions with glycated collagen and their relevance to delayed diabetic wound healing. Biomaterials 2009;30(9): 1689–96.
31. Bagdade JD, Root RK, Bulger RJ. Impaired leukocyte function in patients with poorly controlled diabetes. Diabetes 1974;23(1):9–15.
32. Halkos ME, Thourani VH, Lattouf OM, et al. Preoperative hemoglobin A1c predicts sternal wound infection after coronary artery bypass surgery with bilateral versus single internal thoracic artery grafts. Innovations 2008;3(3):131–8.
33. Stryker LS, Abdel MP, Morrey ME, et al. Elevated postoperative blood glucose and preoperative hemoglobin A1C are associated with increased wound complications following total joint arthroplasty. J Bone Joint Surg Am 2013;95(9): 808–14.S1-2.
34. Hikata T, Iwanami A, Hosogane N, et al. High preoperative hemoglobin A1c is a risk factor for surgical site infection after posterior thoracic and lumbar spinal instrumentation surgery. J Orthop Sci 2014;19(2):223–8.
35. Dronge AS, Perkal MF, Kancir S, et al. Long-term glycemic control and postoperative infectious complications. Arch Surg 2006;141(4):375–80 [discussion: 380].
36. Daley J, Khuri SF, Henderson W, et al. Risk adjustment of the postoperative morbidity rate for the comparative assessment of the quality of surgical care: results of the National Veterans Affairs Surgical Risk Study. J Am Coll Surg 1997; 185(4):328–40.
37. Kudsk KA, Tolley EA, DeWitt RC, et al. Preoperative albumin and surgical site identify surgical risk for major postoperative complications. JPEN J Parenter Enteral Nutr 2003;27(1):1–9.
38. Fazio VW, Coutsoftides T, Steiger E. Factors influencing the outcome of treatment of small bowel cutaneous fistula. World J Surg 1983;7(4):481–8.
39. Veterans Affairs Total Parenteral Nutrition Cooperative Study Group. Perioperative total parenteral nutrition in surgical patients. N Engl J Med 1991;325(8): 525–32.
40. Ross H. Operative surgery for enterocutaneous fistula. Clin Colon Rectal Surg 2010;23(3):190–4.
41. Klein S, Kinney J, Jeejeebhoy K, et al. Nutrition support in clinical practice: review of published data and recommendations for future research directions. Summary of a conference sponsored by the National Institutes of Health, American Society for Parenteral and Enteral Nutrition, and American Society for Clinical Nutrition. Am J Clin Nutr 1997;66(3):683–706.
42. Haupt W, Hohenberger W, Mueller R, et al. Association between preoperative acute phase response and postoperative complications. Eur J Surg 1997; 163(1):39–44.
43. Cereda E. Mini nutritional assessment. Curr Opin Clin Nutr Metab Care 2012; 15(1):29–41.
44. Guigoz Y. The Mini Nutritional Assessment (MNA) review of the literature–what does it tell us? J Nutr Health Aging 2006;10(6):466–85 [discussion: 485–7].
45. Simmons SF, Reuben D. Nutritional intake monitoring for nursing home residents: a comparison of staff documentation, direct observation, and photography methods. J Am Geriatr Soc 2000;48(2):209–13.

46. Ochoa JB, Makarenkova V, Bansal V. A rational use of immune enhancing diets: when should we use dietary arginine supplementation? Nutr Clin Pract 2004; 19(3):216–25.
47. Bansal V, Syres KM, Makarenkova V, et al. Interactions between fatty acids and arginine metabolism: implications for the design of immune-enhancing diets. JPEN J Parenter Enteral Nutr 2005;29(1 Suppl):S75–80.
48. Drover JW, Dhaliwal R, Weitzel L, et al. Perioperative use of arginine-supplemented diets: a systematic review of the evidence. J Am Coll Surg 2011;212(3):385–99, 99.e1.
49. Hegazi RA, Hustead DS, Evans DC. Preoperative standard oral nutrition supplements vs immunonutrition: results of a systematic review and meta-analysis. J Am Coll Surg 2014;219(5):1078–87.
50. Bode LG, Kluytmans JA, Wertheim HF, et al. Preventing surgical-site infections in nasal carriers of Staphylococcus aureus. N Engl J Med 2010;362(1):9–17.
51. Huang SS, Septimus E, Kleinman K, et al. Targeted versus universal decolonization to prevent ICU infection. N Engl J Med 2013;368(24):2255–65.
52. Baucom RB, Ousley J, Oyefule OO, et al. Evaluation of long-term surgical site occurrences in ventral hernia repair: implications of preoperative site independent MRSA infection. Hernia 2016;20(5):701–10.
53. Kapadia BH, Zhou PL, Jauregui JJ, et al. Does preadmission cutaneous chlorhexidine preparation reduce surgical site infections after total knee arthroplasty? Clin Orthop Relat Res 2016;474(7):1592–8.
54. Webster J, Osborne S. Preoperative bathing or showering with skin antiseptics to prevent surgical site infection. Cochrane Database Syst Rev 2015;(2):CD004985.
55. McDonald D, Ackermann G, Khailova L, et al. Extreme dysbiosis of the microbiome in critical illness. mSphere 2016;1(4) [pii:e00199-16].
56. Cogen AL, Yamasaki K, Sanchez KM, et al. Selective antimicrobial action is provided by phenol-soluble modulins derived from Staphylococcus epidermidis, a normal resident of the skin. J Invest Dermatol 2010;130(1):192–200.
57. Cogen AL, Yamasaki K, Muto J, et al. Staphylococcus epidermidis antimicrobial delta-toxin (phenol-soluble modulin-gamma) cooperates with host antimicrobial peptides to kill group A Streptococcus. PLoS One 2010;5(1):e8557.
58. Valkenet K, van de Port IG, Dronkers JJ, et al. The effects of preoperative exercise therapy on postoperative outcome: a systematic review. Clin Rehabil 2011; 25(2):99–111.
59. Moran J, Guinan E, McCormick P, et al. The ability of prehabilitation to influence postoperative outcome after intra-abdominal operation: a systematic review and meta-analysis. Surgery 2016;160(5):1189–201.
60. Krpata DM, Haskins IN, Phillips S, et al. Does preoperative bowel preparation reduce surgical site infections during elective ventral hernia repair? J Am Coll Surg 2017;224(2):204–11.
61. Scarborough JE, Mantyh CR, Sun Z, et al. Combined mechanical and oral antibiotic bowel preparation reduces incisional surgical site infection and anastomotic leak rates after elective colorectal resection: an analysis of colectomy-targeted ACS NSQIP. Ann Surg 2015;262(2):331–7.
62. Moores N, Rosenblatt S, Prabhu A, et al. Do iodine-impregnated adhesive surgical drapes reduce surgical site infections during open ventral hernia repair? A Comparative analysis. Am Surg 2017;83(6):617–22.
63. Webster J, Alghamdi A. Use of plastic adhesive drapes during surgery for preventing surgical site infection. Cochrane Database Syst Rev 2013;(1):CD006353.

64. Prabhu AS, Krpata DM, Perez A, et al. Is it time to reconsider postoperative epidural analgesia in patients undergoing elective ventral hernia repair?: an AHSQC analysis. Ann Surg 2017. [Epub ahead of print].
65. Pratt WB, Steinbrook RA, Maithel SK, et al. Epidural analgesia for pancreatoduodenectomy: a critical appraisal. J Gastrointest Surg 2008;12(7):1207–20.
66. Axelrod TM, Mendez BM, Abood GJ, et al. Peri-operative epidural may not be the preferred form of analgesia in select patients undergoing pancreaticoduodenectomy. J Surg Oncol 2015;111(3):306–10.
67. Cox TC, Blair LJ, Huntington CR, et al. The cost of preventable comorbidities on wound complications in open ventral hernia repair. J Surg Res 2016;206(1): 214–22.

Enhanced Recovery After Surgery Protocols
Rationale and Components

Kyle L. Kleppe, MD[a], Jacob A. Greenberg, MD, EdM[b],*

KEYWORDS

- Enhanced recovery after surgery • ERAS • Hernia • Abdominal wall reconstruction
- Multimodal

KEY POINTS

- Enhanced recovery after surgery (ERAS) represents a multimodal, multidisciplinary approach to enhance surgical outcomes and improve value for the patient and the health care system.
- ERAS protocols seek to minimize surgical stress and its effects through use of evidence-based protocols.
- ERAS protocols include the entire cycle of patient care, including preoperative assessment and optimization, intraoperative technique, and postoperative care.

INTRODUCTION

Enhanced recovery after surgery (ERAS) protocols have been gaining in popularity after their widespread adoption and success in the colorectal literature.[1,2] The initial development and implementation of ERAS protocols has been widely published, and largely successful in improving certain perioperative outcomes and decreasing hospital length of stay.[3,4] These successes have led other fields to explore development and implementation of ERAS protocols for a wide variety of surgical diseases, including abdominal wall reconstruction.[5–8]

ERAS protocols were developed to combat growing health care expenditures by providing a more efficient utilization of health care resources. These protocols have 2 main goals: improving patient outcomes and reducing costs.[2] Pathway elements

Disclosures: J.A. Greenberg receives research support from Bard-Davol and has served as a consultant for Ariste Medical. Dr K.L. Kleppe has nothing to disclose.
[a] Department of Surgery, University of Wisconsin–Madison, School of Medicine and Public Health, K4/739 CSC, 600 Highland Avenue, Madison, WI 53792-7375, USA; [b] Department of Surgery, University of Wisconsin–Madison, School of Medicine and Public Health, J4/703 CSC, 600 Highland Avenue, Madison, WI 53792-7375, USA
* Corresponding author.
E-mail address: greenbergj@surgery.wisc.edu

0039-6109/18/© 2018 Elsevier Inc. All rights reserved.

were selected based on existing literature and applied through a multimodal approach to reduce the effects of surgical stress and to enhance postoperative recovery.[1] The application of various individual elements into organized protocols allowed for significant overall improvement in the care of the surgical patient and evolved into the ERAS movement.

The success in colorectal surgery has led to development of protocols in a wide variety of surgical fields. A meta-analysis performed by Visioni[9] examined ERAS for noncolorectal surgery patients, including 6511 patients, over an array of abdominal procedures. Despite the procedural heterogeneity, there was a reduction in the length of stay by 2.5 days overall and 2.6 days in the randomized controlled trials (RCTs) group. Regarding the other primary outcome of complications, the estimated mean odds ratio (OR) was 0.70 (95% CI 0.56–0.86, $P = .001$), indicating a reduction of complications in the ERAS group. However, this reduction did not reach statistical significance in the RCTs group with an OR of 0.68 (95% CI 0.43–1.10, $P = .12$). Secondary outcomes, including readmission, were similar between groups. Cost data were available in 10 of the studies examined, all of which were RCTs, and demonstrated a mean reduction in cost of $5109.10 (95% CI $5852.40–$4365.80, $P<.001$). The investigators attributed these savings entirely to the decreased length of stay.

There are few studies that directly investigate ERAS protocols when applied to the hernia population.[6–8,10] ERAS protocols are mostly targeted at patients undergoing open abdominal wall reconstruction because these patients are hospitalized postoperatively. Macedo and colleagues[10] published a systematic review on ERAS protocols in ventral hernias in 2016; only 2 studies met inclusion criteria.[6,8] The protocols between the 2 studies were significantly different and are compared in **Table 1**. Despite this, they demonstrated a mean reduction in length of stay of 2.07 days (95% CI −2.6 to −1.5, $P<.0001$) and a trend toward decreased readmission rates in the ERAS group with an OR of 0.46 (95% CI 0.2–1.0, $P = .07$).[10]

Jensen and colleagues[6] examined 32 consecutive subjects undergoing giant ventral hernia repair (VHR). ERAS protocols were implemented and compared retrospectively to a standard care control group. All but 3 patients underwent bilateral endoscopic anterior component separation in addition to laparotomy for reconstruction. The main emphasis in the ERAS protocol included preoperative high-dose glucocorticoid administration (methylprednisolone 125 mg intravenous [IV]) in an effort to attenuate the inflammatory response and lead to low scores of pain, fatigue, and nausea. Other elements differing from the standard pathway included preoperative education on the pathway and expectations of discharge, twice daily discharge assessments, and more aggressive bowel regimens, including gum chewing and scheduled enemas. The complete ERAS protocol is listed in **Table 1**. The primary endpoint of length of stay was decreased after implementation (median 3.0 vs 5.5 days, $P = .003$). There were no statistically significant differences between the 2 groups with respect to rates of readmission ($P = .394$), postoperative complications ($P = .458$), or reoperation ($P = .172$).

Majumder and colleagues[8] also examined the implementation of their ERAS protocol for subjects undergoing major open VHR. The technique of choice was retromuscular VHR with posterior component separation via the transversus abdominis muscle release. ERAS protocols were developed and focused on preoperative subject selection and optimization, multimodal pain control, and intestinal recovery. Their complete ERAS protocol is listed in **Table 1**. The ERAS study cohort began accumulation when there was complete implementation of the protocol; comparison was made with a historical control group of subjects undergoing the same technique of repair. Subjects in the ERAS group demonstrated earlier functional recovery as measured by time to flatus,

Table 1
Comparison of included elements in hernia-specific enhanced recovery after surgery protocols

Protocol Elements	Jensen et al,[6] 2016	Majumder et al,[8] 2016
Preoperative	Information about expected discharge and discharge criteria	Weight loss counseling Diabetic control (hemoglobin A1c <8) Smoking cessation (≥4 wk) OSA screening IMPACT preoperative nutrition shake MRSA screening
Perioperative (Intraoperative)	High-dose glucocorticoid Oral analgesics: paracetamol 1 g, ibuprofen 400 mg, gabapentin 600 mg	SQ heparin 5000 units × 1 dose + SCDs PO alvimopan 12 mg × 1 dose PO gabapentin 100–300 mg × 1 dose First-generation cephalosporin + vancomycin for positive MRSA screen Minimization of intraoperative narcotics and paralytics Intraoperative TAP block, liposomal bupivacaine
Postoperative	Oral analgesics: paracetamol 1 g × 4, ibuprofen 400 mg × 3 Required daily assessment of discharge criteria Duration of epidural analgesia (2 d or less vs 3 d standard) Immediate early oral feeding Immediate pulmonary physiotherapy Supplemental oxygen therapy during first 48 h Gum chewing until bowel function Urinary catheter removed 24 h Enema 48 h, if no bowel function Drains removed when daily output in each drain is <60 mL (30 mL control)	IV hydromorphone PCA PO oxycodone 5–10 mg q 4 h prn after PCA PO acetaminophen 650 mg q 6 h PO gabapentin 100–300 mg tid IV or PO diazepam 5 mg q 6 h prn PO nonsteroidal antiinflammatory drugs 600–800 mg q 6–8 h prn No routine nasogastric tube placement npo except meds on operative day Scheduled diet advancement: postoperative day (POD)-1 limited clears, POD2 clear liquid ad lib, POD3 regular diet PO alvimopan 12 mg bid until discharge or POD 7 Fluid conservative strategy

Abbreviations: OSA, obstructive sleep apnea, PCA, patient-controlled analgesia, SCD, sequential compression device; SQ, subcutaneous, TAP, transversus abdominus plane.

bowel movement, and toleration of solid food (3.1 vs 3.9 days, 3.6 vs 5.2 days, and 3.4 vs 4.8 days, respectively; $P<.001$). This allowed for earlier transition to oral narcotics (2.2 vs 3.6 days; $P<.001$), as well as shorter length of stay (4.0 vs 6.1 days; $P<.001$). The 90-day readmission rate was also significantly lower at 4% versus 16% ($P = .008$).

RATIONALE OF ENHANCED RECOVERY AFTER SURGERY IMPLEMENTATION

For many surgeons, ERAS has been synonymous with fast-track pathways. This mindset inappropriately creates the goal of speeding recovery and decreasing length of stay as the primary endpoint of ERAS protocols. Instead, ERAS protocols focus on creating an environment for the patient to have an optimal perioperative experience.

Given these conditions, patients are likely to recover more expeditiously and, therefore, may have an associated decrease in length of stay.

Some investigators have stated the goals of ERAS are to optimize pain management and accelerate intestinal recovery.[7,8] These are certainly important areas of focus with regard to patients undergoing abdominal operations. These 2 goals are, in fact, intertwined and interdependent. However, the overall goal of ERAS protocols extends beyond these 2 pillars on which many enhanced recovery protocols were created. The underlying process in enhancing a patient's recovery is minimizing and mitigating the effects of surgical stress. Surgical stress can be influenced by many factors, such as pain, catabolism, immune dysfunction, nausea or vomiting, ileus, impaired pulmonary function, increased cardiac demands, coagulation-fibrinolytic dysfunction, cerebral dysfunction, alterations in fluid homeostasis, sleep disturbances, and fatigue.[1] These factors can be managed through a variety of approaches, including alterations in surgical technique, preoperative and postoperative practices, and pharmacologic interventions. Reduction of stress during elective surgical procedures by attenuation of the neurohormonal response to the operation allows for increased recovery and diminishes the risk of organ dysfunction and complications.[1]

The ultimate aim of ERAS protocols should be to improve the value of the care provided to the patient and the health care system as a whole. Health care value is influenced by quality, patient-reported outcomes, safety, and cost of the care delivered.[11] With the changes in reimbursement models, value of care will become increasingly important for health care to be effective in the future. All of these factors should be accounted for in developing hernia-related ERAS protocols.

Care of the hernia patient is complex, and the multiple dynamics that contribute to and have significant interplay in the recovery of the patient are not yet fully understood. Care must be taken in developing protocols that have short-term goals, such as reduction of length of stay, without investigating the impact on the larger recovery of the patient. Improvement in any area without regard to the overall process may lead to suboptimization and unintended consequences are likely to follow. Examples of this have included increased incidence of postoperative nausea and vomiting in the recovery room as a result of increased opioid administration to provide improvements in perioperative pain control.[11] As new ERAS protocols are created, unintended consequences could affect outcomes such as hernia recurrence,[5] chronic pain incidence, and other long-term consequences.[11] Therefore, long-term follow-up is needed for patients enrolled in ERAS protocols to assure that there are no delayed consequences of their implementation. Thus far, the benefits of ERAS protocol implementation have been tangible and ERAS protocols have demonstrated decreased length of stay and cost without increasing complications or readmission rates.[9]

PATIENT SELECTION FOR ENHANCED RECOVERY AFTER SURGERY PROTOCOLS

Hernias of the abdominal wall represent a wide spectrum of disease. The severity ranges from clinically asymptomatic to potentially life-threatening. Although the spectrum of hernia disease includes inguinal, femoral, ventral, incisional, parastomal, and recurrent hernias, most ERAS protocols in hernia surgery should largely focus on surgical repairs associated with longer lengths of stay. This would include primary and recurrent ventral, incisional, and parastomal hernias. There is minimal literature to support the identification of appropriate patient populations for enrollment in ERAS hernia protocols. In studies examining hernia-specific ERAS protocols, it is not entirely clear which patient populations are appropriate for enrollment into ERAS pathways. Although the protocol described by Majumder and colleagues[8] demonstrated benefits from ERAS, 38% of subjects were excluded based on intestinal resection, ostomy manipulation, placement of biologic mesh due to contaminated fields, and other potential sequelae requiring prolonged hospital stay.

The colorectal literature suggests that these protocols should be considered in primarily healthy individuals with no prior abdominal surgeries and with low American Society of Anesthesiologists scores, and who are undergoing straightforward procedures.[12] Patients undergoing abdominal wall reconstruction may not meet the enrollment criteria set forth in these studies from other areas in surgery. Future studies would benefit from inclusion of all subjects followed by subgroup analyses to determine appropriate patients for inclusion in hernia-specific ERAS protocols moving forward.

Additionally, just as hernia is a diverse disease process, so is the local environment in which these procedures take place. Patient demographics may be disparate and a particular intervention may not be effective from 1 patient population to another. Certain equipment, techniques, or medications may not be available in every hospital setting. Thus, individual programs need to identify specific interventions and opportunities for improvement with subsequent evaluation of specific outcomes. Establishment of clinical quality improvement programs is an excellent way to develop means to track and improve outcomes. This tool allows individual programs to interpret interventions in all patients and apply those interventions only to those who will receive the greatest benefit.[11,13]

COMPONENTS OF ENHANCED RECOVERY AFTER SURGERY PROTOCOLS

As previously mentioned, components of ERAS protocols are aimed at minimizing surgical stress and mitigating the subsequent response. These factors can be managed through a variety of approaches, including alterations in surgical technique, preoperative and postoperative protocols, and pharmacologic interventions. Following is an overview of some of the more commonly examined elements and those that have been specifically incorporated into published protocols specific for hernia patients.

Preoperative Practices

ERAS protocols should be developed that include the whole cycle of patient care. This begins with appropriate patient counseling, selection, and preparation during their preoperative visits. This brings up the concept of prehabilitation, which involves the assessment of patient candidacy for surgery and optimization of comorbid conditions before definitive repair. Many patients have concurrent medical problems, such as smoking, obesity, diabetes, and methicillin-resistant *Staphylococcus aureus* (MRSA) colonization, which can have a negative impact on their outcomes for hernia repair surgery.[2,14] It is important to optimize these conditions by working with their primary care providers or other specialists. With regard to diabetes, there is an increased risk of complications in patients with a hemoglobin A1C less than 6.5% and it is recommended to not undertake elective repair without intervention at this level, and a level greater than 8.0% should be prohibitive.[14] Majumder and colleagues[8] also screened for obstructive sleep apnea and MRSA nasal colonization, and instituted corrective interventions as appropriate.

Other modifiable risk factors that affect outcomes should be evaluated and addressed. This begins with an evaluation of overall functional status. Improvement in physical stamina and endurance should be achieved through increased physical activity. All patients should be encouraged to increase their activity even if they have limited mobility. Excess body weight (body mass index ≥ 30 kg/m^2) is associated with worse outcomes after VHR and weight loss is often sought before elective hernia operations.[14] Consultation with specialty services such as nutrition and bariatric services may be warranted. Nutritional status should be assessed and optimized through supplementation and immunomodulation to improve wound healing potential.[14] Majumder and colleagues[8] gave all patients arginine and omega-3 supplementation drinks (IMPACT Advanced Recovery, Nestle) 3 times per day for 5 days before the operation as part of their ERAS protocol. Even administering a carbohydrate load the morning of surgery has been shown to reduce insulin resistance and attenuate catabolism.[15] Smoking is associated with increased risk of complications such as surgical site infection and recurrence. Avoidance of elective surgery on current smokers and cessation for a minimum of 4 weeks is recommended before repair.[14] Some centers require nicotine screening tests before scheduling surgery. Chronic pain management is also an issue frequently encountered in the hernia population. Efforts to reduce preoperative opioid consumption or optimize pain regimens may improve postoperative pain metrics.

Cognitive and behavior disorders should also be addressed. Some patients do not have the skills to cope with a large surgery, especially if they do not have an appropriate social support structure. This may hinder their ability to care for themselves in the perioperative and early postoperative period.[2] Additionally, many patients may have concomitant psychiatric disorders and altered psychological states secondary to chronic pain or failed prior interventions, thus appropriately aligning patient expectations with goals of the operation is of paramount importance. Patients should also be informed of the expected postoperative course and discharge criteria. Jensen and colleagues[6] advised their patients that they expected a 3-day length of stay and continually reinforced this point during the perioperative period.

Patients undergoing colorectal resection who underwent 1 month of prehabilitation, including preoperative exercise, anxiety-reducing strategies, and protein supplementation, were found to have improved postoperative physical activity metrics such as walking distance.[16] Physical conditioning can be accomplished with simple walking and breathing exercises that may be more effective than cycling and strength training.[17] Regardless of the modality, preoperative health interventions have been found to improve recovery in the postoperative period and may improve long-term outcomes as well.[18]

Perioperative Practices, Intraoperative Practices, and Surgical Techniques

Although there is clearly a role for preoperative optimization for patients undergoing hernia surgery, most ERAS protocol elements begin in the immediate perioperative and intraoperative period. Multimodal pain therapy, judicious use of fluids, and attenuation of the stress response to surgery are all aspects of ERAS protocols that have been shown to be effective in achieving the goals of ERAS previously described.

When surgical injury is induced, afferent neuronal impulses are generated at the site of injury and travel to the medulla and the hypothalamus, causing a release of hormones, which results in a shift to catabolism, activation of the sympathetic nervous system, and release of catecholamines.[2] Preemptive blockade of these initial signals at the site of injury through local or systemically applied medications can reduce release of these mediators. Neuraxial blockade through use of epidural catheters has been published in the hernia literature[19–21] and was used in the study by Jensen and colleagues[6]; however, there have been mixed results. Some studies have shown epidural catheter use to be associated with a reduction in postoperative complications, cost,[19] and opioid consumption[21] when applied to the hernia population. Effect on length of stay has been highly variable. One recent study demonstrated no alteration in length of stay[21] and another showed prolonged length of stay associated with the use of epidural catheters.[20] Use of systemic infusions, including lidocaine or ketamine, as part of a multimodal approach to pain control have been demonstrated to decrease the time of intestinal recovery and length of stay in colorectal[22] and open ventral hernia.[21] Local or regional anesthesia has been used with increasing frequency and preoperative blocks can be performed with use of short-acting or long-acting local anesthetics, such as liposomal bupivacaine. Infiltration of local anesthetics in the transversus abdominis plane has been used with increasing frequency in abdominal operations, and has been associated with a reduction in opioid consumption and improved pain scores, as well as length of stay.[2,23,24] The techniques described include preoperative injections via landmark approaches or under ultrasound guidance,[23] as well as infiltration intraoperatively under direct visualization of the abdominal wall.[7,8,10,13,24]

In colorectal surgery, high-dose glucocorticoids have been shown to attenuate the postoperative inflammatory response, resulting in decreased complications and length of stay without an associated increase in wound complications.[25,26] Administration of IV methylprednisolone 125 mg at the time of surgery has been examined as part of an ERAS protocol in giant ventral hernias.[5,27] Other medications have been administered preoperatively to aid in postoperative pain control, including paracetamol, ibuprofen, gabapentin, celecoxib, and extended release oxycodone.[6,8,21] Gabapentin administration, even in a single dose, preoperatively has been shown to decrease the intensity of acute postoperative pain, tramadol consumption, and the incidence and intensity of pain in the first 6 months after inguinal herniorrhaphy.[28]

Minimally invasive techniques reduce wound size, which can decrease the inflammatory response, pain, and catabolism. In several studies, laparoscopy has been identified as the only independent predictive factor for reduction of hospital length of stay and morbidity in colon resections even as compared with open procedures in which ERAS protocols were in place.[29,30] For this reason, a laparoscopic approach is advocated as the preferred technique for patients undergoing colectomy in the setting of ERAS.[12] Minimally invasive techniques, such as endoscopic component separation for ventral hernias, reduce the number of wound complications.[31] Posterior component separation to avoid large skin flaps can also aid in decreasing wound complications.[8,13,23] Addition of other techniques, such as wide skin and soft tissue excision including excision of the umbilicus, and the use of layered quilting sutures to eliminate dead space and reduce tension on skin closure, has been reported to reduce the rate of wound complications.[13,32]

Standard fluid management in colorectal surgery historically involved liberal fluid administration intraoperatively and during the postoperative periods. However, concerns about excess fluid administration leading to increased interstitial fluid accumulation and its subsequent effects on ambulation difficulty, cardiopulmonary dysfunction, impaired tissue oxygenation, anastomotic breakdown, and wound infections led to investigations of restricted fluid administration. A meta-analysis demonstrated significant reduction in morbidity when restrictive goal-directed therapies were used during the operation and continuing into the postoperative period.[33]

Postoperative Practices

Intestinal recovery

Postoperative ileus can be a common finding after abdominal surgeries. There are several strategies to try and speed recovery of the gastrointestinal tract, allowing for resumption of regular diet and effective use of oral medications. Early enteral feeding and avoidance of nasogastric tube placement after surgery is supported in the colorectal surgery literature, which demonstrates that it is well-tolerated and results in earlier return of bowel function, earlier hospital discharge, decreased risk of infection, and improved hyperglycemic control.[34] The optimum strategy for early enteral feeding, which is often defined as less than 24 hours after surgery, has not been clearly defined. The diet regimen is significantly different in the hernia-specific ERAS protocols. Jensen and colleagues[6] allowed for subject regulation of an unrestricted regular diet. A more regimented progression of diet was described by Majumder and colleagues,[8] with subjects remaining at a nothing by mouth status on postoperative day (POD)-0, progression to limited clear liquids (≤250 mL/8 h) on POD1, unlimited clear liquids on POD2, and resumption of regular diet on POD3.[7] With the implementation of a scheduled diet advancement, Majumder and colleagues[8] found that enteral nutrition was introduced significantly earlier in the ERAS group without an increase in the rate of emesis. Measures of intestinal recovery, including time to flatus and bowel movement, were 3.1 versus 3.9 days and 3.6 versus 5.2 days, respectively (P<.001).[8]

Alvimopan, a μ-opioid antagonist, has been demonstrated to reduce time to gastrointestinal function and time to discharge in patients undergoing bowel resection.[35–37] Alvimopan was incorporated in 1 reported hernia-specific ERAS protocol to date.[8]

Multimodal pain control

Optimal pain management through a multimodal approach can lead to reduced opioid consumption, resulting in decreased opioid-related adverse outcomes; for example, nausea, vomiting, sedation, respiratory depression, ileus, and dependence.[38] Medications that should be continued in the postoperative setting to reduce opioid use include nonsteroidal antiinflammatory drug, acetaminophen, gabapentin, long-acting anesthetic blocks, and potentially ketamine.[21] Continued postoperative IV infusion of lidocaine can significantly reduce postoperative morphine consumption and improve pain scores.[39] IV acetaminophen has been studied in patients undergoing laparoscopic abdominal procedures, including hernia repair, with significantly greater pain relief over 24 hours compared with placebo.[40] It has a more rapid and predictable onset, a 70% higher peak plasma concentration compared with equivalent oral and rectal doses, and can be administered to patients who are not tolerating oral medications.[8] As part of a hernia ERAS protocol, its administration has been typically limited to the first postoperative 48 hours, or until tolerance of diet, and then transitioned to oral medication.[7]

Perioperative pain control is highly variable and individualized because not all patients respond to pain medications in a similar fashion. Senagore and colleagues[41] investigated the impact of genetic variants on medication responses in hernia patients. Patients underwent pharmacogenetic testing before the procedure and, based on the findings of specific genes, the analgesic selection was altered. Specific genes analyzed included the cytochrome P450 family, COMT, ACCB1, and OPRM1. Use of pharmacogenetics in this population resulted in a 50% reduction in opioid consumption and a reduced incidence of analgesic-related side effects.

Supportive care

Patients undergoing ventral hernia surgery were also found to have decreased peripheral capillary oxygen saturation in the postoperative period and supplemental oxygen administration has been advocated for in ERAS protocols.[6] Use of postoperative abdominal binders was included in 1 study with some potential benefit.[6] However, a systematic review of the use of abdominal binders in the perioperative period did not reach any significant decrease in postoperative pain or seroma formation after ventral hernia surgery.[42]

DEVELOPING AND IMPLEMENTING AN ENHANCED RECOVERY AFTER SURGERY PROTOCOL

Several of the studies previously discussed have created specific ERAS protocols for the care of patients with abdominal wall defects. The successful implementation of these protocols requires significant surgeon and institutional support. A multidisciplinary approach with support from anesthesia, nursing, and various other ancillary services is necessary for the successful implementation of a hernia-specific ERAS protocol. Additionally, it is important to apply said ERAS protocols to an appropriate patient population, which may vary significantly between institutions.

Despite these variabilities, there has been a call for standardization of protocols across institutions.[10] Although this may help with investigation of ERAS protocols in population-based studies, it does not allow for protocols to be tailored to specific environments or patients. Notably, it is not the aim of standardization to achieve absolute uniformity. Standardization should be a flexible, dynamic process that brings benefits to all those involved. The results should be that of an optimum variety, and not by any means uniformity, rigidity, and hostility to innovation.[43]

ERAS protocols in hernia surgery may potentially lead to significant improvements in a variety of patient outcomes following the repair of abdominal wall defects. Tailored ERAS protocols should be developed and applied with the individual patient and practice setting in mind. ERAS protocols with a focus on pharmacokinetics in metabolism of pain medications, judicious use of IV fluids, and early reintroduction of nutrition may all support improved patient outcomes following hernia surgery. Allowing for flexibility in protocols and identifying patients who will benefit from particular interventions may lead to further improvements in patient outcomes following abdominal wall reconstruction. Further research into hernia-specific ERAS protocols are currently ongoing and should lead to guidelines that can be implemented on a broad scale to improve outcomes for patients undergoing abdominal wall reconstruction.

SUMMARY

ERAS protocols make up a collection of evidence-based practices that are implemented with the goal of improving the value of patient care. ERAS protocols seek to standardize a framework for care of specific patients, rather than the highly individualized and diverse care plans of individual surgeons.[8] As more programs implement ERAS protocols, there should be continued efforts to study the outcomes of ERAS protocols so that surgeons may continue to improve the care provided to patients with defects of the abdominal wall.

REFERENCES

1. Kehlet H, Wilmore D. Evidence-based surgical care and the evolution of fast-track surgery. Ann Surg 2008;24(2):189–98.
2. DeBarros M, Steele SR. Perioperative protocols in colorectal surgery. Clin Colon Rectal Surg 2013;26:139–45.
3. Spanjersberg WR, Reurings J, Keus F, et al. Fast track surgery versus conventional recovery strategies for colorectal surgery. Cochrane Database Syst Rev 2011;(2):CD007635.
4. Nicholson A, Lowe MC, Parker J, et al. Systematic review and meta-analysis of enhanced recovery programmes in surgical patients. Br J Surg 2014;101(3):172–88.
5. Jensen KK. Recovery after abdominal wall reconstruction. Dan Med J 2017;64(3) [pii:B5349].

6. Jensen KK, Brondum TL, Harling H, et al. Enhanced recovery after giant ventral hernia repair. Hernia 2016;20:249–56.

7. Fayezizadeh M, Petro CC, Rosen MJ, et al. Enhanced recovery after surgery pathway for abdominal wall reconstruction: pilot study and preliminary outcomes. Plast Reconstr Surg 2014;134(4 Suppl 2):151S–9S.

8. Majumder A, Fayezizadeh M, Neupane R, et al. Benefits of multimodal enhanced recovery pathway in patients undergoing open ventral hernia repair. J Am Coll Surg 2016;222(6):1106–15.

9. Visioni A. Enhanced recovery after surgery for noncolorectal surgery? A systematic review and meta-analysis of major abdominal surgery. Ann Surg 2017;267(1): 57–65.

10. Macedo FI, Mittal VK. Does enhanced recovery pathways affect outcomes in open ventral hernia repair? Hernia 2016;21(5):817–8.

11. Ramshaw B. Discussion: enhanced recovery after surgery pathway for abdominal wall reconstruction: pilot study and preliminary outcomes. Plast Reconstr Surg 2014;134(4 Suppl 2):160S–1S.

12. Chestovich PJ, Lin AY, Yoo J. Fast-track pathways in colorectal surgery. Surg Clin North Am 2013;93:21–32.

13. Kleppe K, Ramshaw B. The application of complex systems science to healthcare and hernia disease. In: LeBlanc KA, Kingsnorth A, Sanders DL, editors. Management of abdominal hernias. Switzerland: Springer; 2018.

14. Liang MK, Holihan JL, Itani K, et al. Ventral hernia management: expert consensus guided by systematic review. Ann Surg 2017;265(1):80–9.

15. Viganò J, Cereda E, Caccialanza R, et al. Effects of preoperative oral carbohydrate supplementation on postoperative metabolic stress response of patients undergoing elective abdominal surgery. World J Surg 2012;36(8):1738–43.

16. Gillis C, Li C, Lee L, et al. Prehabilitation versus rehabilitation: a randomized control trial in patients undergoing colorectal resection for cancer. Anesthesiology 2014;121:937–47.

17. Carli F, Charlebois P, Stein B, et al. Randomized clinical trial of prehabilitation in colorectal surgery. Br J Surg 2010;97(8):1187–97.

18. Shanahan JL, Leissner KB. Prehabilitation for the enhanced recovery after surgery patient. J Laparoendosc Adv Surg Tech A 2017;27(9):880–2.

19. Fischer JP, Nelson JA, Wes AM, et al. The use of epidurals in abdominal wall reconstruction: an analysis of outcomes and cost. Plast Reconstr Surg 2014; 133(3):687–99.

20. Prabhu AS, Krpata DM, Perez A, et al. Is it time to reconsider postoperative epidural analgesia in patients undergoing elective ventral hernia repair?: an AHSQC analysis. Ann Surg 2017. [Epub ahead of print].

21. Warren JA, Stoddard C, Hunter AL, et al. Effect of multimodal analgesia on opioid use after open ventral hernia repair. J Gastrointest Surg 2017;21(10):1692–9.

22. Herroeder S, Pecher S, Schonherr ME, et al. Systemic lidocaine shortens length of hospital stay after colorectal surgery; a double-blinded, randomized, placebo-controlled trial. Ann Surg 2007;246(2):192–200.

23. Young MJ, Gorlin AW, Modest VE, et al. Clinical implications of the transversus abdominis plane block in adults. Anesthesiol Res Pract 2012;2012:731645.

24. Ramshaw B, Forman BR, Moore K, et al. Real-world clinical quality improvement for complex abdominal wall reconstruction. Surg Technol Int 2017;30:155–64.

25. Schulze S, Andersen J, Overgaard H, et al. Effect of prednisolone on the systemic response and wound healing after colonic surgery. Arch Surg 1997;132:129–35.

26. Srinivasa S, Kahokehr AA, Yu TC, et al. Preoperative glucocorticoid use in major abdominal surgery: systematic review and meta-analysis of randomized trials. Ann Surg 2011;254:183–91.
27. Jensen KK, Brøndum TL, Belhage B, et al. Preoperative steroid in abdominal wall reconstruction: protocol for a randomised trial. Dan Med J 2016;63(8) [pii:A5260].
28. Sen H, Sizlan A, Yanarates O, et al. The effects of gabapentin on acute and chronic pain after inguinal herniorrhaphy. Eur J Anaesthesiol 2009;26:772–6.
29. Vlug MS, Wind J, Hollmann MW, et al, LAFA study group. Laparoscopy in combination with fast track multimodal management is the best perioperative strategy in patients undergoing colonic surgery: a randomized clinical trial (LAFA-study). Ann Surg 2011;254(6):868–75.
30. Kennedy RH, Francis EA, Wharton R, et al. Multicenter randomized controlled trial of conventional versus laparoscopic surgery for colorectal cancer within an enhanced recovery programme: EnROL. J Clin Oncol 2014;32(17):1804–11.
31. Jensen KK, Henriksen NA, Jorgensen LN. Endoscopic component separation for ventral hernia causes fewer wound complications compared to open components separation: a systematic review and meta-analysis. Surg Endosc 2014;28:3046–52.
32. Ramshaw B, Dean J, Forman B, et al. Can abdominal wall reconstruction be safely performed without drains? Am Surg 2016;82(8):707–12.
33. Rahbari NN, Zimmermann JB, Schmidt T, et al. Meta-analysis of standard, restrictive and supplemental fluid administration in colorectal surgery. Br J Surg 2009;96:331–41.
34. Bauer VP. The evidence against prophylactic nasogastric intubation and oral restriction. Clin Colon Rectal Surg 2013;26:182–5.
35. Tan EK, Cornish J, Darzi AW, et al. Meta-analysis: alvimopan vs. placebo in the treatment of post-operative ileus. Aliment Pharmacol Ther 2007;25:47–57.
36. Ludwig K, Enker WE, Delaney CP, et al. Gastrointestinal tract recovery in patients undergoing bowel resection: results of a randomized trial of alvimopan and placebo with a standardized accelerated postoperative care pathway. Arch Surg 2008;143:1098–105.
37. Delaney CP, Craver C, Gibbons MM, et al. Evaluation of clinical outcomes with alvimopan in clinical practice: a national matched-cohort study in patients undergoing bowel resection. Ann Surg 2012;255:731–8.
38. Mariano ER. Management of acute postoperative pain. Waltham (MA): UpToDate; 2017.
39. Tauzin-Fin P, Bernard O, Sesay M, et al. Benefits of intravenous lidocaine on postoperative pain and acute rehabilitation after laparoscopic nephrectomy. J Anaesthesiol Clin Pharmacol 2014;30:366.
40. Wininger SJ, Miller H, Minkowitz HS, et al. A randomized, double-blind, placebo-controlled, multicenter, repeat dose study of two intravenous acetaminophen dosing regimens for the treatment of pain after abdominal laparoscopic surgery. Clin Ther 2010;32:2348–69.
41. Senagore AJ, Champagne BJ, Dosokey E, et al. Pharmacogenetics-guided analgesics in major abdominal surgery: further benefits within an enhanced recovery protocol. Am J Surg 2017;213(3):467–72.
42. Rothman JP, Gunnarsson U, Bisgaard T. Abdominal binders may reduce pain and improve physical function after major abdominal surgery – a systematic review. Dan Med J 2014;61:A4941.
43. Hesser I. Introduction to standards and standardization. Berlin: Beuth Verlag GmbH; 1998.

Incisional Hernia Repair
Open Retromuscular Approaches

Luciano Tastaldi, MD*, Hemasat Alkhatib, MD

KEYWORDS

- Incisional hernia • Component separation • Rives-Stoppa • Perforator sparing
- TAR • Abdominal wall reconstruction

KEY POINTS

- Incisional hernias are a common complication after abdominal surgery.
- Hernia surgery is constantly evolving; innovations in techniques, materials, and patient management have revolutionized the way hernias are repaired.
- The advent of the Rives Stoppa technique contributed to decreased recurrence and wound complications, providing a well-vascularized space for mesh placement.
- Abdominal wall reconstructive techniques have been successfully implemented into the surgical armamentarium to repair large and complex incisional hernias.
- Complex incisional hernias will increasingly be part of the general surgeon's practice, making imperative a profound knowledge of the abdominal wall anatomy and surgical techniques for hernia repair.

INTRODUCTION

Hernia repair has undergone vast evolution in the last 5 decades. Surgeons have embarked on an incessant search for the "optimal approach" to repair incisional hernias, driven perhaps by their patients' frustration as well as their own when faced with a failed repair after what initially looked like the "perfect surgery." These efforts have led to remarkable accomplishments in hernia surgery.

With the unacceptable rates of hernia recurrence seen with primary fascial repairs, the first revolution in hernia surgery came with the concept of the tension-free fascial closure with mesh. Soon enough, mesh repair became the gold standard for elective ventral hernia repair. The second revolution came later when, still uncomfortable with persisting high rates of recurrence despite the use of mesh, Drs Rene Stoppa, Jean Rives, and George Wantz explored the retromuscular and preperitoneal planes of the abdominal wall, contributing to significant refinements in surgical techniques. Mesh now could be placed in a space that was well-vascularized and entirely

Disclosure Statement: The authors have nothing to disclose.
Comprehensive Hernia Center, Digestive Disease and Surgery Institute, Cleveland Clinic Foundation, 9500 Euclid Avenue, A10-133, Cleveland, OH 44195, USA
* Corresponding author.
E-mail address: tastall@ccf.org

excluded from the bowel. This technique, although unknown at that time, was the first true myofascial release, because it involved releasing the rectus muscle from its fascial compartment and provided 5 cm of medial advancement on each side of the abdomen.[1] Although the Rives-Stoppa retromuscular repair has gained popularity and became the global "standard approach" for incisional hernia repairs, it still was not sufficient to adequately fix larger and more complex defects.

Dr Oscar Ramirez was responsible for starting the third revolution in hernia surgery by describing the anatomic components separation of the abdominal wall,[2] which became what is now known as "abdominal wall reconstruction." He described the anterior components separation that involved the release of the external oblique muscle and fascia to achieve medial advancement. Subsequent modification of this technique arose, each with its own set of disadvantages. Most recently, a new development in hernia repair was described with initially promising results: the posterior component separation with transversus abdominis release (TAR). This technique allowed for significant myofascial advancement and wide mesh overlap in the sublay position, while preserving blood supply to subcutaneous tissue and skin.

The so-called optimal approach for hernia repair is yet to be defined, and further innovations are still essential to address the quality of life for hernia patients. We aim in this article to summarize the open retromuscular techniques available in the current surgical armamentarium to repair an incisional hernia.

RIVES-STOPPA RETROMUSCULAR REPAIR

Developed by Drs Jean Rives and Rene Stoppa in the 1960s, and later popularized by Dr George Wantz, the Rives-Stoppa retromuscular repair remains the gold standard open approach for incisional hernia repair owing to its superior durability and lower wound complications rates when compared with other open approaches.[1] The principles of placing the mesh in a well-vascularized space favoring mesh incorporation, and in addition completely excluding the prosthesis from intraabdominal contents mitigating mesh-related complications have leveraged the adoption of this technique. In addition, having intraabdominal pressure forcing the prosthesis against the rectus muscle and, thus, supporting mesh incorporation into the abdominal wall was also the biomechanical principle involved in the rationale of this technique to decrease hernia recurrence.[1]

A retromuscular hernia repair is primarily based on freeing the rectus muscle from its fascial compartment by releasing the posterior rectus sheath from its dorsal insertion into the linea alba, and sequentially dissecting the muscle off the fascia laterally. This procedure ultimately allows for a medial advancement of the linea alba of up to 5 cm at the level of the umbilicus and 3 cm above and below the umbilicus. Without any further complicated component separation, this simple myofascial release of the rectus muscle should be enough to adequately provide a tension-free fascial closure for defects of maximum 10 cm in width. In addition, the creation of a retrorectus pocket provides adequate space for mesh positioning secluded from intraabdominal contents. By closing the anterior fascia on top of the mesh, the prosthesis is protected from the more superficial layers of the wound, decreasing risk for mesh infection.[1,3] More important, the Rives-Stoppa retromuscular repair does not require the creation of subcutaneous flaps and, therefore, can help to minimize wound complications and mesh exposure in case of wound breakdown.

Preoperative Planning

During the preoperative visit, the surgeon should conduct a comprehensive clinical evaluation, considering patient and hernia aspects that can influence the outcomes of hernia repair. Preoperative planning and optimization of the hernia patient are discussed in depth in elsewhere in this issue. It is important to obtain an imaging study to aid in surgical planning, and an abdominal computed tomography scan without intravenous contrast should be appropriate for the majority of the cases. This imaging modality provides valuable information, including the integrity of the abdominal wall musculature, defect dimensions, associated defects, prior meshes, and other aspects of previous repairs if dealing with a recurrent hernia. The preoperative imaging also helps to evaluate hernia characteristics that might limit hernia repair by means of a Rives-Stoppa technique.

Hernia width is the first factor that should be analyzed when planning for a Rives-Stoppa retromuscular repair. As stated, this technique can provide significant medialization of the linea alba and should be sufficient to repair defects that are no larger than 10 cm. Nevertheless, evaluating only hernia width might be insufficient to predict fascial closure. Another crucial aspect to be considered is how wide the rectus muscles and their fascial compartments are. Disruption of the linea alba as a consequence of hernia formation unloads the muscles of the lateral abdominal wall, resulting in disuse atrophy. Such atrophy results in a lateral retraction of the lateral abdominal wall musculature. In addition, the rectus muscles can also experience atrophic changes, which present as fibrosis and fat deposition. Ultimately, these structural changes result in decreased abdominal wall compliance and, therefore, simple retrorectus dissection might be insufficient to ensure a tension-free fascial closure, even if the hernia width is appropriate. Finally, an atrophic/fibrotic rectus muscle will seem to be contracted and cylindrical as opposed to broad and elliptical on a computed tomography scan, suggesting that the retrorectus space might be insufficient for adequate mesh overlap in such instances.

Figs. 1 and **2** illustrate 2 cases where such aspects are evaluated on preoperative imaging.

Patient Preparation and Positioning

Patient preparation and positioning are standard for all the open retromuscular approaches as well as the postoperative care discussed elsewhere in this article. Patients are positioned supine with arms out. The procedure is performed under general anesthesia, and the bladder and stomach are decompressed by insertion of a Foley catheter and orogastric tube after anesthesia induction. Hair is clipped, and

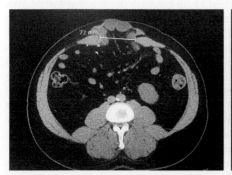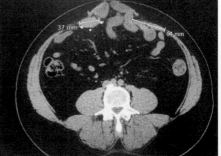

Fig. 1. Preoperative computed tomography scan. In this patient, although the hernia width measured above the umbilicus is 7 cm, there is significant atrophy and narrowing on the left rectus muscle (3.7 cm) when compared with the right side (6.4 cm). This feature will significantly limit medial advancement and mesh overlap.

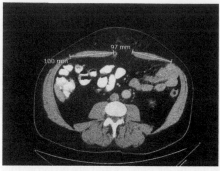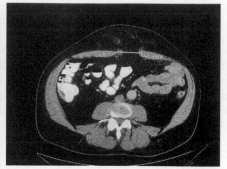

Fig. 2. In this patient with a hernia width measured to be 5.5 cm right above the umbilicus, the rectus muscles are sufficiently wide bilaterally not only to provide adequate advancement, but also to ensure wide mesh overlap.

skin prep is performed using a solution of 2% chlorhexidine gluconate in 70% isopropyl alcohol.[4,5] Antibiotics are administered within 1 hour of incision, sequential compression devices are applied intraoperatively, and confirmation that the patient has received a preoperative dose of unfractionated heparin is obtained during the operative time out.

Operative Steps: Rives-Stoppa Retromuscular Repair

1. The operation begins with a midline laparotomy, extending at least 5 cm above and below the defect. We choose to excise the prior scar for a better cosmetic outcome routinely.
2. The subcutaneous tissue is divided using a mix of electrocautery dissection and manual lateral traction as a way to minimize energy use and excessive lipolysis. Upon reaching the hernia sac, it should be opened in the midline and preserved at this moment, because this structure can be useful later to recreate the visceral sac.
3. Upon entering the abdomen, we routinely perform a full inspection of the intraabdominal contents along with a complete adhesiolysis of omentum and bowel that are adhered to the anterior abdominal wall. This step will not only result in a safer dissection minimizing the risk of injuries to the bowel, but will also be necessary to optimize the medial advancement of the linea alba. Interloop adhesions are not necessarily lysed unless they are deemed to be causing obstructive symptoms. It is critical that this adhesiolysis is performed carefully and painstakingly, and almost exclusively using sharp dissection (scissors and a no. 15 blade). This step minimizes the risk of an inadvertent enterotomy. Upon taking down all adhesions, a thorough inspection of the bowel should be performed to ensure that no serosal injuries or full-thickness enterotomies are being left behind. When present, we try to remove all prior meshes completely. There should be a balance between attempting to remove prior meshes in their entirety and not causing significant damage to the peritoneum and posterior rectus sheath. Usually, intraperitoneal polypropylene and polytetrafluoroethylene meshes can be removed without major damage to the peritoneum.[4] Last, attention can be turned to the abdominal wall. We place a moist blue towel in the abdomen covering all quadrants to protect the viscera during dissection.
4. We initiate the retromuscular dissection by incising the posterior rectus sheath one-half of a centimeter below the linea alba. This step can be performed with a knife or using electrocautery. When incising the posterior rectus sheath, the

rectus muscle fibers should be identified before extending the incision, confirming that we are in the correct plane. This incision is carried cranially and caudally until the posterior sheath has been incised in all its length, completely releasing the posterior sheath from its midline insertion in the linea alba **Fig. 3**.

5. The next step is to fully release the posterior sheath from the rectus muscle, which is accomplished by carrying a lateral dissection in the direction of the linea semi-lunaris. To facilitate this dissection, it is important that the surgeon and his or her assistant work together, adequately using traction and countertraction. We initially place 3 or 4 Kocher clamps on the posterior sheath, and the surgeon will hold those with their left hand, maintaining traction in the direction of midline. The assistant will also place 3 or 4 Kocher clamps in the linea alba and will keep those tractioned in an upward direction (toward the ceiling). Using electrocautery, the surgeon will dissect the posterior sheath off the rectus muscle. This dissection is carried laterally in the direction of linea semilunaris while identifying and preserving the deep inferior epigastric vessels running on an intramuscular plane on the rectus muscle. In this fashion, the rectus muscle and the inferior epigastric vessels go up, and only the posterior rectus sheath goes down. Medial to the linea semi-lunaris, the intercostal neurovascular bundles are encountered, perforating the posterior sheath. It is critical that those bundles are adequately identified and preserved, because inadvertent injury results in denervation and laxity of the abdominal wall **Figs. 4** and **5**.

6. Retrorectus dissection is performed in the same manner on the contralateral side. It is important to ensure that such release is performed at least 5 to 8 cm cranial and caudal to the defect to create a sufficient pocket for mesh placement. Also, extending this release cranial and caudal to the defect will ensure that all the potential medial advancement is reached. Upon finishing the retrorectus dissection on both sides, the dissection planes must be joined on the cranial and caudal edges of the abdomen, allowing the retrorectus space to communicate across the midline. This maneuver requires a pelvic dissection into the space of Retzius, and release of the posterior sheath from its insertion into the xiphoid, as detailed.

7. Pelvic dissection: Below the arcuate line, there is a transition where the posterior rectus sheath does not exist anymore, and the posterior layer is formed by the transversalis fascia and the peritoneum. By retracting the rectus muscles superiorly with the aid of 2 Richardson retractors with the patient in the Trendelenburg position, and by retracting the posterior rectus sheaths inferiorly using 2 Kocher clamps, the insertion of the posterior sheaths into the linea alba is released. Blunt dissection is now used to develop a preperitoneal pocket in the pelvis. This step is very similar to the dissection that is performed during a laparoscopic

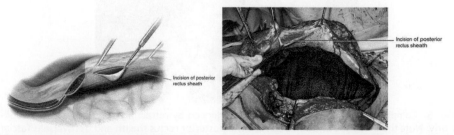

Fig. 3. Incision of the posterior rectus sheath exposing rectus muscle fibers. (*From* Rosen MJ. Posterior component separation with transversus abdominis muscle release. In: Atlas of abdominal wall reconstruction. 2nd edition. Elsevier; 2017. p. 87; with permission.)

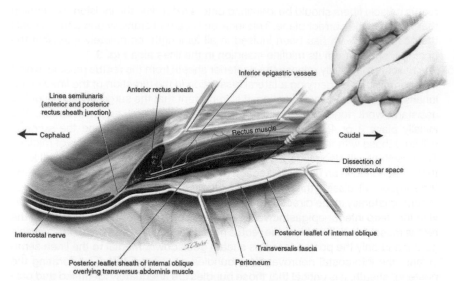

Fig. 4. Retromuscular dissection. Note the evident extension from the posterior lamella of the internal oblique and transversus abdominis muscles across the linea semilunaris. (*From* Rosen MJ. Posterior component separation with transversus abdominis muscle release. In: Atlas of abdominal wall reconstruction. 2nd edition. Elsevier; 2017. p. 89; with permission.)

transabdominal preperitoneal inguinal hernia repair, and the same anatomic landmarks should be used to guide this dissection.[4] The pubis and both of Cooper's ligaments are identified medially, and the spermatic cord structures are skeletonized (or the round ligament is divided if the patient is female). The deep inferior epigastric vessels are identified, preserved, and kept in their anatomic bed superiorly in the abdominal wall. Laterally and inferiorly, the medial border of the psoas muscle is identified and marks the end of lateral dissection **Fig. 6**.

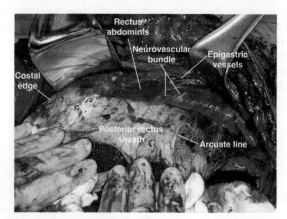

Fig. 5. Completed retromuscular dissection, evidenced by retracting the rectus muscles superiorly. Note the evident transition between the posterior rectus sheath and transversalis fascia/peritoneum on the level of the arcuate line. (*From* Rosen MJ. Posterior component separation with transversus abdominis muscle release. In: Atlas of abdominal wall reconstruction. 2nd edition. Elsevier; 2017. p. 89; with permission.)

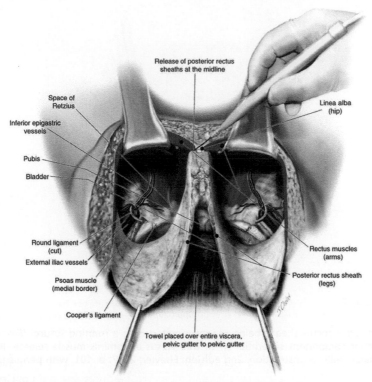

Release of posterior rectus
sheaths at the midline

Space of
Retzius

Inferior epigastric
vessels

Pubis

Bladder

Round ligament
(cut)

External iliac vessels

Psoas muscle
(medial border)

Cooper's ligament

Towel placed over entire viscera,
pelvic gutter to pelvic gutter

Linea alba
(hip)

Rectus muscles
(arms)

Posterior rectus sheath
(legs)

Fig. 6. Pelvic dissection. (*From* Rosen MJ. Posterior component separation with transversus abdominis muscle release. In: Atlas of abdominal wall reconstruction. 2nd edition. Elsevier; 2017. p. 91; with permission.)

8. Subxiphoid dissection: Retroxiphoid exposure will only be needed when the defect extends next to the bony prominence of the costal margin. This cranial dissection is performed by releasing the posterior sheath from its insertion into the xiphoid and entering a preperitoneal plane below the xiphoid. Note that for defects in lower or mid abdomen, as stated before, a 5- to 8-cm dissection above the defect should be sufficient.

9. Posterior sheath closure: Here it is important to assess whether the retromuscular dissection is enough to guarantee that both the posterior and anterior fascia can be closed without tension. This assessment can be easily performed by bringing the linea alba to midline with the aid of Kocher clamps. If this can be done without tension, the posterior sheath can now be reapproximated with a running 2-0 absorbable suture. It is important to close the posterior sheath completely to avoid mesh exposure to the bowel and also to prevent internal herniation of the intestine into the retrorectus space. At this point, if the posterior sheath cannot be reapproximated without tension, the best next step is to add a posterior component separation with TAR, which is further detailed elsewhere in this article **Fig. 7**.

10. Mesh placement and fixation: A standard piece of uncoated, large pore, medium weight polypropylene mesh, trimmed to occupy all of the retrorectus space, might be appropriate for the great majority of the cases. Nevertheless, other types of prostheses like a biologic scaffold might be suitable when considering a multitude of patient, hernia, and intraoperative variables, especially the

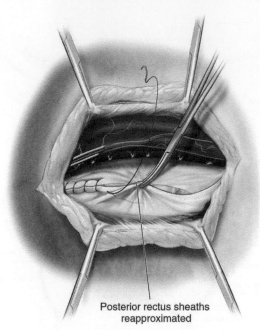

Fig. 7. Posterior rectus sheath being reapproximated with a running suture. (*From* Rosen MJ. Posterior component separation with transversus abdominis muscle release. In: Atlas of abdominal wall reconstruction. 2nd edition. Elsevier; 2017. p. 101; with permission.)

presence of contamination. We fixate the mesh circumferentially using full-thickness transfascial sutures with no. 1 slowly absorbable monofilament sutures. This is performed with the aid of a Carter-Thomason (CooperSurgical, Trumbull, CT) suture passer. The suture is placed through the mesh with a 1-cm bite; a small stab wound is made on the skin with a no. 11 blade, through which the suture passer is introduced to grab the suture ends. The sutures are tied, and the knot lies in the subcutaneous tissue. In addition, inferiorly, the mesh is secured to Cooper's ligaments bilaterally with interrupted stitches and superiorly to the xiphoid and costal margins if the dissection was carried out to this level. The mesh should lay flat on the posterior layer without wrinkles that could impair its incorporation to the abdominal wall. These authors prefer to place sutures sequentially without tying them, but having assistants place tension on them, to help ensure that forces are equally distributed and the mesh will ultimately lay flat in the retrorectus space **Fig. 8**.

11. Midline reconstruction by approximating the anterior fascia: Upon completing mesh fixation, 2 large closed suction drains are placed above the mesh (one on each side) and exteriorized through separate skin incisions. Midline can be now restored with running or figure-of-8 sutures, also using no. 1 slowly absorbable sutures. Sometimes, the anterior fascia cannot be closed. At that point, the preferred strategy is to perform a TAR. Some surgeons would perform concomitant anterior components separation at this point; however, our group prefers to avoid combining anterior and posterior components separation, because it may lead to a destabilization injury of the lateral abdominal wall. Although theoretically undesirable, one other possible approach is to leave the anterior fascia open and close the subcutaneous tissue and skin on top of the mesh, which is referred to as a bridged repair. To date,

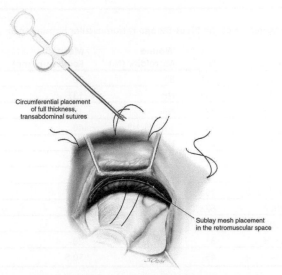

Circumferential placement
of full thickness,
transabdominal sutures

Sublay mesh placement
in the retromuscular space

Fig. 8. Mesh placement and lateral fixation with transfascial sutures. (*From* Rosen MJ. Posterior component separation with transversus abdominis muscle release. In: Atlas of abdominal wall reconstruction. 2nd edition. Elsevier; 2017. p. 103; with permission.)

there is insufficient evidence to speak that this might result in increased chance of recurrence.[3] Nevertheless, it is better, when possible, to completely close the anterior fascia to avoid mesh exposure in case of wound breakdown and, therefore, minimize the chance of mesh infection.[3]

12. Upon closing the anterior fascia, we reapproximate the subcutaneous tissue and skin with subcuticular absorbable sutures. If there is tension on the skin, we use nylon vertical mattress sutures.[1,4,5]

Clinical results in the literature

Table 1 summarizes published outcomes of the Rives-Stoppa retromuscular repair. Overall, results in the literature consistently show that the standard open Rives-Stoppa retromuscular repair is efficient in providing a safe and durable repair for small to moderate sized midline incisional hernias.

ANTERIOR COMPONENTS SEPARATION

Dr Ramirez has revolutionized the field of hernia surgery with the development of components separation. Dr Ramirez described in his original publication[2] that, by performing a longitudinal external oblique fasciotomy on both sides of the abdomen and dissecting the avascular plane between the external and internal oblique muscles, a medial advancement of 5 cm at the epigastrium, 10 cm in the waist, and 3 cm in the suprapubic region could be achieved per side.[17,18] In addition, his anatomic study stunningly demonstrates that the standard retromuscular dissection, as described by Stoppa and Rives, would confer additional advancement of the abdominal wall into midline if needed. He then reported his initial experience applying the described technique on 11 patients with complex incisional hernias. This was the historical landmark that established the concepts of abdominal wall reconstructive techniques as they are known today.

Table 1				
Clinical results in literature of the Rives-Stoppa retromuscular hernia repair				
Author, Reference	N	Wound Morbidity (%)	Mean Follow-up (mo)	Recurrence Rate (%)
Petersen et al,[3] 2004	175	8[a]	20	9
Rogmark et al,[6] 2017	217	NR	137	8.1
Israelsson et al,[7] 2006	123	NR	12–24	7.3 (9 of 123)
Maman et al,[8] 2012	89	11.9/(5.1)[b]	40	1.7
Helgstrand et al,[9] 2013	323	NR	48	12.1
Iqbal et al,[10] 2007	254	13	70	5
McLanahan et al,[11] 1997	106	18	24	3.5
Martin-Dulce et al,[12] 2001	152	25	72	1.3
Flament et al,[13] 2002	623	4.3	NR	6.7
Ferranti et al,[14] 2003	35	14.2	NR	2.8
Novitsky et al,[15] 2006	32	12.5	28	3.1
Fischer et al,[16] 2014	45	33.3	10.5	0

Abbreviation: NR, not reported.
[a] Deep mesh infections.
[b] Mesh infection requiring removal of the mesh.
Data from Refs.[1,3,5–16]

Unfortunately, this technique as originally described was associated with significant wound morbidity.[17,18] The extensive subcutaneous dissection needed to expose the linea semilunaris and perform the external oblique release, especially in large hernias, resulted in significant destruction of the blood supply to the skin and subcutaneous tissue, exposing patients to an increased risk for skin necrosis and wound disruption. The large area of dead space created as consequence of subcutaneous flaps elevation predisposed to a variety of wound complications, including seromas, hematomas, and wound infections. Furthermore, the original idea of Dr Ramirez was that his technique provided the opportunity of anatomic reconstruction of midline without tension and, therefore, could obviate the need for mesh.[17] Unfortunately, reproduction of the technique without a prosthesis was still associated with high recurrences rates in the long term (**Table 2**).

To overcome its drawbacks, the anterior component separation underwent important technical modifications by other investigators. First, routine mesh was implemented. Several series reported the use of synthetic and biologic meshes, in either onlay or underlay positions, which has contributed to decreasing recurrence rates. Furthermore, Dumanian and colleagues[25–27] modified the original technique to minimize skin and subcutaneous tissue devascularization. While maintaining the technical aspects of the Ramirez technique, dissection of subcutaneous tissue was limited by the creation of skin flaps only above the umbilicus, preserving the periumbilical perforators and decreasing the amount of skin undermining.[25] This modification, as demonstrated in a cohort of 66 patients, has resulted in a decrease in wound complications from 20% (original anterior component separation) to 2% (periumbilical perforator sparing technique).[26] A minimally invasive approach was later implemented to perform the external oblique release laparoscopically, the endoscopic component separation, which is discussed elsewhere in this issue.

The anterior components separation and its variants continue to be useful tools in the surgical armamentarium and are still used globally by a significant number of surgeons.

Operative Steps: Open Periumbilical Perforator–Sparing Component Separation with Retromuscular Mesh Placement

1. Laparotomy and adhesiolysis are performed as previously described in this article.[27]
2. A transverse incision of 6 to 8 cm is made below the costal margins right above the linea semilunaris. Subcutaneous tissue is dissected while the assistant retracts the incision superiorly and inferiorly until the linea semilunaris is exposed. Using blunt dissection, a tunnel that extends from the costal margin to the anterior superior iliac spine is dissected, fully exposing the medial aspect of the external oblique aponeurosis in its junction to form linea semilunaris **Fig. 9**.
3. With electrocautery, the external oblique fascia and muscle are divided laterally to the linea semilunaris. It is critical to adequately identify the linea semilunaris and incise the external oblique aponeurosis at least 1 to 2 cm away to avoid iatrogenic disruption of the linea semilunaris. This fasciotomy should extend superiorly above the ribs to decrease the tension in the midline **Fig. 10**.
4. Using blunt dissection, a tunnel that extends from the suprapubic region (in the lower aspect of the laparotomy) to the anterior superior iliac spine is created. This opening communicates with the lateral tunnel that was used for external oblique release. On this inferior tunnel, additional fibers and fascia of the external oblique are divided up to the inferior limit, the inguinal ligament. This dissection should be repeated in the same manner on the contralateral side **Fig. 11**.
5. A bilateral retrorectus dissection is performed as previously detailed in this article.
6. Mesh is placed in the retrorectus space and fixed with transfascial sutures after the posterior rectus sheath has been closed. Two large closed suction drains are placed above the mesh. Additional closed suction drains are placed in the lateral tunnels created for the external oblique release (**Fig. 12**).
7. The anterior fascia can now be closed with running or figure-of-8 sutures made with no. 1 slowly absorbable material (**Fig. 13**).
8. Subcutaneous tissue and skin are closed with subcuticular, absorbable sutures, or nylon vertical mattress sutures if there is tension on the skin.

Table 2
Clinical results in literature of the anterior component separation without mesh

Author, Reference	N	Wound Morbidity (%)	Mean Follow-up (mo)	Recurrence Rate (%)
Ramirez et al,[2] 1990[a]	11	NR	4–42	0
Girotto et al,[19] 1999[b]	37	30.0	21	6.1
De Vries Reilingh et al,[20] 2003	43	32.6	15.6	32.0
De Vries Reilingh et al,[21] 2007	19	53	36	53.0
Jernigan et al,[22] 2003[b]	73 (66 without mesh)	NR	24	5.5
Lowe et al,[23] 2003[b]	30 (20 without mesh)	35.0	9.5	10.0
Clarke,[24] 2010	63 (29 without mesh)	28.5	35	19.0

Abbreviation: NR, not reported.
[a] Data from Ref.[5]
[b] Data from Ref.[18]

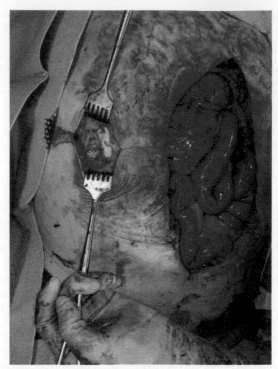

Fig. 9. Lateral incision exposing the linea semilunaris. (*From* Dumanian GA. Periumbilical perforator sparing component separation. In: Rosen MJ, editor. Atlas of abdominal wall reconstruction. Philadelphia: Elsevier; 2017. p. 172; with permission.)

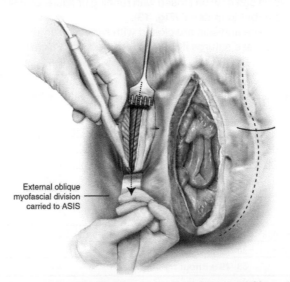

External oblique myofascial division carried to ASIS

Fig. 10. External oblique release by division of external fascia and fibers. (*From* Dumanian GA. Periumbilical perforator sparing component separation. In: Rosen MJ, editor. Atlas of abdominal wall reconstruction. Philadelphia: Elsevier; 2017. p. 173; with permission.)

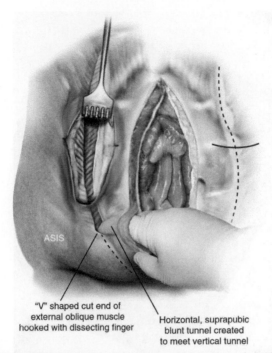

"V" shaped cut end of
external oblique muscle
hooked with dissecting finger

Horizontal, suprapubic
blunt tunnel created
to meet vertical tunnel

Fig. 11. Creation of a tunnel communicating the inferior edge of the laparotomy and the interior edge of the external oblique release. ASIS, anterior superior iliac spine. (*From* Dumanian GA. Periumbilical perforator sparing component separation. In: Rosen MJ, editor. Atlas of abdominal wall reconstruction. Philadelphia: Elsevier; 2017. p. 175; with permission.)

Clinical results in the literature
Tables 2–4 summarize the published outcomes of anterior component separation without mesh, anterior component separation with mesh, and periumbilical perforators sparing anterior component separation.

POSTERIOR COMPONENT SEPARATION WITH TRANSVERSUS ABDOMINIS RELEASE

The increasing popularity of the posterior component separation with TAR can be easily explained by its inherent ability to overcome the weaknesses of the previously mentioned reconstructive techniques. The possibility of obtaining significant medialization of the abdominal wall by incising the posterior lamella of the internal oblique and dividing the transversus abdominis fibers has addressed the problem of insufficient advancement for larger hernias with the standard retromuscular dissection. Additionally, by extending dissection of the retromuscular space into the preperitoneal and retroperitoneal spaces, an enormous sublay pocket for mesh placement can be created to guarantee sufficient mesh overlap for the majority of incisional hernias. The dissection beyond the linea semilunaris and release of the anterior fascia from its posterior attachments made the TAR a versatile reconstructive technique that is, able to address subxiphoid and nonmidline defects. Last, because TAR precludes any type of subcutaneous dissection, minimally invasive or not, a decrease in wound complications related to extensive subcutaneous dissection could be expected.

TAR began to be performed in 2006 at a single institution in Cleveland where it was developed, and the initial results were published by Novitsky and associates in 2012,[39]

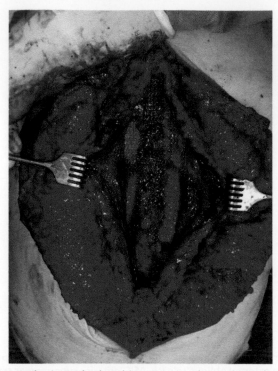

Fig. 12. Permanent synthetic mesh placed in retromuscular position. (*From* Dumanian GA. Periumbilical perforator sparing component separation. In: Rosen MJ, editor. Atlas of abdominal wall reconstruction. Philadelphia: Elsevier; 2017. p. 177; with permission.)

creating great enthusiasm in the surgical community. Initial experience showed a deep surgical site infection rate of 7% and a recurrence rate of 4.7% after a median 26 months of follow-up. In the same year, Krpata and colleagues[40] compared the TAR retrospectively with open anterior component separation with sublay mesh, and showed that the TAR could achieve equivalent rates of fascial closure when compared with anterior component separation, but with a significantly lower rate of wound complications. Although recurrence rates were higher in the anterior component separation group, this difference was not sufficient to reach statistical significance, and the median follow-up period was relatively short. Since then, the procedure has gained great popularity, and several other series have been published reporting consistent outcomes. **Table 5** summarizes published outcomes of TAR.[41–48] In fact, the safety and feasibility of the technique have been tested in challenging patient cohorts like those with complex parastomal hernias,[45,48] hernias after open abdomen,[41] and hernias after kidney transplantation.[42] The latest innovation in TAR involved minimally invasive approaches, especially with the robotic platform.[49–53] Robotic-assisted TAR seems to result in a shorter duration of hospital stay when compared with the traditional open approach. However, until the date of this publication, there are insufficient data to draw meaningful conclusions and surgeons are still overcoming the learning curve of the robotic TAR as evidenced by the significantly longer operative times.[49–51]

Anatomic Concepts of Posterior Component Separation with Transversus Abdominis Release

The rationale for TAR is based on the anatomic observation in the upper third of the abdomen; both the posterior lamella of the internal oblique and the transversus

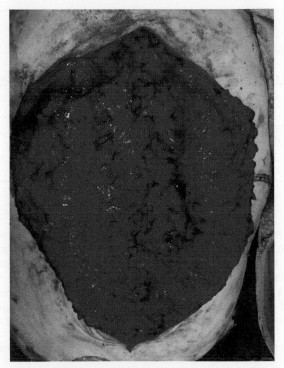

Fig. 13. Anterior fascia reapproximated on top of the mesh. (*From* Dumanian GA. Perium-bilical perforator sparing component separation. In: Rosen MJ, editor. Atlas of abdominal wall reconstruction. Philadelphia: Elsevier; 2017. p. 177; with permission.)

Table 3
Clinical results in literature of the anterior component separation with mesh

Author, Reference	N	Wound Morbidity (%)	Mean Follow-up (mo)	Recurrence Rate (%)
Girotto et al,[28] 2003[a,b]	96 (onlay)	26	26	22
Gonzalez et al,[29] 2005[b]	42 (onlay)	33	16	7
Espinosa-de-los-Monteros et al,[30] 2007[a]	39 (onlay with acellular human dermal matrix)	26	15	5
DiBello & Moore,[31] 1996[c]	35 (onlay)	14	22	8.5
Diaz et al,[32] 2009[a]	31 (onlay with acellular human dermal matrix)	42	10.5	6.5
Garvey et al,[33] 2016	151 (underlay of acellular dermal matrix)	25	53	13.6
Sailes et al,[34] 2010[b]	545 (onlay with various types of mesh)	7.5	NR	18.3

[a] Data from Ref.[5]
[b] Data from Ref.[18]
[c] Data from Ref.[35]

Table 4
Clinical results in literature of the periumbilical perforator sparing anterior component separation

Author, Reference	N	Wound Morbidity (%)	Mean Follow-up (mo)	Recurrence Rate (%)
Saulis,[26,a]	41	4	NR	8
Clarke,[24,a,b]	65	3.0	38	13.8
Butler & Campbell,[36] 2011	38	27.0	12.4	3.0
Patel et al,[37] 2012[b]	41 (34 perforator sparing)	24.4	15.8	0
Ghali et al,[38] 2012	57	14.0	15.2	4.0

[a] Data from Ref.[5]
[b] Data from Ref.[35]

abdominis muscle fibers extend medially to the linea semilunaris. Such extension allows the surgeon to gain access to the preperitoneal space of the lateral abdominal wall and perform the 2 operative steps responsible for obtaining the desired advancement: (1) by releasing the posterior lamella of the internal oblique, midline fascia is released from its posterior attachments and can be advanced, and (2) by dividing the medial fibers of the transversus abdominis muscle, the peritoneum and posterior components can be advanced to recreate the visceral sac in midline without tension.

Operative Steps: Open Posterior Component Separation with Transversus Abdominis Release

1. The procedure begins with a generous midline laparotomy, and the abdomen is entered sharply.[4,5]
2. Adhesiolysis is performed in the same manner described before, using sharp dissection. Because with TAR the dissection is extended beyond linea semilunaris into the preperitoneal and retroperitoneal spaces, we would reinforce the importance of performing a full adhesiolysis. As stated, a safer dissection can be

Table 5
Clinical results in literature of the open posterior component separation with transversus abdominis release

Author, Reference	N	Wound Morbidity (%)	Mean Follow-up (mo)	Recurrence Rate (%)
Novitsky et al,[39] 2012	42	24.0	26	4.7
Krpata et al,[40] 2012	55	25.0	7	3.6
Petro et al,[41] 2015[a]	34	35.0	18	14.7
Petro et al,[42] 2015[b]	11	27.0	12	9.0
Winder et al,[43] 2016	37	5.4	21	2.7
Raigani et al,[44] 2014[c]	48	43.8	13	11.0
Pauli et al,[45] 2016	29	45.0	11	3.0
Fayezizadeh et al,[46] 2016	77	43.0	28	12.5
Novitsky et al,[47] 2016	428	18.7	31.5	3.7
Tastaldi et al,[48] 2017[c]	38	13.0	13	11.0

[a] Complex hernias after open abdomen.
[b] Complex hernia after kidney transplantation.
[c] Complex parastomal hernias.

performed knowing that no bowel is plastered underneath the posterior sheath and peritoneum. In addition, medialization of the fascia is optimized when there are no adherent intraabdominal contents. In such cases, we do prefer to lyse the most significant interloop adhesions to decrease the chance of reoperation owing to a small bowel obstruction. However, this more intense bowel manipulation can indeed result in longer times for return of bowel function.

3. We routinely try to remove all prior intraperitoneal meshes to enhance incorporation of the new prosthesis into the abdominal wall.

4. Retromuscular dissection, pelvic dissection, and subxiphoid exposure are performed as described in the operative steps section of the Rives-Stoppa procedure. Again, it is extremely important to identify and preserve the neurovascular bundles that supply the rectus muscle; they are encountered perforating the posterior sheath medial to the linea semilunaris.

5. When performing an abdominal wall reconstruction, the plan is always to first complete the Rives-Stoppa repair dissection, including the pelvic dissection into the space of Retzius. At this point, we assess if (1) the advancement achieved is enough to close the posterior sheath without tension, and (2) tension on midline is not excessive when bringing the anterior fascia together. Although it might be determined in the majority of cases preoperatively that a Rives-Stoppa repair would not suffice, we consider it particularly important for the surgeon to exercise this stepwise strategy. We believe patients should undergo only the myofascial release that is necessary to adequately repair their hernias and nothing beyond that. Many times, a substantial amount of advancement can be achieved in certain patients who tend to have a more compliant abdominal wall. Therefore, always exercising this approach will avoid huge TAR dissections in patients where a more conservative release would be satisfactory for the repair.

6. If it is decided that a TAR will be needed, the next step is to incise the posterior lamella of the internal oblique. This incision is performed longitudinally along the posterior sheath, immediately medial to where the neurovascular bundles are seen. We recommend beginning the release in the lower third of the abdomen, below the arcuate line, because no posterior sheath exists at this level and the preperitoneal space can be more easily accessed. However, this is not a rule, and the release can be started in the upper abdomen as well. We do not recommend starting this initial step next to the umbilicus because the absence of transversus abdominis fibers across the linea semilunaris at this level makes the identification of the surgical planes more difficult. If choosing to start the release in the upper abdomen, the transversus abdominis fibers must be identified right underneath the posterior sheath to confirm the correct plane. The posterior lamella is incised with electrocautery while keeping the posterior rectus sheath under tension, because it facilitates dissection and exposure of the anatomic plane (**Fig. 14**).

7. With the aid of a right-angle clamp, we dissect the transversus abdominis fibers off the peritoneum and divide them using electrocautery (**Fig. 15**).

8. After the posterior lamella of the internal oblique and the transversus abdominis fibers have been divided, the next step is to extend the dissection into the preperitoneal space laterally. With blunt dissection (best performed with the aid of a Kittner dissector), the plane between the transversalis fascia and the peritoneum can be developed laterally in the direction of the retroperitoneum. The medial border of the psoas muscle should mark the end of the lateral dissection (**Fig. 16**).

9. Cranially, the insertions of the posterior sheath into the xiphoid can be released, and the peritoneum can be cleared of the diaphragm all the way to the central

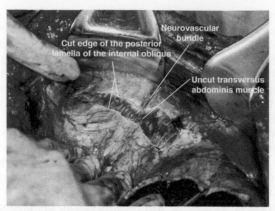

Fig. 14. Incised posterior lamella of the internal oblique evidencing underlying transversus abdominis muscle fibers. (*From* Rosen MJ. Posterior component separation with transversus abdominis muscle release. In: Atlas of abdominal wall reconstruction. 2nd edition. Elsevier; 2017. p. 95; with permission.)

tendon. Dissection of the retroxiphoid space on a preperitoneal level allows extending the mesh well above the costal margins and ensuring wide mesh overlap for hernias of the upper abdomen that extend on to the thoracoabdominal transition (**Fig. 17**).

10. The same dissection is performed on the contralateral side.
11. The posterior sheath is now reapproximated on midline with running, 2-0 absorbable suture recreating the visceral sac. If any accidental holes were made in the peritoneum during dissection, they should be sutured with absorbable sutures to ensure that the mesh will not be exposed to the bowel, and to avoid the herniation of loops through these defects, causing bowel obstruction in the postoperative period. In the rare instances where the posterior sheath cannot be closed, either omentum or an absorbable synthetic mesh can be used to bridge this gap and exclude the intraabdominal contents from the synthetic material that will be placed on top of it.

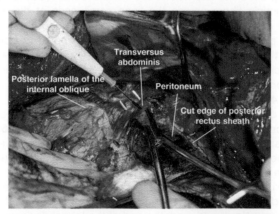

Fig. 15. Division of the transversus abdominis muscle fibers. (*From* Rosen MJ. Posterior component separation with transversus abdominis muscle release. In: Atlas of abdominal wall reconstruction. 2nd edition. Elsevier; 2017. p. 97; with permission.)

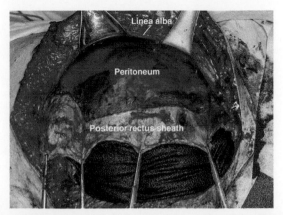

Fig. 16. Final aspect of lateral dissection all the way down to the retroperitoneum. (*From* Rosen MJ. Posterior component separation with transversus abdominis muscle release. In: Atlas of abdominal wall reconstruction. 2nd edition. Elsevier; 2017. p. 99; with permission.)

12. Similar to what was discussed for the Rives-Stoppa repair, a standard piece of macroporous medium-weight polypropylene is usually adequate for the majority of the cases. In massive hernias with loss of domain, we tend to prefer a heavy-weight polypropylene mesh, although there is to date no evidence suggesting the superiority of such material with respect to recurrence or pain.

13. The mesh is placed in sublay position in a diamond configuration, occupying all the retromuscular, preperitoneal, and retroperitoneal spaces. The inferior aspect of the mesh is secured to both of Cooper's ligaments and the pubis with interrupted sutures of no. 1 slowly absorbable material. Superiorly, the mesh is secured with 2 interrupted sutures around the xiphoid and on each costal margin. The lateral aspects are fixed circumferentially with full-thickness transfascial sutures with the aid of a suture passer (**Fig. 18**).

14. Two large closed suction drains are placed above the mesh. After that, the anterior fascia can be reapproximated in the midline with running or figure-of-8 no.1 slowly absorbable sutures.

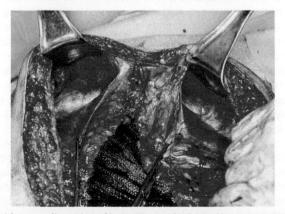

Fig. 17. Subxiphoid space dissection. (*From* Rosen MJ. Posterior component separation with transversus abdominis muscle release. In: Atlas of abdominal wall reconstruction. 2nd edition. Elsevier; 2017. p. 93; with permission.)

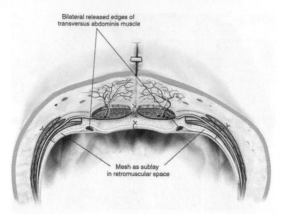

Fig. 18. Mesh placed in sublay position covering retromuscular space and the preperitoneal and retroperitoneal spaces of the lateral abdominal wall. (*From* Rosen MJ. Posterior component separation with transversus abdominis muscle release. In: Atlas of abdominal wall reconstruction. 2nd edition. Elsevier; 2017. p. 103; with permission.)

15. Upon closing the anterior fascia, reapproximate the subcutaneous tissue and skin with subcuticular absorbable sutures. Nylon vertical mattress sutures are preferred when there is tension on the skin.

Immediate Postoperative Care

- Pain management: We have gradually abandoned the use of epidurals for analgesia on ventral hernia repair after a recent analysis of the Americas Hernia Society Quality Collaborative showed that patients receiving epidurals experienced lengthier hospital durations of stay and higher pain scores when compared with patients who did not receive epidurals.[54] Those findings were concordant with clinical observations from our group, noting unpredictable pain control with epidurals. As of late, we have developed an enhanced recovery after surgery pathway for ventral hernia repair at our institution, for which a multimodal approach for pain management is a pivotal component. Instead of epidurals, we now perform transversus abdominis plane blocks with long-lasting bupivacaine. This step is performed intraoperatively under direct visualization by the surgeon on 5 levels (T7 through T11). Additionally, with the objective of decreasing opioid use, all patients receive different classes of pain medications postoperatively. Nevertheless, because significant pain can be expected after an open retromuscular hernia repair, all patients receive a patient-controlled analgesia device to ensure adequate pain control during the entire duration of their hospital stay. The role of this approach is under current study in our institution.
- Antibiotics are discontinued 24 hours postoperatively
- Sequential compression devices are maintained during the entire hospital stay and daily doses of low-molecular-weight heparin are prescribed.
- Dietary: Early feeding is encouraged when possible. Usually, a liquid diet is introduced on postoperative day 1 and progressed according to patient tolerance. It should be noted that ileus frequently complicates the postoperative period of such patients and surgeons should remain vigilant.
- Drains remain in place until output is less than 40 mL/d. If output remains high on the day of hospital discharge, they are kept in place and patients are educated on

how to manage drains at home. Patients are instructed to record daily drain output and an earlier postoperative visit is scheduled.

Other Important Considerations

It should be noted that TAR is a challenging operation and a thorough knowledge of the anatomy of the abdominal wall is mandatory to adequately perform this procedure.[4,5,43] Occasionally, the normal anatomy of the abdominal wall is severely distorted by the hernia itself, prior meshes, exuberant scar tissue, and a multitude of other factors that might complicate the intraoperative recognition of the correct anatomic planes. Therefore, before embarking on the "TAR world," surgeons should be aware that mastering TAR takes time, effort, and adequate mentoring. Deep immersion into a surgical atlas, demonstrative videos, scrubbed-in observations of the technique being performed by experts, and hands-on cadaver laboratory practices are useful to construct a solid base, but often those are not enough. To provide a safe and durable repair for patients, we do recommend that surgeons have an experienced proctor in the surgical field for the first cases.

Second, although TAR and the other abdominal wall reconstructive techniques are useful components of the surgical armamentarium for hernia repair, patient selection and identifying those patients who will benefit from such technique is extremely important because (1) not all hernias will need a TAR to be adequately repaired, (2) not all patients need their fascia closed to experience the benefits of hernia repair, and (3) not all surgeons need to be able to offer complex abdominal wall reconstructions. We base these statements on several factors: patients who will likely benefit from abdominal wall reconstruction are those with large and complex defects leading to significant impairment in abdominal wall function and patient quality of life. Patients with smaller hernias do not seem to experience significant impairment in abdominal wall function, with repair having the principal objective of decreasing pain, cosmetic discomfort, and the risk of incarceration/strangulation. In addition, as the available data on defect closure during laparoscopic ventral hernia repairs can illustrate, fascial closure for such smaller defects does not necessarily result in better short-term (wound complications)[55] or long-term (recurrence)[56] outcomes. Overall, data quality about this subject are poor[57] and, with conflicting results, fail to show definitive benefit with defect closure during laparoscopic ventral hernia repair. Although fascial closure logically is desired, bringing the rectus muscles back together should not be the only variable a surgeon considers when deciding that a patient is not a candidate for laparoscopic approach or a Rives-Stoppa retromuscular repair and should undergo a TAR. Functional status, level of activity before the hernia and quality-of-life metrics are important factors that should be considered and discussed with the patient in a shared decision-making process. The idea that routinely closing the fascia might lead to better functional outcomes increasingly influences surgeons to use complex reconstructive techniques to repair hernias that could be repaired through a laparoscopic intraabdominal peritoneal onlay mesh repair or standard retromuscular repair. Last, because surgeon expertise for a determined technique and local resource availability are major factors that influence patient outcomes, it is important for the surgeon to critically appraise the limitations of the center where they are integrated before offering elective repair for the most complex cases.

Mesh Selection

There are different aspects a surgeon must consider when deciding which mesh to use. The type of repair, planned mesh position, wound class, and patient factors can all impact a surgeon's decision. Meshes have different properties that can influence their success in each individual case. A good mesh, theoretically, should be both elastic and durable, and be able to incorporate well into the tissue without causing significant adhesions or infections. Currently, the choice lies between permanent synthetic mesh, biologic mesh, and, most recently, biosynthetic mesh.

For most ventral hernia repairs in clean cases, placing a macroporous medium-weight synthetic mesh in sublay position yields good results in terms of recurrence and wound morbidity. For other wound classes, there has still been no consensus on the ideal mesh.

SUMMARY

Retromuscular approaches are an important component of the surgical armamentarium for incisional hernia repair. Hernia surgery is constantly evolving. Patient characteristics, hernia variables, and surgical technique directly influence outcomes of hernia repair; therefore, a comprehensive preoperative evaluation is the foundation of a successful repair. A Rives-Stoppa repair is adequate for most of the moderate sized defects, providing a durable repair with low rates of wound complications. TAR can be the option for larger and more complex defects, reproducing good surgical results in experienced hands. In instances where there is a contraindication to extend dissection into the retroperitoneum, a periumbilical perforator–sparing component separation remains an acceptable option for the reconstructive surgeon.

REFERENCES

1. Carbonell AM. Rives-Stoppa retromuscular repair. In: Novitsky YW, editor. Hernia surgery: current principles. Switzerland: Springer; 2016.
2. Ramirez OM, Ruas E, Dellon AL. "Components separation" method for closure of abdominal wall defects: method for closure of abdominal wall defects: an anatomic and clinical study. Plast Reconstr Surg 1990;86(3):519–26.
3. Petersen S, Henke G, Zimmerman L, et al. Ventral rectus fascia closure on top of mesh hernia repair in the sublay technique. Plast Reconstr Surg 2004;114(7): 1754–60.
4. Rosen MJ. Posterior component separation with transversus abdominis muscle release. In: Rosen MJ, editor. Atlas of abdominal wall reconstruction. 2nd edition. Philadelphia: Elsevier; 2017. p. 82–109.
5. Pauli EM, Rosen MJ. Open ventral hernia repair with component separation. Surg Clin North Am 2013;93:1111–33.
6. Rogmark P, Smedberg S, Montgomery A. Long-term follow-up of retromuscular incisional hernia repairs: recurrence and quality of life. World J Surg 2017. https://doi.org/10.1007/s00268-017-4268-0.
7. Israelsson LA, Smedberg S, Montgomery A, et al. Incisional hernia repair in Sweden 2002. Hernia 2006;10(3):258–61.
8. Maman D, Greenwald D, Kreniske J, et al. Modified Rives-Stoppa technique for repair of complex incisional hernias in 59 patients. Ann Plast Surg 2012;68(2): 190–3.
9. Helgstrand F, Rosenberg J, Kehlet H, et al. Nationwide prospective study of outcomes after elective incisional hernia repair. J Am Coll Surg 2013;216(2):217–28.
10. Iqbal CW, Pham TH, Joseph A, et al. Long-term outcome of 254 complex incisional hernia repairs using the modified Rives-Stoppa technique. World J Surg 2007;31(12):2398–404.
11. McLanahan D, King LT, Weems C, et al. Retrorectus prosthetic mesh repair of midline abdominal hernia. Am J Surg 1997;173(5):445–9.

12. Martin-Dulce A, Noguerales F, Villeta R, et al. Modifications to Rives technique for midline incisional hernia repair. Hernia 2001;5(2):70–2.
13. Flament JB, Palot JB, Lubrano D, et al. Retromuscular prosthetic repair: experience from France. Chirurg 2002;73(10):1053–8.
14. Ferranti F, Triveri P, Mancini P, et al. The treatment of large midline incisional hernias using a retromuscular prosthetic mesh (Stoppa-Rives technique). Chir Ital 2003;55(1):129–36.
15. Novitsky YW, Porter JR, Rucho ZC, et al. Open preperitoneal retrofascial mesh repair for multiply recurrent ventral incisional hernias. J Am Coll Surg 2006;203(3):283–9.
16. Fischer JP, Vasta MN, Mirzabeigi MN, et al. A comparison of outcomes and cost in VHWG grande II hernia between Rives-Stoppa synthetic mesh hernia repair versus underlay biologic mesh repair. Hernia 2014;18(6):781–9.
17. Heller L, McNichols CH, Ramirez OM. Component separations. Semin Plast Surg 2012;26:25–8.
18. Thompson P, Losken A. Open anterior component separation. In: Novitsky YW, editor. Hernia Surgery: Current Principles. Switzerland: Springer; 2016.
19. Girotto JA, Ko MJ, Muehlberger T, et al. Closure of chronic abdominal wall defects: a long-term evaluation of the components separation method. Ann Plast Surg 1999;42(4):385–94 [discussion: 394–5].
20. De Vries Reilingh TS, van Goor H, Rosman C, et al. "Components separation technique" for the repair of large abdominal wall hernias. J Am Coll Surg 2003; 196(1):32–7.
21. De Vries Reilingh TS, van Goor H, Carbon JA, et al. Repair of giant midline abdominal wall hernias: "components separation technique" versus prosthetic repair. World J Surg 2007;31:756–63.
22. Jernigan TQ, Fabian TC, Croce MA, et al. Staged management of giant abdominal wall defects: acute and long-term results. Ann Surg 2003;238(3):349–55.
23. Lowe JB 3rd, Lowe JB, Baty JD, et al. Risks associated with "components separation" for closure of complex abdominal wall defects. Plast Reconstr Surg 2003; 111(3):1276–83.
24. Clarke JM. Incisional hernia repair by fascial component separation: results in 128 cases and evolution of the technique. Am J Surg 2010;200:2–8.
25. Sukkar SM, Dumanian GA, Szczerba SM, et al. Challenging abdominal wall defects. Am J Surg 2001;181(2):115–21.
26. Saulis AS, Dumanian GA. Periumbilical rectus abdominis perforator preservation significantly reduces superficial wound complications in "separation of parts" hernia repairs. Plast Reconstr Surg 2002;109(7):2275–80.
27. Dumanian GA. Periumbilical perforator sparing component separation. In: Rosen MJ, editor. Atlas of abdominal wall reconstruction. 2nd edition. Philadelphia: Elsevier; 2017. p. 166–80.
28. Girotto JA, Chiaramonte M, Menong NG, et al. Recalcitrant abdominal wall hernias: long-term superiority of autologous tissue repair. Plast Reconstr Surg 2003;112:106–14.
29. Gonzalez R, Rehnke RD, Ramaswamy A, et al. Components separation technique and laparoscopic approach: a comparison of two evolving strategies for ventral hernia repair. Am Surg 2005;71(7):598–605.
30. Espinosa-de-los-Monteros A, de la Torre JI, Marerro I, et al. Utilization of human cadaveric acellular dermis for abdominal hernia reconstruction. Ann Plast Surg 2007;58:264–7.
31. DiBello JN Jr, Moore JH Jr. Sliding myofascial flap of the rectus abdominis muscles for the closure of recurrent ventral hernias. Plast Reconstr Surg 1996;98(3):464–9.

32. Diaz JJ Jr, Conquest AM, Ferzoco SJ, et al. Multi-institutional experience using human acellular dermal matrix for ventral hernia repair in a compromised surgical field. Arch Surg 2009;114:209–15.
33. Garvey PB, Giordano SA, Baumann DP, et al. Long-term outcomes after abdominal wall reconstruction with acellular dermal matrix. J Am Coll Surg 2016;224(3): 341–50.
34. Sailes FC, Walls J, Guelig D, et al. Synthetic and biological mesh in component separation: a 10-year single institution review. Ann Plast Surg 2010;64(5): 696–8.
35. Cornette B, De Bacquer D, Berrevoet F. Component separation technique for giant incisional hernia: a systematic review. Am J Surg 2017. https://doi.org/10. 1016/j.amjsurg.2017.07.032.
36. Butler CE, Campbell KT. Minimally invasive component separation with inlay bioprosthetic mesh (MICSIB) for complex abdominal wall reconstruction. Plast Reconstr Surg 2011;128(3):698–709.
37. Patel KM, Nahabedian MY, Gati M, et al. Indications and outcomes following complex abdominal wall reconstruction with component separation combined with porcine acellular dermal matrix reinforcement. Ann Plast Surg 2012;69(4): 394–8.
38. Ghali S, Turza KC, Baumann DP, et al. Minimally invasive component separation results in fewer wound healing complications than open component separation for large ventral hernia repair. J Am Coll Surg 2012;214(6):981–9.
39. Novitsky YW, Elliott HL, Orenstein SB, et al. Transversus abdominis muscle release: a novel approach to posterior component separation during abdominal wall reconstruction. Am J Surg 2012;204(5):709–16.
40. Krpata DM, Blatnick JA, Novitsky YW, et al. Posterior and open anterior components separation: a comparative analysis. Am J Surg 2012;203(2):318–22.
41. Petro CC, Como JJ, Yee S, et al. Posterior component separation and transversus abdominis muscle release for complex incisional hernia repair in patients with an history of open abdomen. J Trauma Acute Care Surg 2015;78(2):422–9.
42. Petro CC, Orenstein SB, Criss CN, et al. Transversus abdominis muscle release for repair of complex incisional hernias in kidney transplant patients. Am J Surg 2015;210:334–9.
43. Winder JS, Behar BJ, Juza RM, et al. Transversus abdominis release for abdominal wall reconstruction: early experience with a novel technique. J Am Coll Surg 2016;223(2):271–8.
44. Raigani S, Criss CN, Petro CC, et al. Single-center experience with parastomal hernia repair using retromuscular mesh placement. J Gastrointest Surg 2014; 18(9):1673–7.
45. Pauli EM, Wang J, Petro CC, et al. Posterior component separation with transversus abdominis release successfully addresses recurrent ventral hernias following anterior component separation. Hernia 2016;19(2):285–91.
46. Fayezizadeh M, Majumder A, Belyansky I, et al. Outcomes of retromuscular porcine biologic mesh repairs using transversus abdominis release reconstruction. J Am Coll Surg 2016;223(3):461–8.
47. Novitsky YW, Fayezizadeh M, Majumder A, et al. Outcomes of posterior component separation with transversus abdominis muscle release and synthetic mesh sublay reinforcement. Ann Surg 2016;264(2):226–32.
48. Tastaldi L, Haskins IN, Perez AJ, et al. Single-center experience with the modified retromuscular Sugarbaker technique for parastomal hernia repair. Hernia 2017; 21(6):941–9.

49. Halka JT, Vasyluk A, DeMare AM, et al. Robotic and hybrid robotic transversus abdominis release may be performed with low length of stay and wound morbidity. Am J Surg 2017. https://doi.org/10.1016/j.amjsurg.2017.10.053.
50. Carbonell AM, Warren JA, Prabhu AS, et al. reducing length of stay using a robotic-assisted approach for retromuscular ventral hernia repair: a comparative analysis from the Americas Hernia Society Quality Collaborative. Am J Surg 2018; 267(2):210-7.
51. Bittner JG 4th, Alrefai S, Vy M, et al. Comparative analysis of open and robotic transversus abdominis release for ventral hernia repair. Surg Endosc 2018; 32(2):727-34.
52. Martin-del-Campo LA, Weltz AS, Belyansky I, et al. Comparative analysis of perioperative outcomes of robotic versus open transversus abdominis release for ventral hernia repair. Surg Endosc 2018;32(2):840-5.
53. Amaral MVFD, Guimaraes JR, Volpe P, et al. Robotic transversus abdominis release (TAR): is it possible to offer minimally invasive surgery for abdominal wall complex defects? Rev Col Bras Cir 2017;44(2):216-9.
54. Prabhu AS, Krpata DM, Perez A, et al. Is it time to reconsider postoperative epidural analgesia in patients undergoing elective ventral hernia repair? An AHSQC analysis. Ann Surg 2017. https://doi.org/10.1097/SLA.0000000000002214.
55. Papageorge CM, Funk LM, Poulose BK, et al. Primary fascial closure during laparoscopic ventral hernia repair does not reduce 30-day wound complications. Surg Endosc 2017;31(11):4551-7.
56. Wennergren JE, Askenasy EP, Greenberg JA, et al. Laparoscopic ventral hernia repair with primary fascial closure versus bridged repair: a risk-adjusted comparative study. Surg Endosc 2016;30(8):3231-8.
57. Nguyen DH, Nguyen MT, Askenasy EP, et al. Primary fascial closure with laparoscopic ventral hernia repair: systematic review. World J Surg 2014;38(12): 3097-104.

Incisional Hernia Repair
Minimally Invasive Approaches

Jeremy A. Warren, MD[a,b,*], Michael Love, MD[c]

KEYWORDS

- Minimally invasive hernia repair • Laparoscopic hernia repair • Robotic hernia repair
- Robotic retromuscular hernia repair • Robotic transversus abdominis release

KEY POINTS

- Minimally invasive repair of ventral incisional hernias decreases the risk of wound morbidity compared with open hernia repair.
- Controversy in various technical aspects of laparoscopic hernia repair, particularly mesh selection, fixation technique, and defect closure, are discussed in detail.
- Placement of mesh in the peritoneal cavity does carry a small but significant long-term risk of complications, particularly in the event of subsequent abdominal operations.
- Robotic ventral hernia repair is rapidly disseminating, with the potential benefits of reliable hernia defect closure and decreased pain associated with mesh fixation.
- Advanced robotic and laparoscopic techniques allow complete abdominal wall reconstruction through rectus abdominis and transversus abdominis myofascial release and extraperitoneal mesh placement.

INTRODUCTION

Minimally invasive surgery has revolutionized surgical treatment of disease for a variety of pathologic conditions. Shortened hospitalizations, less pain, decreased recovery time, faster return to work or activity, improved cosmesis, and reduction in wound morbidity are clear advantages of laparoscopic surgery. Laparoscopic incisional ventral hernia repair (VHR) was first described by LeBlanc and Booth.[1] Using

---

Disclosure Statement: Dr J.A. Warren receives honoraria for education, consulting, and speaking from Maquet Surgical and Intuitive Surgical. Dr M. Love has no disclosures.
[a] Division of Minimal Access, Department of Surgery, Greenville Health System, University of South Carolina School of Medicine Greenville, 701 Grove Road, Suite 3, Greenville, SC 29605, USA; [b] Division of Bariatric Surgery, Department of Surgery, Greenville Health System, University of South Carolina School of Medicine Greenville, 701 Grove Road, Suite 3, Greenville, SC 29605, USA; [c] Department of Surgery, Greenville Health System, 701 Grove Road, Suite 3, Greenville, SC 29605, USA
* Corresponding author. Division of Minimal Access, Department of Surgery, Greenville Health System, University of South Carolina School of Medicine Greenville, 701 Grove Road, Suite 3, Greenville, SC 29605.
E-mail address: jwarrenmd@ghs.org

Surg Clin N Am 98 (2018) 537–559
https://doi.org/10.1016/j.suc.2018.01.008
0039-6109/18/© 2018 Elsevier Inc. All rights reserved.

intraperitoneal placement of expanded polytetrafluoroethylene (ePTFE) mesh, secured to the abdominal wall and bridging the hernia defect, they demonstrated the safety and feasibility of laparoscopic VHR (LVHR). As this approach disseminated, the reduction in wound morbidity compared with open VHR (OVHR) became clear. However, not all patients are candidates for this approach owing to comorbid conditions and hernia morphology. Potential long-term complications related to intraperitoneal mesh placement and bridging of hernia defects has also limited its application in some cases. Additionally, long-term follow-up has revealed recurrence rates to be similar to OVHR.

Modifications in technique, such as defect closure and extraperitoneal mesh placement, along with technological advances in mesh and fixation constructs, have sought to address the weaknesses of LVHR. Most recently, robotic VHR (RVHR) has gained immense popularity. Despite these advances, there remains a lack of consensus regarding the optimal approach for hernia repair. This article provides a summary of reported outcomes of both LVHR and RVHR. Various aspects of technique are reviewed in detail. Finally, the article looks ahead to the future possibilities of minimally invasive hernia repair.

TECHNICAL OVERVIEW OF LAPAROSCOPIC VENTRAL HERNIA REPAIR

Some variation in technique exists for LVHR. The choice of mesh, the method of fixation, the decision to close the hernia defect under tension or maintain a tension-free repair, and the position of the mesh remain somewhat controversial (see later discussion). However, several universal principles apply to LVHR[2]:

1. Patient positioned supine, arms tucked at the side (**Fig. 1**A)
   - This may vary for nonmidline or atypical hernias
2. Safe peritoneal entry
   - The authors prefer optical trocar entry along the right costal margin
   - Veress needle or open Hasson technique along either costal margin is also appropriate
3. Trocar placement
   - Peripherally away from the defect, separated and positioned to allow triangulation of the camera and working instruments (**Fig. 1**B)
   - The authors recommend at least 3 trocars, with at least 1 contralateral for ease of tack fixation
   - A 30° or 45° laparoscope improves visualization of the abdominal wall
4. Adhesiolysis
   - Should be performed sharply or bluntly
   - Minimize cautery to decrease potential thermal injury to bowel
   - All herniated contents should be reduced and the abdominal wall must be cleared to allow adequate mesh overlap
   - Extensive adhesiolysis beyond what is necessary for reduction and mesh placement increases the risk of enterotomy and should be avoided
   - Falciform ligament and/or supravesical fat should be taken down to allow mesh overlap (**Fig. 2**), extending to the space of Retzius to expose Cooper's ligaments if needed[3]
5. Defect measurement
   - Accurate measurement necessary to determine appropriate mesh size
   - The authors recommend intracorporeal measurement, which negates the thickness of the abdominal wall, minimizes the effect of pneumoperitoneum, and centers the mesh over the defect (**Fig. 3**)

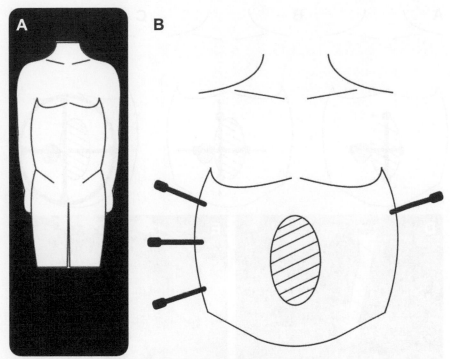

Fig. 1. Setup. (*A*) Patient positioned supine with arms tucked at the side. (*B*) Trocars placed laterally, away from the hernia defect. Triangulate camera and working trocars. Recommend at least 1 contralateral trocar for tacking purposes.

6. Mesh selection
   • A barrier-coated mesh should be used for intraperitoneal placement to minimize the risk of adhesions (see later discussion)
7. Mesh size and overlap
   • Mesh should overlap the hernia defect onto the abdominal wall a minimum of 5 cm in every direction (see later discussion)
8. Mesh fixation (**Fig. 4**)

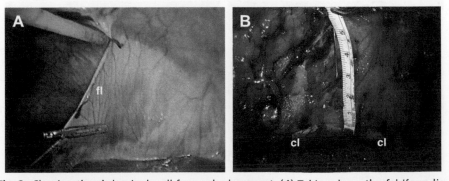

Fig. 2. Clearing the abdominal wall for mesh placement. (*A*) Taking down the falciform ligament (fl) for mesh placement in the upper abdomen. (*B*) Space of Retzius, with Coopers ligaments (cl) exposed for mesh fixation.

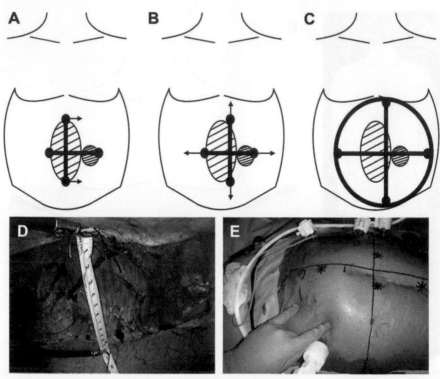

Fig. 3. Measuring and sizing mesh. (*A*) Spinal needles (*black dots*) are placed at the superior, inferior, and lateral-most (*arrows*) extent of the hernia defects. (*B*) Needles are moved (*arrows*) to the midpoint of the horizontal and vertical lines, connecting them to find the center of the defects. (*C*) Needles are moved 5 cm outward, corresponding to the size of the mesh needed for placement. (*D*) Metric ruler used to measure distance between spinal needles intracorporeally. (*E*) Grid is drawn on the abdominal wall, marking the borders of the hernia defect, the center of the defects, and the periphery of the mesh.

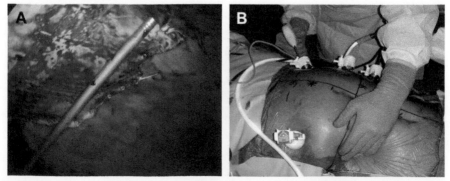

Fig. 4. Mesh fixation. (*A*) Permanent tack fixation circumferentially at the periphery of the mesh. (*B*) External counterpressure ensures adequate penetration through the mesh into the abdominal wall.

- Fixation of intraperitoneal mesh is mandatory
- The authors recommend permanent fixation with 2 to 4 transfascial sutures and double-crown of tacks
- Significant debate exists regarding fixation (see later discussion).

MESH SELECTION

A rapid proliferation of new barrier-coated meshes and fixation constructs followed the advent of LVHR (**Fig. 5**). Despite the breadth of options, there is a dearth of high-level evidence to guide mesh selection, leaving this mainly to the judgment of the surgeon. Although biologic and absorbable synthetic materials have been used for LVHR, evidence is lacking to recommend their routine use.[4–6] Three materials form the backbone of permanent synthetic mesh: polypropylene, polyester, and expanded ePTFE. Polypropylene and polyester within the peritoneal cavity are adhesiogenic, and various antiadhesive barriers have been used to limit visceral adhesions. Permanent barrier materials include silicone and ePTFE. A variety of absorbable barriers provide protection against adhesions (see **Fig. 5**). No material is entirely resistant to adhesions, although ePTFE and omega 3 fatty acids have been shown to have the lowest area and least tenacious adhesions in both animal models and clinical studies[7–10] (see later discussion).

MESH OVERLAP

Appropriate mesh size is critically important to successful LVHR. Current guidelines recommend at least 3 to 4 cm mesh overlap (grade B recommendation), although greater than 5 cm overlap, particularly for larger defects without transfascial fixation, may be preferred (grade C recommendation).[2] A recent meta-analysis of almost 9000

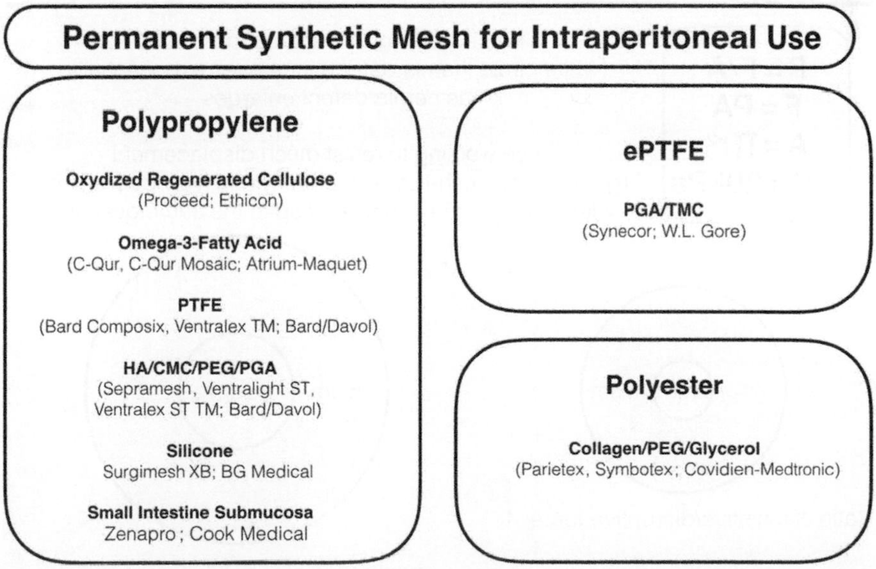

Permanent Synthetic Mesh for Intraperitoneal Use

Polypropylene

Oxydized Regenerated Cellulose
(Proceed; Ethicon)

Omega-3-Fatty Acid
(C-Qur, C-Qur Mosaic; Atrium-Maquet)

PTFE
(Bard Composix, Ventralex TM; Bard/Davol)

HA/CMC/PEG/PGA
(Sepramesh, Ventralight ST,
Ventralex ST TM; Bard/Davol)

Silicone
Surgimesh XB; BG Medical

Small Intestine Submucosa
Zenapro ; Cook Medical

ePTFE

PGA/TMC
(Synecor; W.L. Gore)

Polyester

Collagen/PEG/Glycerol
(Parietex, Symbotex; Covidien-Medtronic)

Fig. 5. Permanent synthetic, barrier-coated mesh options for intraperitoneal use. CMC, carboxymethylcellulose; HA, hyaluronic acid; PEG, polyethylene glycol; PGA, polyglycolic acid; TMC, trimethyl carbonate.

LVHR subjects demonstrated a reduction in hernia recurrence from 8.6% to 1.4% using a 5 cm overlap compared with less than 3 cm overlap.[11] The choice of mesh fixation also affects mesh overlap, with transfascial suture fixation improving recurrence rates with smaller overlap, and greater overlap required with tack fixation alone.[2,12–14]

Applying a simple standard length of overlap to all hernias, however, likely fails to address the underlying etiologic factors of hernia recurrence after LVHR. Intraabdominal pressure creates a constant force against the mesh, which is unopposed centrally when the hernia defect is bridged. Force is proportional to the area over which the force is applied, thus the larger the hernia defect, the greater the displacing force. Mesh overlap, tissue ingrowth of the mesh into the abdominal wall, and mesh fixation all work to resist this displacing force.[15] Consequently, mesh size should increase in proportion to the hernia defect size rather than at a set distance overlap (**Fig. 6**). A recent clinical evaluation of 213 LVHRs demonstrated that a mesh/defect area ratio (M/D) less than or equal to 12 was an independent risk factor for recurrence; an M/D of less than or equal to 8 resulted in 70% recurrence. Practically, this requires a significantly larger diameter mesh as hernia defect size increases, with a 5 cm hernia defect requiring at least an 18 cm diameter mesh (6.5 cm overlap in all directions) and an 8 cm defect requiring at least a 29 cm mesh (10.5 cm overlap).[16] The impact of defect closure on mesh overlap is not known.

DEFECT CLOSURE

The concept of a tension-free repair is a guiding principle in hernia repair. Standard LVHR accomplishes this by bridging the hernia defect with mesh. However, many surgeons now advocate routine closure of the hernia defect along with LVHR (**Fig. 7**).

Physics of Hernia Repair

$$P = F/A$$
$$F = PA$$
$$A = \Pi r^2$$
$$IAP = 20kPa$$

Force working to displace the mesh (white circle; hernia defect) increases exponentially as hernia defect enlarges

Force working to resist mesh displacement (gray circle; mesh-tissue interface) relatively decreases with increasing hernia size despite the same overlap

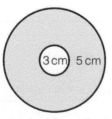

Ratio of resistive/disruptive force: 17

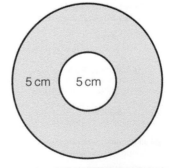

Ratio of resistive/disruptive force: 8

Fig. 6. Physics of laparoscopic hernia repair. A, area; F, force; IAP, intraabdominal pressure; kPa, kilopascal; P, pressure.

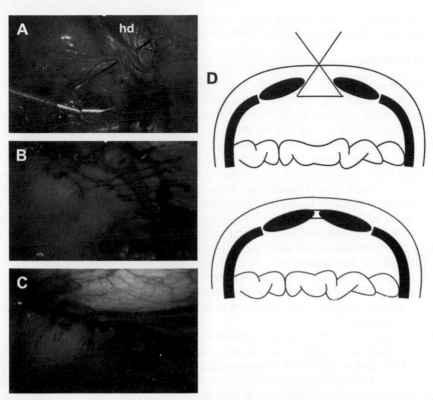

Fig. 7. Closure of the hernia defect (hd). (*A*) Suture passed through stab incisions in the abdominal wall in a figure-8 fashion. (*B*) Multiple sutures used for complete closure. (*C*) Pneumoperitoneum is decreased when tying sutures. (*D*) Transcutaneous defect closure.

Intuitively, this is appealing because it restores abdominal wall anatomy and augments repair rather than simply bridging the defect. Although evidence for this approach is still emerging, its popularity has grown rapidly and is a major factor driving the proliferation of RVHR. In a recent study of the Americas Hernia Society Quality Collaborative (AHSQC), defect closure was performed in 69% of LVHRs.[17] Several studies have demonstrated the benefit of defect closure. Franklin and colleagues[18] reported recurrence in 2.9% of subjects with a mean 47-month follow-up. Similarly, with a 78-month follow-up, Chelala and colleagues[19] reported 4.7% recurrence with routine closure of the fascial defect. Clapp and colleagues[20] noted a decrease in seroma from 27.8% to 5.6%, and a decrease in recurrence from 16.7% to 0% with 24-month follow-up. Meta-analysis of 16 LVHR trials evaluating the impact of defect closure demonstrated a significantly lower rate of adverse events (4.9 v 22.3%), including eventration and recurrence, when the defect was closed compared with bridging repair.[21]

The difficulty with this approach is the tension required for closure of larger defects. Orenstein and colleagues[22] used a so-called shoelacing technique for closure, using transfascial sutures placed 2 cm from the midline on each side of the closed hernia defect to offset the tension along the midline. No recurrences were noted in 47 subjects with a mean follow-up of 16 months. Chelala and colleagues[19] incised the anterior rectus fascia to facilitate closure in select cases. Endoscopic component separation (see later discussion) allows a greater degree of midline medialization.

Current guidelines recommend defect closure when possible, including adjunctive measures to offset tension (grade C recommendation).[2]

MESH FIXATION

Intraperitoneal placement requires mesh fixation to ensure appropriate positioning and prevent mesh migration within the abdominal cavity. The choice of fixation is widely debated, with no clear consensus among experts or in the literature. Transfascial sutures placed around the periphery of the mesh through the abdominal wall were long considered necessary. However, a recent meta-analysis failed to clearly demonstrate a difference in fixation techniques with regard to hernia recurrence,[13] although there was significant heterogeneity in technique and materials used in the studies reviewed. The International Endohernia Society guidelines recommend fixation with sutures or tacks; the recurrence rate does not seem to be related to the choice of fixation technique.[2] A prospective randomized controlled trial by Muysoms and colleagues[23] comparing double-crown permanent tack fixation to suture plus tack fixation, showed no difference in recurrence at 24 months. Additionally, the use of transfascial sutures may contribute to postoperative pain. In this study, double-crown fixation alone resulted in significantly decreased pain out to 3 months postoperatively. However, the affect of fixation construct on postoperative pain is variably reported, and current guidelines make no clear distinction between fixation constructs.[2,14]

Permanent fixation is generally recommended and should be spaced every 1 to 1.5 cm.[2] Purely absorbable fixation is associated with higher rates of recurrent hernia after LVHR[24] and no significant differences in postoperative or chronic pain have been shown.[2,24,25] Finally, biologic adhesives may be used for mesh fixation. Several small trials have demonstrated reduction in postoperative pain compared with permanent tack fixation. However, current data are limited to relatively small hernia defects with short-term follow-up.[2,26,27] Despite the lack of high-quality evidence, popular opinion seems to implicate transfascial suture fixation and permanent tack fixation as a significant cause of pain after LVHR. This is another contributing factor in the proliferation of RVHR: mesh can more easily be secured with circumferential sutures than with transfascial sutures or penetrating tacks.

INNOVATIONS IN TECHNIQUE

Several innovative modifications of standard LVHR have been described. These techniques primarily serve to facilitate defect closure and/or extraperitoneal mesh placement.

TRANSABDOMINAL PREPERITONEAL REPAIR

Transabdominal preperitoneal (TAPP) repair has long been used for inguinal hernia repair and is now being applied to VHR. The peritoneum is dissected free from the abdominal wall surrounding the hernia defect, creating a large pocket for mesh placement. After closure of the defect, mesh is placed against the abdominal wall, and the peritoneum closed over the mesh (**Fig. 8**). Reported outcomes for TAPP LVHR are comparable to standard LVHR, with lower cost associated with a preperitoneal approach.[28,29] Potential advantages of TAPP VHR include

- Decreased adhesions with peritoneal coverage of mesh
- Less mesh fixation required because mesh is confined within the layers of the abdominal wall and intraabdominal forces act to hold mesh in place

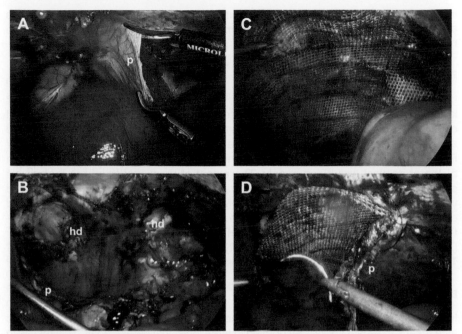

Fig. 8. Laparoscopic preperitoneal repair. (*A*) Incise the peritoneum (p) at least 5 cm from the hernia defect. (*B*) Peritoneal flap fully dissected, exposing the hernia defects. (*C*) Defects closed and mesh placed into preperitoneal space. (*D*) Peritoneal flap closed over the mesh.

- Less pain due to mesh fixation
- Lower mesh cost because more expensive barrier-coated mesh is unnecessary.

LAPAROSCOPIC RETROMUSCULAR REPAIR

As with TAPP LVHR, laparoscopic retromuscular repair excludes mesh from the abdominal cavity and provides the added benefit of myofascial release to offset tension on the midline defect closure. First described in 2002[30] using a totally extraperitoneal approach, 15 subjects were repaired with retromuscular placement of mesh but without closure of the hernia defect. One subject recurred with short (<6 months) follow-up. Schroeder and colleagues[31] reported laparoscopic retromuscular hernia repair in 43 subjects compared with 50 open retromuscular VHRs, with comparable outcomes and no recurrent hernias at 17-month follow-up. A variation on this approach was reported by Costa and colleagues[32] in 15 subjects. After gaining optical access to the peritoneum through a 5 mm trocar, the retromuscular space is entered below the umbilicus with trocars in a suprapubic position. Retromuscular dissection is completed on each, up to the level of the costal margin. A linear cutting stapler is then used to simultaneously plicate the posterior sheath, close the hernia defect, and create the common space across the midline for mesh reinforcement. No recurrences were reported with a mean follow-up of 17 months. Most recently, Belyansky and colleagues[33] reported a totally extraperitoneal retromuscular repair for VHR, commonly termed extended totally extraperitoneal. This added to the techniques previously described by fully closing the hernia defect and remaining entirely outside of the abdominal cavity, fully exploiting the myofascial release and retromuscular position in the manner of the Rives-Stoppa repair with the addition of laparoscopic transversus abdominis release (TAR) to allow greater mobilization of the midline fascia and wide mesh overlap.

ENDOSCOPIC COMPONENT SEPARATION

Initially described by Lowe and colleagues,[34] endoscopic component separation uses laparoscopic balloon dissection of the interparietal plane between the internal and external oblique musculature, followed by incision of the external oblique muscle and fascia. This effectively duplicates the musculofascial release as described by Ramirez and colleagues[35] but eliminates the subcutaneous dissection and disruption of the abdominal wall blood supply. The extent of medialization of the rectus was shown to be 86% of that achieved using traditional open technique.[36] This technique was initially used to augment open VHR, resulting in significantly decreased wound complications in multiple series.[37–39] More recently, endoscopic component separation has been combined with standard LVHR for a totally laparoscopic approach.[40,41] Despite encouraging results, the popularity of this technique has waned in favor of TAR and the desire for extraperitoneal mesh placement.

BOTULINUM TOXIN A

Injection of botulinum toxin A (BTA) into the oblique musculature has also been used as a means to regain abdominal domain in large incisional hernia repair. This results in decreased oblique thickness, increased oblique length, and decreased width of the hernia defect, allowing more reliable abdominal wall closure.[42–44] A new report used BTA injection before LVHR, achieving a totally laparoscopic closure in 41 subjects with a mean hernia width of 12 cm.[45] Head-to-head comparisons of BTA with other methods of abdominal closure, such as components separation, are currently lacking. There is also a paucity of long-term data regarding this technique for hernia repair. Further studies are necessary to delineate the indications and/or patient candidates for this procedure.

OUTCOMES OF LAPAROSCOPIC VENTRAL HERNIA REPAIR
Surgical Site and Prosthetic Mesh Infection

The preponderance of the literature demonstrates reduction in surgical site infection (SSI) as among the primary benefits of LVHR. Most studies report the rate of SSI at less than 3% (**Table 1**).[17–19,23,46–48] Trials comparing LVHR with OVHR show the rates of SSI significantly lower in most studies (**Table 2**).[49–52] A recent study of more than 25,000 subjects from the National Surgical Quality Improvement Project (NSQIP) showed that open repair conferred a 3-fold increased risk of SSI.[53]

Notably, interpretation of the hernia literature can be quite difficult due to the variation in reporting of wound complications and the disparity in surgical techniques used across studies. For example, Itani and colleagues[51] demonstrated a higher rate of wound infection with OVHR, resulting in early termination of the trial. However, this compared an open technique at arguably the highest risk for wound complications, an onlay repair, with laparoscopy. Although compelling, NSQIP data cannot discriminate among the various open techniques that may have been used, nor the litany of factors that may have required an open approach.[54] Hernia-specific data that can account for the granular details of surgical technique and track outcomes using a clearly defined set of criteria are necessary to truly determine the optimal hernia repair.

Table 1
Outcomes of laparoscopic ventral hernia repair (select studies)

Author, Year	Study Design	Number of Subjects	Follow-up (mo)	SSI (%)	Recurrence (%)
Toy et al,[86] 1998	P	144	7.3	3.0	4.0
Chowbey et al,[48] 2000	R	202	34	2.5	1.0
Berger et al,[3] 2002	R	150	15	0.0	2.7
Rosen et al,[47] 2003	R	100	30	5.3	17.0
Heniford et al,[46] 2003	R	850	20	1.8	4.7
Franklin et al,[18] 2004	R	384	47	1.1	2.9
Orenstein et al,[22] 2011	R	47	16.2	0.0	0.0
Muysoms et al,[23] 2013	PRCT	76	24	0.0	6.5
Clapp et al,[20] 2013	R	72	24	11.0	16.7
Liang et al,[63] 2013	R	122	24	16.4	14.7
Chelala et al,[19] 2016	R	1326	78	0.5	3.2
Picazo-Yeste et al,[87] 2017	P	124	30	2.6	2.6

Surgical Site Occurrences

Surgical site occurrences (SSOs) encompass any wound event, including SSI, although it is commonly used to denote wound complications that do not meet criteria for SSI. This includes seroma, hematoma, skin or fascial disruption, chronic wounds, skin necrosis, and cellulitis, among others. Seroma is the most common SSO following hernia repair and occurs in about 30% of cases, although it can be detected in virtually all patients with imaging.[17,19,55] Almost all resolve spontaneously. There is some evidence that closure of the fascial defect may decrease the seroma rate but this remains disputed in the literature.[17,19–21] A more appropriate measure is an SSO requiring procedural intervention, which more accurately captures the clinical significance of an SSO.

Recurrence, Pseudorecurrence, and Quality of Life

Recurrence rates after LVHR are similar to OVHR and range from 1% to 17% (see **Tables 1** and **2**). Risk is increased by a variety of modifiable and nonmodifiable factors, including obesity, smoking, number of prior repairs, wound complications, hernia size, and subsequent abdominal operations.[46,47,55] Hernias greater than 10 cm are more likely to recur after standard LVHR.[49] Recurrence may also occur due to inadequate mesh fixation,[13,24] inadequate mesh overlap,[2,11,55,56] or mesh failure[57,58]; or occur at tack or transfascial suture sites (**Fig. 9**).[59,60] The effect of defect closure requires greater long-term follow-up but initial results are encouraging.[19,21,22,61]

Aside from true hernia recurrence, eventration of mesh through the hernia defect following standard bridging LVHR can result in impaired quality of life from poor cosmesis and chronic pain. Sometimes termed pseudorecurrence, eventration occurs in as many as 20% of cases.[20,49,62] Patients who reported poor satisfaction are more likely to complain of eventration and less likely to have had the defect closed.[20,63] Eventration is more likely with bridging of larger hernia defects. Repeat repair is indicated in cases of significant symptoms.[55]

Table 2
Laparoscopic versus open ventral hernia repair (select studies)

Author, Year	Study Design	Number of Subjects	Open Technique	SSI (%)		Recurrence		Follow-up
				Open	Laparoscopic	Open	Laparoscopic	
Olmi et al,[50] 2007	PRCT	170	RM	7.1	1.1	1.1	2.3	24
Itani et al,[51] 2010	PRCT	146	Onlay	23.3	5.6	8.2	12.5	24
Kurmann et al,[49] 2011	P	125	RM	26.8	5.8	18.0	16.0	32.5
Colavita et al,[52] 2012	P	710	Mixed	3.2	0.3	6.0	5.2	12
Lee et al,[88] 2013	NIS	47,661	Varied	1.5	0.1	NR	NR	NR
Eker et al,[89] 2013	PRCT	194	RM	5	4.0	14.0	18.0	35
Kaoutzanis et al,[53] 2013	National Surgical Quality Improvement Project	26,766	Mixed	5.8	1.5	NR	NR	NR
Neupane et al,[90] 2017	R	263	Mixed	11.7	1.1	9.5	7.1	24

Abbreviations: NIS, National Inpatient Sample; NR, not reported; P, prospective; PRCT, Prospective Randomized Control Trial; R, retrospective; RM, retromuscular.

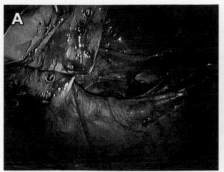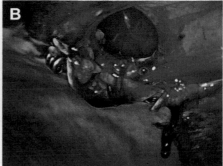

Fig. 9. Recurrence after LVHR. (*A*) Mesh migration due to inadequate fixation. (*B*) Transfascial suture site hernia.

Complications of Intraperitoneal Mesh

The position of mesh in the peritoneal cavity with standard LVHR is potentially problematic. Reoperative surgery, whether for recurrent hernia, complications of hernia repair, or a completely distinct intraabdominal pathologic condition, may be complicated by the presence of intraperitoneal prosthesis. As many as 25% of patients will require some subsequent abdominal operation following LVHR.[10,64,65] Adhesions to intraperitoneal mesh are present to some degree in most patients,[9,66] increasing the risk of visceral injury to between 4% and 21% during subsequent abdominal operation.[10,64,67,68] This should be considered for patients who may be at a higher risk of subsequent abdominal operations before proceeding with standard LVHR. Though rare, there is also a risk of spontaneous erosion of mesh into the viscera, creating an enteroprosthetic, enteroprosthetic-cutaneous, or vesicocutaneous fistula (**Fig. 10**).[69–73] Finally, although the rate of mesh infection is quite low, intraperitoneal mesh is typically not salvageable and requires complete removal when infected, particularly if ePTFE or multifilament mesh is involved (**Fig. 11**).[55]

ROBOTIC VENTRAL HERNIA REPAIR

Robotic-assisted surgery is the latest technological advance in minimally invasive surgery. This platform enhances visualization of the operative field with 10-times magnification and 3-dimensional imaging. The instruments articulate with a degree of freedom greater than the human wrist. Surgeon ergonomics are improved over many standard laparoscopic procedures. RVHR has grown exponentially, fueled by several factors, including surgeon preference, surgeon comfort, and dissatisfaction of various aspects of traditional OVHR and LVHR. In particular, acute and chronic pain is often associated with tack and transfascial suture fixation of mesh. The growing trend toward hernia defect closure makes robotic RVHR appealing because intracorporeal suturing is much less technically challenging robotically compared with laparoscopically, and anecdotally less painful than percutaneous closure. Additionally, the technological advantages of the robot enable fine preperitoneal dissection and myofascial release to more easily facilitate extraperitoneal mesh placement.

To date, there are limited data regarding RVHR. This was first described by Ballantyne and colleagues[74] using a standard IPOM (intraperitoneal onlay of mesh)

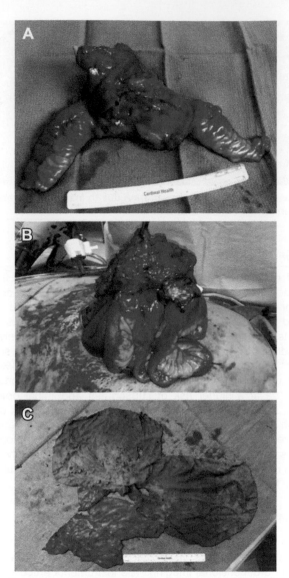

Fig. 10. Complications of intraperitoneal mesh. (*A*) Enteroprosthetic fistula: Specimen of mesh eroding into small bowel. (*B*) Multiple loops of small bowel densely adherent to intraperitoneal mesh. (*C*) Mesh explanted due to erosion into small bowel, colon, and vagina.

repair; however, this approach gained little traction until recent years. This is changing rapidly, with 7 publications in the last year alone.[75–81] A variety of techniques has been used, although most are a variation of standard laparoscopy with the addition of defect closure and intracorporeal suture fixation of the mesh. Kudsi and colleagues[82] reported 106 consecutive RVHRs with a variety of mesh types using this approach. Two subjects (1.8%) recurred at 6-month follow-up, with only 1 reported SSI and 1 seroma requiring drainage. In the largest series to date, 368 subjects were repaired robotically. Nearly 70% achieved fascial closure, with a 1.4% rate of SSI, 0.8% conversion rate, and only 1 recurrence.[81]

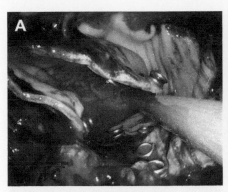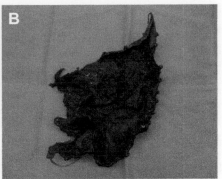

Fig. 11. Infected intraperitoneal mesh. (*A*) Laparoscopic view of infected ePTFE mesh. (*B*) Explanted mesh.

The feasibility of retromuscular mesh placement during RVHR was first demonstrated by Abdalla and colleagues.[83] This led directly to the authors' experience with this technique, which was first reported in 2015. Comparing our first 21 robotic cases to case-matched OVHR, the authors found a significant decrease in hospital LOS (4.2 vs 2.3 days; $P = .046$) and trend toward lower rate of SSI (0 vs 9.8%; $P = .488$) despite the longer operative times.[84] The authors subsequently compared our first 53 robotic retromuscular VHRs to standard LVHR, noting a shorter median length of stay (LOS) but a longer operative time and a greater number of simple seromas.[75] Analysis of 111 robotic repairs compared with a propensity-matched group of similar subjects undergoing open repair from the AHSQC demonstrated a significantly shorter median LOS (3 vs 2 days).[76] In 2 studies published this year, RVHR with TAR was compared with open TAR, both demonstrating shorter LOS after RVHR with TAR, with a trend toward lower rate of infection.[77,78]

The technique for robotic retromuscular VHR with TAR is demonstrated in **Fig. 12** and has also been reported in detail elsewhere.[85] Peritoneal access, trocar placement, and adhesiolysis follow similar principles to those previously outlined for LVHR. The case then progresses as follows:

- Retromuscular dissection begins by incising the posterior sheath just lateral to the linea alba at the level of the hernia defect.
- Blunt dissection separates the posterior sheath from rectus muscle, extending the dissection laterally to the semilunar line.
- Semilunar line is identified by
  - Identification of the intercostal neurovascular bundles that penetrate the lateral posterior sheath to innervate the rectus muscle
  - Visualizing the thicker fascial condensation just beyond the rectus muscle, which typically appears bright white
  - Downward retraction of the posterior sheath, revealing vertical stretch fibers along the linea semilunaris.
- Retromuscular dissection extends at least 5 cm above and below the defect.
- The peritoneum is incised transversely at superior and inferior borders of the hernia, and the preperitoneal space separated from the intact linea alba, leaving the peritoneum attached to the posterior sheath.
- The posterior sheath is divided above and below the defect after the preperitoneal space and retromuscular spaces are opened. This is the first step in creating

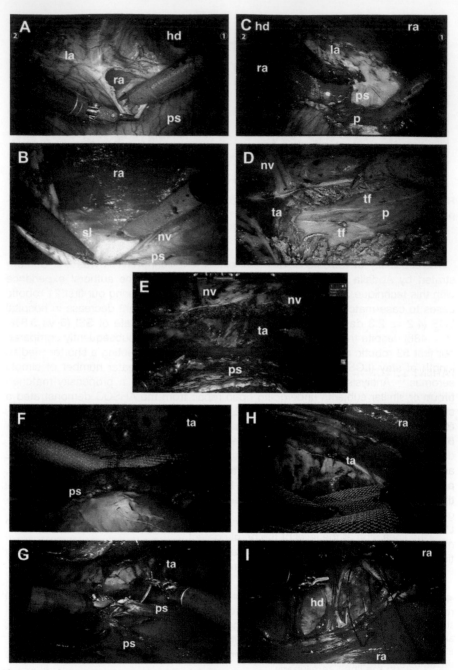

Fig. 12. Robotic retromuscular VHR. (*A*) Opening the retromuscular space by incising the posterior sheath just lateral to the linea alba. (*B*) Retromuscular space dissected laterally to the semilunar line. Intercostal neurovascular bundles are seen entering the lateral aspect of the rectus sheath to innervate the rectus muscle. (*C*) Midline dissection above or below the hernia defect. The peritoneum is taken down from the intact linea alba, leaving it attached to the posterior sheath. The incision of the posterior sheath continues to create a continuous space from the retromuscular space across the midline to the contralateral

a continuous space between the preperitoneal and retromuscular compartments for mesh overlap.

- TAR is initiated in upper portion of the rectus sheath by incising the posterior lamella of the internal oblique and dividing the transversus abdominis muscle to enter the preperitoneal or pretransversal space. Either plane is suitable for TAR.
- Preperitoneal dissection continues laterally until the posterior flap is lying flat across the viscera, at approximately the level of the midaxillary line.
- Three new trocars are placed into the dissected space in mirror image to the initially placed trocars.
- Hernia defect and dissected space are measured. Vertical space corresponds to length of the mesh needed. Width of mesh is estimated by placing a spinal needle through the far edge of the hernia defect, creating a right angle with the ruler lying flat across the peritoneal flap. This will be half the total mesh width needed.
- Mesh is cut to size, rolled, and fixated lateral to the newly placed trocars.
- The robot is redocked on the contralateral side and retromuscular dissection and TAR are completed, bringing the initially placed trocars into the preperitoneal space.
- The posterior sheath is closed with an absorbable, self-fixating suture.
- Mesh is retrieved and deployed across the closed posterior sheath, then fixated on the far side.
- The hernia defect is closed with an absorbable, self-fixating suture.

PATIENT SELECTION

Minimally invasive repair is particularly appealing for patients at higher risk for wound complications. Patients who are obese, have chronic obstructive pulmonary disease or diabetes, or who smoke particularly benefit from LVHR or RVHR. However, many other factors come in to play. Given the potential risk of intraperitoneal mesh, a standard IPOM approach may be less desirable for a patient at higher risk for subsequent abdominal operations, such as younger patients, or those with known gastrointestinal pathologic conditions. Because no gold-standard for VHR has been clearly identified, the surgeon is left to his or her best judgment in selecting the optimal hernia repair for a given patient. Surgeon experience is paramount. Any surgeon endeavoring to perform LVHR or RVHR must have adequate experience with complex minimally invasive techniques and intimate knowledge of abdominal wall anatomy. Absolute contraindications to minimally invasive surgery VHR include

---

retromuscular space above and below the hernia defect for mesh placement. (*D*) TAR is started by incising the posterior lamella of the internal oblique fascia and the transversus abdominis muscle. Two layers lie below the muscle: the transversalis fascia and peritoneum. Either the pretransversal or the preperitoneal planes are acceptable for TAR. (*E*) Completed retromuscular dissection and TAR. (*F*) Contralateral trocars are placed and the mesh is cut to size, rolled, and placed along the contralateral abdominal wall. (*G*) The posterior sheath is closed with a running, absorbable self-fixating suture. (*H*) Mesh is deployed across the closed posterior sheath and fixated to the lateral abdominal wall. (*I*) Hernia defect closed using running, absorbable self-fixating suture. Inclusion of bites of the hernia sac serves to imbricate the deadspace, potentially decreasing seroma formation. la, linea alba; nv, neurovascular bundle; ps, posterior sheath; ra, rectus abdominis; sl, semilunar line; ta, transversus abdominis; tf, transversalis fascia.

- Open abdominal wound
- Enterocutaneous fistula
- Prior abdominal wall skin graft after open abdomen
- Inability to tolerate general anesthesia.

Relative contraindications to minimally invasive surgery VHR include

- Multiple previous abdominal operations or a so-called hostile abdomen
- Acute incarceration or strangulation
- Larger (>10–15 cm) hernias
- Surgeon experience.

Potential benefits of robotic repair include

- Improved ability to close the defect, with or without added myofascial release
- Improved ability to place mesh in extraperitoneal position
- Preperitoneal or retromuscular mesh requires less fixation, potentially decreasing pain
- Shorter LOS.

SUMMARY

Minimally invasive VHR is a desirable approach for correction of abdominal wall defects. Wound morbidity is significantly decreased, with comparable recurrence rates compared with open surgery. Patient selection is critical because hernia morphology, patient comorbidities, skin integrity, and surgeon experience play important roles in outcomes. Undesirable long-term outcomes, including chronic pain, eventration following bridging repair, and potential complications with intraperitoneal mesh, cannot be ignored. Advances in technique and technology are being used to address these issues, with increasing focus on defect closure and alternative fixation techniques. In particular, the application of robotic surgery to hernia repair is disseminating rapidly. The ease of defect closure and ability to secure mesh intracorporeally without transfascial or tack fixation is appealing to many surgeons, although its true efficacy is yet to be rigorously studied. Robotic retromuscular repair with TAR is a promising procedure to address many of the complications of both open and laparoscopic repair. Wound complications are minimized, mesh is placed in an extraperitoneal position and requires minimal fixation, and complete restoration of abdominal wall anatomy and function is more easily achieved. Without question, minimally invasive surgery for VHR and abdominal wall reconstruction will continue to evolve in the pursuit of optimal patient outcomes in this common and complex disease.

REFERENCES

1. LeBlanc KA, Booth WV. Laparoscopic repair of incisional abdominal hernias using expanded polytetrafluoroethylene: preliminary findings. Surg Laparosc Endosc 1993;3(1):39–41.

2. Bittner R, Bingener-Casey J, Dietz U, et al. Guidelines for laparoscopic treatment of ventral and incisional abdominal wall hernias International Endohernia Society (IEHS)-part 1. Surg Endosc 2014;28(1):2–29.

3. Berger D, Bientzle M, Müller A. Postoperative complications after laparoscopic incisional hernia repair. Incidence and treatment. Surg Endosc 2002;16(12):1720–3.

4. Bellows CF, Smith A, Malsbury J, et al. Repair of incisional hernias with biological prosthesis: a systematic review of current evidence. Am J Surg 2013;205(1): 85–101.

5. Bittner R, Bingener-Casey J, Dietz U, et al. Guidelines for laparoscopic treatment of ventral and incisional abdominal wall hernias (International Endohernia Society [IEHS])-Part III. Surg Endosc 2014;28(2):380–404.

6. Catena F, Coccolini F, Ansaloni L, et al. Closure of the LAPSIS trial. Br J Surg 2010;97(10):1598.

7. Pierce RA, Perrone JM, Nimeri A, et al. 120-day comparative analysis of adhesion grade and quantity, mesh contraction, and tissue response to a novel omega-3 fatty acid bioabsorbable barrier macroporous mesh after intraperitoneal placement. Surg Innov 2009;16(1):46–54.

8. Deeken CR, Faucher KM, Matthews BD. A review of the composition, characteristics, and effectiveness of barrier mesh prostheses utilized for laparoscopic ventral hernia repair. Surg Endosc 2012;26(2):566–75.

9. Jenkins ED, Yom V, Melman L, et al. Prospective evaluation of adhesion characteristics to intraperitoneal mesh and adhesiolysis-related complications during laparoscopic re-exploration after prior ventral hernia repair. Surg Endosc 2010; 24(12):3002–7.

10. Snyder CW, Graham LA, Gray SH, et al. Effect of mesh type and position on subsequent abdominal operations after incisional hernia repair. J Am Coll Surg 2011; 212(4):496–502.

11. LeBlanc K. Proper mesh overlap is a key determinant in hernia recurrence following laparoscopic ventral and incisional hernia repair. Hernia 2016;20(1): 85–99.

12. Vorst AL, Kaoutzanis C, Carbonell AM, et al. Evolution and advances in laparoscopic ventral and incisional hernia repair. World J Gastrointest Surg 2015; 7(11):293–305.

13. LeBlanc KA. Laparoscopic incisional hernia repair: are transfascial sutures necessary? A review of the literature. Surg Endosc 2007;21(4):508–13.

14. Silecchia G, Campanile FC, Sanchez L, et al. Laparoscopic ventral/incisional hernia repair: updated Consensus Development Conference based guidelines. Surg Endosc 2015;29(9):2463–84.

15. Tulloh B, de Beaux A. Defects and donuts: the importance of the mesh:defect area ratio. Hernia 2017;20(6):893–5.

16. Hauters P, Desmet J, Gherardi D, et al. Assessment of predictive factors for recurrence in laparoscopic ventral hernia repair using a bridging technique. Surg Endosc 2017;38(5):2233–8.

17. Papageorge CM, Funk LM, Poulose BK, et al. Primary fascial closure during laparoscopic ventral hernia repair does not reduce 30-day wound complications. Surg Endosc 2017;149(5 Suppl):e3–7.

18. Franklin ME, Gonzalez JJ, Glass JL, et al. Laparoscopic ventral and incisional hernia repair: an 11-year experience. Hernia 2004;8(1):23–7.

19. Chelala E, Baraké H, Estievenart J, et al. Long-term outcomes of 1326 laparoscopic incisional and ventral hernia repair with the routine suturing concept: a single institution experience. Hernia 2016;20(1):101–10.

20. Clapp ML, Hicks SC, Awad SS, et al. Trans-cutaneous Closure of Central Defects (TCCD) in laparoscopic ventral hernia repairs (LVHR). World J Surg 2013;37(1): 42–51.

21. Tandon A, Pathak S, Lyons NJR, et al. Meta-analysis of closure of the fascial defect during laparoscopic incisional and ventral hernia repair. Br J Surg 2016; 103(12):1598–607.

22. Orenstein SB, Dumeer JL, Monteagudo J, et al. Outcomes of laparoscopic ventral hernia repair with routine defect closure using "shoelacing" technique. Surg Endosc 2011;25(5):1452–7.

23. Muysoms F, Vander Mijnsbrugge G, Pletinckx P, et al. Randomized clinical trial of mesh fixation with "double crown" versus "sutures and tackers" in laparoscopic ventral hernia repair. Hernia 2013;17(5):603–12.

24. Christoffersen MW, Brandt E, Helgstrand F, et al. Recurrence rate after absorbable tack fixation of mesh in laparoscopic incisional hernia repair. Br J Surg 2015;102(5):541–7.

25. Bansal VK, Asuri K, Panaiyadiyan S, et al. Comparison of absorbable versus nonabsorbable tackers in terms of long-term outcomes, chronic pain, and quality of life after laparoscopic incisional hernia repair: a randomized study. Surg Laparosc Endosc Percutan Tech 2016;26(6):476–83.

26. Fortelny RH, Petter-Puchner AH, Glaser KS, et al. Use of fibrin sealant (Tisseel/Tissucol) in hernia repair: a systematic review. Surg Endosc 2012;26(7):1803–12.

27. Eriksen JR, Bisgaard T, Assaadzadeh S, et al. Randomized clinical trial of fibrin sealant versus titanium tacks for mesh fixation in laparoscopic umbilical hernia repair. Br J Surg 2011;98(11):1537–45.

28. Hilling DE, Koppert LB, Keijzer R, et al. Laparoscopic correction of umbilical hernias using a transabdominal preperitoneal approach: results of a pilot study. Surg Endosc 2009;23(8):1740–4.

29. Prasad P, Tantia O, Patle NM, et al. Laparoscopic transabdominal preperitoneal repair of ventral hernia: a step towards physiological repair. Indian J Surg 2011; 73(6):403–8.

30. Miserez M, Penninckx F. Endoscopic totally preperitoneal ventral hernia repair. Surg Endosc 2002;16(8):1207–13.

31. Schroeder AD, Debus ES, Schroeder M, et al. Laparoscopic transperitoneal sublay mesh repair: a new technique for the cure of ventral and incisional hernias. Surg Endosc 2012;27(2):648–54.

32. Costa TN, Abdalla RZ, Santo MA, et al. Transabdominal midline reconstruction by minimally invasive surgery: technique and results. Hernia 2016;20(2):257–65.

33. Belyansky I, Zahiri HR, Park A. Laparoscopic transversus abdominis release, a novel minimally invasive approach to complex abdominal wall reconstruction. Surg Innov 2016;23(2):134–41.

34. Lowe JB, Garza JR, Bowman JL, et al. Endoscopically assisted "components separation" for closure of abdominal wall defects. Plast Reconstr Surg 2000; 105(2):720.

35. Ramirez OM, Ruas E, Dellon AL. "Components separation" method for closure of abdominal-wall defects: an anatomic and clinical study. Plast Reconstr Surg 1990;86(3):519.

36. Rosen MJ, Williams C, Jin J, et al. Laparoscopic versus open-component separation: a comparative analysis in a porcine model. Am J Surg 2007;194(3):385–9.

37. Harth KC, Rosen MJ. Endoscopic versus open component separation in complex abdominal wall reconstruction. Am J Surg 2010;199(3):342–6.

38. Fox M, Cannon RM, Egger M, et al. Laparoscopic component separation reduces postoperative wound complications but does not alter recurrence rates in complex hernia repairs. Am J Surg 2013;206(6):869–74.

39. Albright E, Diaz D, Davenport D. The component separation technique for hernia repair: a comparison of open and endoscopic techniques. Am Surg 2011;77(7): 839–43.

40. Daes J, Dennis RJ. Endoscopic subcutaneous component separation as an adjunct to abdominal wall reconstruction. Surg Endosc 2017;31(2):872–6.

41. Moazzez A, Mason RJ, Darehzereshki A, et al. Totally laparoscopic abdominal wall reconstruction: lessons learned and results of a short-term follow-up. Hernia 2013;17(5):633–8.

42. Ibarra-Hurtado TR, Nuño-Guzmán CM, Miranda-Díaz AG, et al. Effect of botulinum toxin type A in lateral abdominal wall muscles thickness and length of patients with midline incisional hernia secondary to open abdomen management. Hernia 2014;18(5):647–52.

43. Ibarra-Hurtado TR, Nuño-Guzmán CM, Echeagaray-Herrera JE, et al. Use of botulinum toxin type a before abdominal wall hernia reconstruction. World J Surg 2009;33(12):2553–6.

44. Zendejas B, Khasawneh MA, Srvantstyan B, et al. Outcomes of chemical component paralysis using botulinum toxin for incisional hernia repairs. World J Surg 2013;37(12):2830–7.

45. Rodriguez-Acevedo O, Elstner KE, Jacombs ASW, et al. Preoperative Botulinum toxin A enabling defect closure and laparoscopic repair of complex ventral hernia. Surg Endosc 2018;32(2):831–9.

46. Henlford BT, Park A, Ramshaw BJ, et al. Laparoscopic repair of ventral hernias: nine years' experience with 850 consecutive hernias. Ann Surg 2003;238(3): 391–9 [discussion: 399–400].

47. Rosen M, Brody F, Ponsky J, et al. Recurrence after laparoscopic ventral hernia repair. Surg Endosc 2003;17(1):123–8.

48. Chowbey PK, Sharma A, Khullar R, et al. Laparoscopic ventral hernia repair. J Laparoendosc Adv Surg Tech A 2000;10(2):79–84.

49. Kurmann A, Visth E, Candinas D, et al. Long-term follow-up of open and laparoscopic repair of large incisional hernias. World J Surg 2011;35(2):297–301.

50. Olmi S, Scaini A, Cesana GC, et al. Laparoscopic versus open incisional hernia repair: an open randomized controlled study. Surg Endosc 2007;21(4):555–9.

51. Itani K, Hur K, Kim LT, et al. Comparison of laparoscopic and open repair with mesh for the treatment of ventral incisional hernia: a randomized trial. Arch Surg 2010;145(4):322–8.

52. Colavita PD, Tsirline VB, Belyansky I, et al. Prospective, long-term comparison of quality of life in laparoscopic versus open ventral hernia repair. Ann Surg 2012; 256(5):714–22.

53. Kaoutzanis C, Leichtle SW, Mouawad NJ, et al. Postoperative surgical site infections after ventral/incisional hernia repair: a comparison of open and laparoscopic outcomes. Surg Endosc 2013;27(6):2221–30.

54. Kaoutzanis C, Leichtle SW, Mouawad NJ, et al. Risk factors for postoperative wound infections and prolonged hospitalization after ventral/incisional hernia repair. Hernia 2015;19(1):113–23.

55. Bittner R, Bingener-Casey J, Dietz U, et al. Guidelines for laparoscopic treatment of ventral and incisional abdominal wall hernias (International Endohernia Society [IEHS])—Part 2. Surg Endosc 2014;28(2):353–79.

56. Moreno-Egea A, Bustos JAC, Girela E, et al. Long-term results of laparoscopic repair of incisional hernias using an intraperitoneal composite mesh. Surg Endosc 2010;24(2):359–65.

57. Petro CC, Nahabet EH, Criss CN, et al. Central failures of lightweight monofilament polyester mesh causing hernia recurrence: a cautionary note. Hernia 2015;19(1):155–9.
58. Cobb WS, Warren JA, Ewing JA, et al. Open retromuscular mesh repair of complex incisional hernia: predictors of wound events and recurrence. J Am Coll Surg 2015;220(4):606–13.
59. LeBlanc KA. Tack hernia: a new entity. JSLS 2003;7(4):383–7.
60. Barzana D, Johnson K, Clancy TV, et al. Hernia recurrence through a composite mesh secondary to transfascial suture holes. Hernia 2012;16(2):219–21.
61. Banerjee A, Beck C, Narula VK, et al. Laparoscopic ventral hernia repair: does primary repair in addition to placement of mesh decrease recurrence? Surg Endosc 2012;26(5):1264–8.
62. Carter SA, Hicks SC, Brahmbhatt R, et al. Recurrence and pseudorecurrence after laparoscopic ventral hernia repair: predictors and patient-focused outcomes. Am Surg 2014;80(2):138–48.
63. Liang MK, Clapp M, Li LT, et al. Patient Satisfaction, chronic pain, and functional status following laparoscopic ventral hernia repair. World J Surg 2013;37(3):530–7.
64. Patel PP, Love MW, Ewing JA, et al. Risks of subsequent abdominal operations after laparoscopic ventral hernia repair. Surg Endosc 2017;31(2):823–8.
65. Liang MK, Li LT, Nguyen MT, et al. Abdominal reoperation and mesh explantation following open ventral hernia repair with mesh. Am J Surg 2014;208(4):670–6.
66. Chelala E, Debardemaeker Y, Elias B, et al. Eighty-five redo surgeries after 733 laparoscopic treatments for ventral and incisional hernia: adhesion and recurrence analysis. Hernia 2010;14(2):123–9.
67. Halm JA, De Wall LL, Steyerberg EW, et al. Intraperitoneal polypropylene mesh hernia repair complicates subsequent abdominal surgery. World J Surg 2007;31(2):423–9.
68. Gray SH, Vick CC, Graham LA, et al. Risk of complications from enterotomy or unplanned bowel resection during elective hernia repair. Arch Surg 2008;143(6):582–6.
69. Leber GE, Garb JL, Alexander AI. Long-term complications associated with prosthetic repair of incisional hernias. Arch Surg 1998;133(4):378–82.
70. Steinhagen E, Khaitov S, Steinhagen RM. Intraluminal migration of mesh following incisional hernia repair. Hernia 2010;14(6):659–62.
71. Riaz AA, Ismail M, Barsam A, et al. Mesh erosion into the bladder: a late complication of incisional hernia repair. A case report and review of the literature. Hernia 2004;8(2):158–9.
72. Voisard G, Feldman LS. An unusual cause of chronic anemia and abdominal pain caused by transmural mesh migration in the small bowel after laparoscopic incisional hernia repair. Hernia 2013;17(5):673–7.
73. Nelson EC, Vidovszky TJ. Composite mesh migration into the sigmoid colon following ventral hernia repair. Hernia 2011;15(1):101–3.
74. Ballantyne GH, Hourmont K, Wasielewski A. Telerobotic laparoscopic repair of incisional ventral hernias using intraperitoneal prosthetic mesh. JSLS 2003;7(1):7–14.
75. Warren JA, Cobb WS, Ewing JA, et al. Standard laparoscopic versus robotic retromuscular ventral hernia repair. Surg Endosc 2017;31(1):324–32.
76. Carbonell AM, Warren JA, Prabhu AS, et al. Reducing length of stay using a robotic-assisted approach for retromuscular ventral hernia repair: a comparative

analysis from the Americas Hernia Society Quality Collaborative. Ann Surg 2018; 267(2):210–7.

77. Bittner JG, Alrefai S, Vy M, et al. Comparative analysis of open and robotic transversus abdominis release for ventral hernia repair. Surg Endosc 2018;32:727–34.

78. Martin-del-Campo LA, Weltz AS, Belyansky I, et al. Comparative analysis of perioperative outcomes of robotic versus open transversus abdominis release. Surg Endosc 2018;32:840–5.

79. Oviedo RJ, Robertson JC, Alrajhi S. First 101 robotic general surgery cases in a community hospital. JSLS 2016;20(3) [pii:e2016.00056].

80. Chen YJ, Huynh D, Nguyen S, et al. Outcomes of robot-assisted versus laparoscopic repair of small-sized ventral hernias. Surg Endosc 2017;31(3):1275–9.

81. Gonzalez A, Escobar E, Romero R, et al. Robotic-assisted ventral hernia repair: a multicenter evaluation of clinical outcomes. Surg Endosc 2017;31(3):1342–9.

82. Kudsi OY, Paluvoi N, Bhurtel P, et al. Robotic repair of ventral hernias: preliminary findings of a case series of 106 consecutive cases. Am J Robot Surg 2015;2(1): 22–6.

83. Abdalla RZ, Garcia RB, Costa R, et al. Procedimento de Rives/Stoppa modificado robô-assistido para correção de hérnias ventrais da linha média. Arq Bras Cir Dig 2012;25(2):129–32.

84. Warren J, Cobb W, Ewing J, et al. Prospective observational cohort study of robotic vs open Rives-Stoppa retrorectus incisional hernia repair. Hernia 2015; 19(1):S181.

85. Warren JA, Carbonell AM. Robotic ventral hernia repair. In: Hope WW, Cobb WS, Adrales GL, editors. Textbook of hernia. New York: Springer; 2017. p. 381–93.

86. Toy FK, Balley RW, Carey S, et al. Prospective, multicenter study of laparoscopic ventral hernioplasty. Preliminary results. Surg Endosc 1998;12(7):955–9.

87. Picazo-Yeste J, Moreno-Sanz C, Sedano-Vizcaíno C, et al. Outcomes after laparoscopic ventral hernia repair: does the number of previous recurrences matter? A prospective study. Surg Endosc 2017;72:70–8.

88. Lee J, Mabardy A, Kermani R, et al. Laparoscopic vs open ventral hernia repair in the era of obesity. JAMA Surg 2013;148(8):723–6.

89. Eker HH, Hansson BME, Buunen M, et al. Laparoscopic vs. open incisional hernia repair: a randomized clinical trial. JAMA Surg 2013;148(3):259–63.

90. Neupane R, Fayezizadeh M, Majumder A, et al. Is old age a contraindication to elective ventral hernia repair? Surg Endosc 2017;31(11):4425–30.

Umbilical Hernia Repair
Overview of Approaches and Review of Literature

Paul W. Appleby, MD, Tasha A. Martin, MD,
William W. Hope, MD*

KEYWORDS

- Umbilical • Hernia • Repair • Mesh • Primary • Laparoscopic • Robotic • Open

KEY POINTS

- Although umbilical hernias are often thought of as simple to repair, long-term recurrences and chronic complaints occur.
- Multiple treatment options exist for umbilical hernias, ranging from watchful waiting to surgical repair.
- Open, laparoscopic, and robotic repairs of umbilical hernias have been described and should be tailored based on clinical characteristics.
- In general, mesh use has been shown to decrease recurrence rates in umbilical hernia repair, however, mesh can result in an increase in surgical site infections/occurrences.

INTRODUCTION

Umbilical hernias are some of the most common hernias encountered by surgeons; approximately 175,000 umbilical hernias are surgically repaired annually in the United States.[1] Although umbilical hernias are often thought of as simple hernias, they can be complex and, if not handled properly, can be irritating to patients and surgeons. A true umbilical hernia is classified as a primary hernia; however, because the umbilicus is often used for laparoscopic access, incisional hernias can occur at the umbilicus, and surgeons should be aware of the distinctions between the 2. Several things make umbilical hernias challenging, including the heterogeneity of presentation, multiple options for repair, and potential for complications, including infection and

Dr W.W. Hope's disclosures: CR Bard: honorarium, speaking, and research support; WL Gore: research support and speaking; Lifecell: consulting; and Intuitive: speaking and consulting. Drs P.W. Appleby and T.A. Martin have nothing to disclose.
Department of Surgery, New Hanover Regional Medical Center, South East Area Health Education Center, 2131 South 17th Street, PO Box 9025, Wilmington, NC 28401, USA
* Corresponding author.
E-mail address: William.Hope@nhrmc.org

Surg Clin N Am 98 (2018) 561–576
https://doi.org/10.1016/j.suc.2018.02.001
0039-6109/18/© 2018 Elsevier Inc. All rights reserved.

surgical.theclinics.com

recurrence (**Figs. 1** and **2**). Debate continues regarding the indications for mesh use for umbilical hernias, optimal techniques for repair, and the role of robotic technology for repair.

OPEN TECHNIQUES AND USE OF MESH

A major decision facing surgeons when planning an open umbilical hernia repair relates to mesh use. The use of mesh and precise indications for mesh and nonmesh repair are debated with no clear consensus. Four prospective randomized trials have evaluated the use of mesh for umbilical hernias; 3 of 4 reported lower recurrence rates with mesh use,[2–5] with the greatest benefit in patients with cirrhosis[4] and patients undergoing emergent repair of incarcerated hernias.[3] A population-based study from the Danish Ventral Hernia Database reported similar findings.[6] Reoperation rates for recurrence were less in patients undergoing mesh repair compared with nonmesh repair in 4786 patients undergoing elective open repair of small (≤2 cm) umbilical or epigastric hernias.[6]

Primary Repair

Despite the fairly conclusive evidence supporting the use of mesh to decrease recurrence rates in open umbilical hernia repair, approximately 50% of elective umbilical hernias in the United States are repaired using a primary (suture) repair, indicating a reluctance among surgeons to use mesh in all cases.[7] The Mayo repair, first described in 1901, was a primary suture repair of umbilical hernias described as a "vest over pants" fascial closure in a transverse orientation using 2 rows of horizontal mattress sutures.[8] Although this technique was popular for many years and is occasionally used today, high long-term recurrence rates have limited its use with most surgeons who use a simple, interrupted or figure-of-8 primary closure in a horizontal fashion (**Fig. 3**).

Techniques of open primary repair vary. In general, however, patients should be prepared similarly to other abdominal operations with general anesthesia and perioperative antibiotics. Most umbilical hernias can be approached through a 3 cm to 4 cm curvilinear infraumbilical incision in the infraumbilical fold. Blunt dissection is begun on either side of the umbilicus to encircle the umbilical stalk and hernia

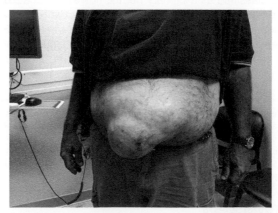

Fig. 1. Large complex primary umbilical hernia. Although umbilical hernias are usually small, they can grow to large sizes and can be difficult to fix.

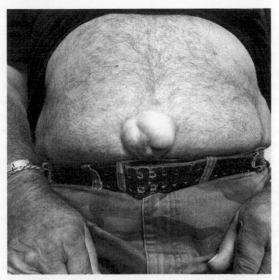

Fig. 2. Moderate-sized umbilical hernia. Umbilical hernias can be difficult due to the heterogeneity of size and associated clinical factors.

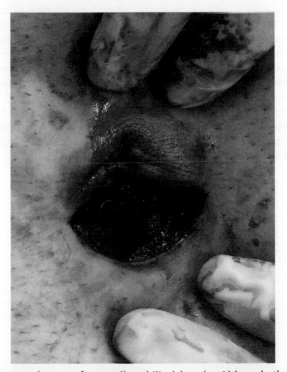

Fig. 3. Primary suture closure of a small umbilical hernia. Although the use of mesh is advised for umbilical hernia repair to decrease recurrences rates, a large number of umbilical hernias are still repaired in this fashion.

sac. Typically, a hemostat is placed above and around the umbilical stalk (**Fig. 4**), and the hernia sac is dissected off the stalk (**Fig. 5**). It is important to avoid button-holing the skin at this juncture of operation. This can be avoided by placing a finger or a blunt instrument in the umbilicus to help identify the junction. After the hernia sac is dissected free, it can be opened to identify the contents. When preperitoneal fat or omentum is present, this can be reduced back into the abdominal cavity or simply excised at the fascial level. At this point, the fascial edges should be clearly identified. Most surgeons dissect approximately 1 cm to 2 cm of subcutaneous tissue off the fascia to ensure clear identification for suturing. Because there are no studies relating to technique of suturing for umbilical hernia repair, this should be left to the discretion of the surgeon and usually involves interrupted or figure-of-8 sutures. Although there is no convincing evidence as to the type of suture material that should be used, based on some data from the Danish Ventral Hernia Database, there seems to be a higher recurrence rate using absorbable sutures compared with nonabsorbable sutures, so this should be considered when repairing umbilical hernias.[9] After the fascia has been closed, the wound is irrigated, and the umbilical stalk is sutured to the anterior fascia to restore the normal umbilical shape. The skin can then be closed with an absorbable suture and dressing applied. When the umbilical skin has been stretched from the hernia, a pressure dressing can be applied to potentially reduce seroma formation.

Mesh-based Repairs

As discussed previously, the decision regarding mesh use is related to many patient factors and hernia characteristics. In some cases, this decision is made at the time of surgery after the hernia defect and integrity of the fascia are examined. When the decision to use mesh is made, the proposed risks and benefits should have been discussed with the patient preoperatively.

After the decision to use mesh is made, the surgeon must choose the best mesh type and placement location. In general, most elective umbilical hernia repairs are clean, so a permanent synthetic mesh is typically recommended. There are few data related to using biologic or bioabsorbable meshes due to the fairly low wound and mesh infectious complications associated with mesh-based umbilical hernia repairs. So these expensive mesh technologies are likely of little benefit and only used for specific indications.

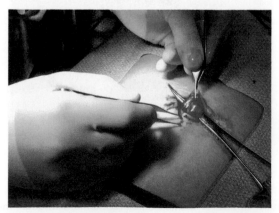

Fig. 4. Blunt dissection is performed to encircle umbilical stalk and hernia sac. Care must be taken not to button-hole the skin when dissecting the hernia sac off the umbilical stalk.

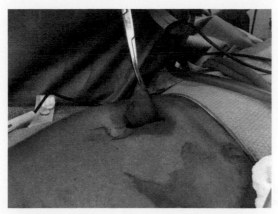

Fig. 5. Hernia sac that has been dissected free containing preperitoneal fat.

Mesh choice should be based on the chosen repair technique. As in other ventral hernia repairs, mesh can be placed as a sublay (an intra-abdominal, preperitoneal, or retrorectus position), an inlay (mesh plug sewn to fascial edges), or an onlay (mesh placed over primarily closed fascia). As with mesh repairs for ventral hernias in general, there is no consensus on the ideal location for mesh placement, and this should be based on the clinical scenario. Knowledge of the potential advantages and disadvantages of different mesh products and mesh locations is essential. In general, inlay techniques have higher recurrence rates and, therefore, should not be routinely used. Sublay techniques have the theoretic advantage of using the body's forces to help hold the mesh in place and potentially allow wider mesh overlap without having to create subcutaneous flaps that may increase wound infection rates. Onlay techniques can be appropriate in some cases but require subcutaneous flap dissection for adequate mesh overlap and can lead to mesh exposure when superficial wound infections occur.

Open umbilical hernia repair using a sublay mesh technique begins as described for a primary suture repair. The patient is prepped/draped and preoperative preparation is per standard abdominal surgery. A curvilinear incision below the umbilicus is made, and the hernia sac is dissected off the umbilical stalk. When the mesh is to be placed in the preperitoneal space, the hernia sac is not opened and can be dissected at the level of the fascia with blunt dissection. This preperitoneal dissection is accomplished circumferentially for several centimeters, and holes in the peritoneum are closed with absorbable sutures. After adequate preperitoneal dissection, mesh of the surgeon's choosing is placed and fixed at the discretion of the surgeon. Although flat sheet meshes can be used for this repair, several commercially available meshes work well for the sublay repairs. These include the Ventralex ST Hernia Patch (CR Bard, Warwick, RI), the PROCEED Ventral Patch (Ethicon, Sommerville, NJ), and the C-QUR V-Patch (Atrium, Hudson, NH) (**Fig. 6**). Theses meshes have a string-like device attached to a flat sheet of coated polypropylene mesh to facilitate easy mesh placement (**Figs. 7** and **8**). Another option for sublay repair involves the intra-abdominal placement of mesh, which is technically simpler than the preperitoneal repair. In this technique, the hernia sac can be opened and contents either reduced or excised if contents are fat or omentum. The hernia sac is excised to the level of the fascia, and blunt dissection intra-abdominally (typically with a finger) circumferentially around the defect is used to ensure no other hernia defects. The mesh is chosen,

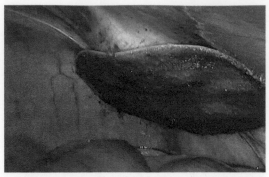

Fig. 6. Laparoscopic view of remote preperitoneal umbilical hernia repair with mesh during nonrelated laparoscopic procedure.

placed intra-abdominally, and fixed to the abdominal wall using sutures (**Fig. 9**). In both of these repairs, the fascia is closed overlying the mesh after the tails of the mesh are cut flush with the fascia. Skin is closured, and dressings are applied. The last option for a sublay repair is the retrorectus repair. This is rarely required for umbilical hernias due to the small size of the defects. In some cases of large umbilical hernias, however, this is a viable option. In this repair, a periumbilical vertical incision is

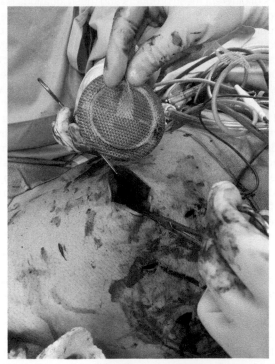

Fig. 7. Mesh prosthetic for umbilical hernia repair in the sublay position (either intra-abdominal or preperitoneal). This mesh made of polypropylene has a tissue separating layer so that it can be placed intra-abdominally.

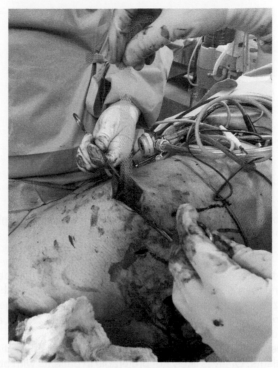

Fig. 8. The mesh has a mesh string to facilitate placement through a small incision and fascial defect.

made, and the hernia sac is dissected off the umbilical stalk and reduced or excised (**Fig. 10**). The posterior rectus sheath is incised on the right and left sides and closed in the midline, excluding the abdominal contents from contact with the mesh. Closing the posterior rectus sheath at the most superior and inferior portion of the incision can be

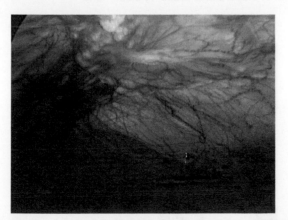

Fig. 9. Laparoscopic view of an umbilical hernia mesh placed intra-abdominally through a small curvilinear periumbilical incision. The mesh is typically fixed using sutures, but in some cases, a hybrid laparoscopic-open repair can be done, and the mesh can be fixed laparoscopically with tacks.

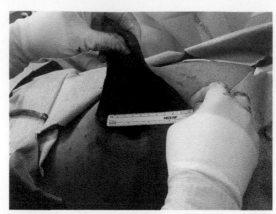

Fig. 10. Large umbilical hernia (approximately 5 cm) approached through a periumbilical midline incision and retrorectus repair.

difficult, because the incision is usually quite small. This can usually be accomplished, however, with continued dissection. After the posterior rectus sheath is closed, a flat sheet of mesh sized appropriately is placed and fixed per the surgeon's discretion, usually with sutures (**Figs. 11** and **12**). The anterior fascia is closed and followed by skin closure and dressing application.

Onlay techniques for mesh repair of umbilical hernia are viable options in appropriately selected patients. Onlay is likely not preferable in patients with obesity, diabetes, or smoking. The umbilical hernia is dissected and repaired, as described for a primary repair. After the fascia is closed, subcutaneous flaps are dissected to allow mesh placement. Close attention should be directed to the width of the subcutaneous dissection, because there is a relationship between wide mesh overlap and infection. The wider the subcutaneous dissection, the more chance for infection. Mesh fixation is left to the discretion of the surgeon. Suture, glue, and tack fixation have been described. After mesh placement, the umbilical stalk can be sutured to the mesh and followed by skin closure and dressing placement.

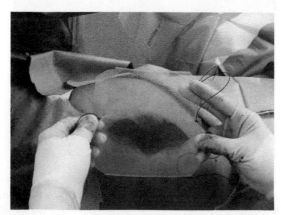

Fig. 11. Synthetic polypropylene mesh chosen for retrorectus repair and fixed using transfacial sutures.

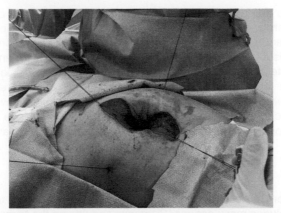

Fig. 12. Mesh placed in the retrorectus space and fixed with 4 sutures. The anterior fascia will be closed overlying the mesh for repair of this large umbilical hernia.

Although there is no definitive literature supporting 1 mesh-based technique for umbilical hernia repair, surgeons should know all the potential options and advantages and disadvantages associated with each repair (**Fig. 13**). Because umbilical hernias are heterogeneous, type and repair technique should be tailored to each clinical scenario.

LAPAROSCOPIC TECHNIQUES

At present, the use of laparoscopy for umbilical hernia repair is fairly low. Studies have indicated that laparoscopy is used in only one-quarter of cases.[7] The American College of Surgeons National Surgery Quality Improvement Program reported a potential decrease in the total and wound morbidity associated with laparoscopic compared with open, elective, primary repair of umbilical hernias.[10] This came at the expense of long operative time and hospital stay, with an increase in respiratory and cardiac complications.[10] After controlling for patient factors, including body mass index, gender, American Society of Anesthesiologists class, and chronic obstructive pulmonary disease, the odds ratio for overall complications favored

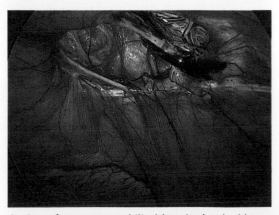

Fig. 13. Laparoscopic view of recurrent umbilical hernia that had been repaired using primary (suture) repair. Mesh has been shown to reduce recurrence rates in most studies and series related to umbilical hernia repair.

the laparoscopic approach, which was driven by reduced wound complications.[10] Laparoscopic hernia repair is indicated for several reasons, including obesity, large fascial defects, and previous hernia repair.[11] The laparoscopic approach allows the surgeon to unmistakably define the margins of the hernia defect and identify additional fascial defects or occult hernias. Some hernias include small facial defects adjacent to the large defect, and, when missed, this can increase recurrence rates.[12] The laparoscopic approach also allows for wider mesh coverage, because the mesh is placed in the intraperitoneal position. This technique has resulted in decreased postoperative pain, shorter return to normal activity, and lower recurrence rates.[13]

PROCEDURE

The technique for laparoscopic repair first involves gaining access to the peritoneal cavity, which includes many options. Surgeons should use the technique for laparoscopic access they feel most comfortable with, because there is no conclusive evidence on the superiority of one technique. The authors place a Veress needle in the left subcostal region followed by placement of an optical trocar after pneumoperitoneum is established. Other options include cutdown technique or optical access without Veress needle. The authors typically place 3 to 5 total ports depending on the size of the defect and adhesions; however, many surgeons complete this repair with 2 ports to 3 ports. The authors' typical port placement involves an 11-mm trocar in the midlateral left side of the abdomen and 2 additional 5-mm trocars in the left upper and lower quadrants laterally. Diagnostic laparoscopy is initially performed, followed by evaluation of the abdominal wall and hernia defect. One potential advantage of the laparoscopic approach is the identification of additional hernia defects along the linea alba above or below the umbilical hernia, that can be laparoscopically repaired. Often, these defects are not identified during an open operation, especially when the umbilical hernia defect is small and does not allow intra-abdominal palpation of the linea alba (**Fig. 14**). The operation is begun by lysing adhesions to the abdominal wall and reducing contents that are present in the umbilical hernia. Although this can be the Achilles heel for the laparoscopic approach to incisional hernia repair, typically adhesions in umbilical hernia repair are not too difficult (**Fig. 15**). After adhesions are

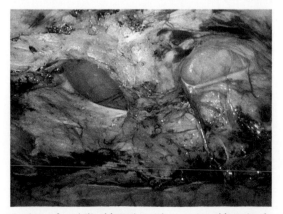

Fig. 14. Laparoscopic view of umbilical hernia with associated hernia above the defect. The ability to see the entire abdominal wall and evaluate additional hernias is one proposed benefit of the laparoscopic repair.

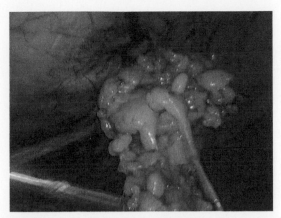

Fig. 15. Often, omentum is in the hernia sac and has to be dissected and reduced to evaluate the size of the defect.

taken down and the hernia is reduced, the hernia defect is measured intracorporeally, and a mesh is chosen that allows at least a 3-cm to 5-cm overlap on all sides (**Fig. 16**).

Type of mesh and methods of fixation for laparoscopic ventral and umbilical hernias remain an ongoing debate with no consensus. Due to this, the choice of mesh and fixation technique are left to the discretion of the surgeon with a few caveats. Because the mesh used is placed intra-abdominally, a mesh suited for intra-abdominal placement should be chosen. Several mesh options include expanded polytetrafluoroethylene–based meshes and the so-called coated meshes that include polypropylene or polyester-based mesh with a tissue separating layer allowing for intra-abdominal placement (**Figs. 17** and **18**).

The mesh should be placed and centered appropriately to allow for wide overlap of the hernia defect. This can be done using sutures or commercially available positioning devices. Mesh can be fixated using sutures, tacks, glue, or a combination of these. Aside from the debate about mesh type and fixation, there is disagreement

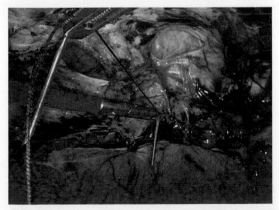

Fig. 16. The hernia defect should be measured intracorporeal to get an exact measurement to help size the mesh. The defect can be measured by placing a ruler intra-abdominally or by simply using a suture that can be stretched across the defect and measured outside of the abdomen.

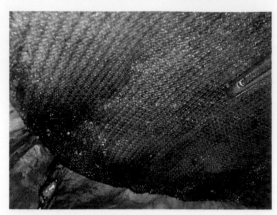

Fig. 17. Mesh placement with wide overlap of the umbilical hernia defect (at least 3–5 cm in all directions). Several tissue separating meshes are available that can be placed intra-abdominally and fixed with a variety of commercially absorbable and nonabsorbable tacks and/or sutures.

regarding whether the hernia defect should be closed in laparoscopic hernia repair in attempts to mimic the open repair and potentially decrease recurrence and seroma rates. Despite the theoretic advantage of fascial closure in laparoscopic hernia repair, there has been no conclusive evidence supporting closure, and further study is needed. When the surgeon decides to close the defect, this can be done using laparoscopic suturing, a suture passer, or a hybrid technique with an open incision to close the defect and laparoscopically place mesh.

ROBOTIC TECHNIQUES

Robotic technology is gaining widespread adoption in many fields of surgery. Initially used in urologic and gynecologic surgery, it has now gained momentum in general surgery, especially hernia surgery. Robotic surgery is similar in many ways to laparoscopic surgery with the proposed advantages of improved visualization, dexterity, and ergonomics for the surgeon.[14]

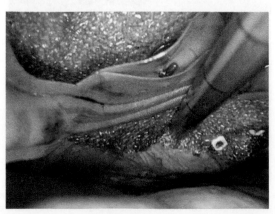

Fig. 18. Mesh fixation using a permanent tacker and the aid of a mesh positioning device to help keep the mesh on the abdominal wall during fixation.

Because robotic technology is an emerging technology in general surgery, there are currently more questions than answers about its use for hernia repair. Despite this, surgeons are increasingly adopting robotic technology for repair of ventral and umbilical hernias. There is little literature to guide discussions related to robotic umbilical hernia repair; however, several issues should be discussed. The use of the robot for umbilical hernia repair at first seems like a waste of resources and time; however, if there are some advantages associated with robotic technology, these should be evaluated in the same fashion as other emerging technologies.

Some of the proposed advantages of using the robot for minimally invasive and umbilical hernia repair include facilitating suture closure of the fascial defect (**Fig. 19**), the ability to place mesh in the preperitoneal or retrorectus position, and the ability to suture fixate mesh without the use of tacks or transfascial sutures (**Fig. 20**). Although these proposed advantages may seem to be a step forward in hernia repair, they require careful evaluation. There is little argument about the improved ability to suture robotically compared with laparoscopically. Currently there is no conclusive evidence, however, that suture closure of the defect in minimally invasive hernia repair significantly improves outcomes. Despite the theoretic advantage of placing mesh in the preperitoneal or retrorectus position, there is no good evidence that this is better than intra-abdominal placement. Lastly, although there are some claims of decreased pain with suturing of mesh compared with transfascial sutures and tacks, this again has not been proved. Further study is warranted to evaluate these potential advantages. Robotic surgery likely will find a place in the realm of minimally invasive hernia repair, but its use should be justified, and it should be used in an economically sustainable way.

REVIEW OF THE LITERATURE

Although umbilical hernias are some of the most commonly repaired hernias in the world, there are still many unanswered questions related to their repair, and the literature on the topic is sparse, with few well done studies.

TREATMENT OPTIONS

Few studies are available to guide the surgeon on the surgical treatment of umbilical hernias. In general surgery, treatment is recommended for symptomatic patients. Two studies evaluated the strategies of surgery and watchful waiting for umbilical hernias

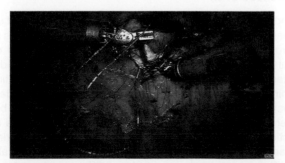

Fig. 19. One proposed potential advantage of robotic hernia repair is the ability to facilitate suture closure of the fascia. Although to date, this has not proved to significantly improve outcomes, many surgeons favor closure of the defect to possibly reduce seromas and produce a more durable repair.

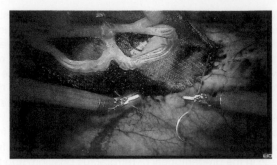

Fig. 20. Due to the improved ability to suture using robotic technology, many surgeons fix mesh during robotic umbilical hernia repair with a running suture, avoiding the use of tack fixation and transfascial sutures. In this case, a mesh positioning device helps to hold the mesh to the abdominal wall to facilitate suturing.

and have differing conclusions.[15,16] Strosberg and colleagues[15] evaluated a large administrative database of 279 employees with umbilical hernias and their treatment of surgery or no surgery. They reported higher financial cost in the surgical group but significantly more days of health care utilization and more estimated work days missed in the no surgery group and recommended early surgical intervention to potentially decrease cost and resource utilization.[15] Kokotovic and colleagues[16] evaluated 569 patients with incisional hernias and 789 patients with umbilical/epigastric hernias. They reported a 16% probability of patients with umbilical/epigastric hernias to require surgery over 5 years and a 4% chance of requiring emergency surgery.[16] The investigators also reported no significant outcome differences between the watchful waiting patients who ultimately required surgery and the patients who underwent surgery initially. They concluded that watchful waiting is a safe strategy in patients with umbilical/epigastric hernias.

MESH

The use of mesh remains a debated topic for umbilical hernia repair. As discussed previously, the evidence is clear that the use of mesh reduces recurrence rates but possibly increases the risk of surgical site infections and occurrences.[2–6,17–19]

LAPAROSCOPIC VERSUS OPEN

There are few good trials comparing laparoscopic and open repair of umbilical hernia. Cassie and colleagues[10] evaluated the American College of Surgeons National Quality Improvement Program comparing outcomes for laparoscopic and open repairs of elective umbilical hernias in 14,652 patients. They reported decreased wound complications associated with the laparoscopic repair but increased operating times, length of stay, and respiratory and cardiac complications. This concept of decreased wound morbidity in laparoscopic hernia repair compared with open has been well documented; however, it should be taken in context for umbilical hernia repair, because the wound infection rate is low. One other randomized controlled trial evaluated the postoperative use of abdominal binders after laparoscopic umbilical and epigastric hernia repair.[20] The investigators reported no difference in outcomes related to pain, movement limitation, fatigue, seroma formation, general well-being, or quality of life in the 56 randomized patients.[20] They reported an improved subjective beneficial effect, however, of using the binder in most patients.[20]

COMPLICATIONS

Although it is generally believed that umbilical hernia repairs are associated with low recurrence and complications rates, there are few studies that evaluate long-term outcomes of this common procedure, and several population-based studies show outcomes that are likely higher than surgeons think. Two studies from Denmark evaluated chronic complaints after repair of umbilical and epigastric hernias.[9,21] Westen and colleagues[9] surveyed 295 patients who underwent suture repair of umbilical and epigastric hernias with a median follow-up of 5 years and reported that 5.5% of patient had chronic complaints, such as pain or work/leisure restrictions, and this could be explained in part by hernia recurrence. Erritzoe-Jervild and colleagues[21] surveyed 132 patients who underwent suture and mesh repair of umbilical and epigastric hernias with a median follow-up of 36 months. They reported 12% of patients had moderate or severe pain and discomfort and a cumulative risk of recurrence of 11.5%.[21] These 2 studies show that umbilical hernias are not simple hernias, and surgeons should work to improve outcomes in these patients.

SUMMARY

Umbilical hernias are common and often thought of as simple hernias; however, they can pose many challenges to the surgeon, and long-term outcomes are still not ideal. Open, laparoscopic, and possibly robotic techniques all have a role in umbilical hernia repair, and their use should be determined by the requirements of the clinical situation. Open techniques are used most often due to the small size of these hernias, and small incisions typically are used for repair. Mesh repairs have been shown to decrease umbilical hernia recurrence rates and should be used in most cases but can result in slightly higher wound morbidity. Laparoscopic repairs are usually well suited for obese patients or patients at high risk for wound complications. Robotic surgery, an emerging technology for hernia repair, may have some potential advantages, but this must be weighed against the cost of this technology. Further study using robotic technology is needed. Surgeons should continue to strive to improve outcomes for patients with umbilical hernias and clarify indications for the use of mesh and various surgical techniques.

REFERENCES

1. Rutkow IM. Epidemiologic, economic, and sociologic aspects of hernia surgery in the United States in the 1990s. Surg Clin North Am 1998;78:941–51, v–vi.

2. Arroyo A, Garcia P, Perez F, et al. Randomized clinical trial comparing suture and mesh repair of umbilical hernia in adults. Br J Surg 2001;88:1321–3.

3. Abdel-Baki NA, Bessa SS, Abdel-Razek AH. Comparison of prosthetic mesh repair and tissue repair in the emergency management of incarcerated paraumbilical hernia: a prospective randomized study. Hernia 2007;11:163–7.

4. Ammar SA. Management of complicated umbilical hernias in cirrhotic patients using permanent mesh: randomized clinical trial. Hernia 2010;14:35–8.

5. Polat C, Dervisoglu A, Senyurek G, et al. Umbilical hernia repair with the prolene hernia system. Am J Surg 2005;190:61–4.

6. Christoffersen MW, Helgstrand F, Rosenberg J, et al. Lower reoperation rate for recurrence after mesh versus sutured elective repair in small umbilical and epigastric hernias. A nationwide register study. World J Surg 2013;37:2548–52.

7. Funk LM, Perry KA, Narula VK, et al. Current national practice patterns for inpatient management of ventral abdominal wall hernia in the United States. Surg Endosc 2013;27:4104–12.

8. Mayo WJ. VI. An operation for the radical cure of umbilical hernia. Ann Surg 1901; 34:276–80.

9. Westen M, Christoffersen MW, Jorgensen LN, et al. Chronic complaints after simple sutured repair for umbilical or epigastric hernias may be related to recurrence. Langenbecks Arch Surg 2014;399:65–9.

10. Cassie S, Okrainec A, Saleh F, et al. Laparoscopic versus open elective repair of primary umbilical hernias: short-term outcomes from the American College of Surgeons National Surgery Quality Improvement Program. Surg Endosc 2014;28: 741–6.

11. Ramshaw BJ, Esartia P, Schwab J, et al. Comparison of laparoscopic and open ventral herniorrhaphy. Am Surg 1999;65:827–31 [discussion: 31–2].

12. Gonzalez R, Mason E, Duncan T, et al. Laparoscopic versus open umbilical hernia repair. JSLS 2003;7:323–8.

13. Bencini L, Sanchez LJ, Bernini M, et al. Predictors of recurrence after laparoscopic ventral hernia repair. Surg Laparosc Endosc Percutan Tech 2009;19: 128–32.

14. Lanfranco AR, Castellanos AE, Desai JP, et al. Robotic surgery: a current perspective. Ann Surg 2004;239:14–21.

15. Strosberg DS, Pittman M, Mikami D. Umbilical hernias: the cost of waiting. Surg Endosc 2017;31:901–6.

16. Kokotovic D, Sjolander H, Gogenur I, et al. Watchful waiting as a treatment strategy for patients with a ventral hernia appears to be safe. Hernia 2016;20:281–7.

17. Nguyen MT, Berger RL, Hicks SC, et al. Comparison of outcomes of synthetic mesh vs suture repair of elective primary ventral herniorrhaphy: a systematic review and meta-analysis. JAMA Surg 2014;149:415–21.

18. Christoffersen MW, Helgstrand F, Rosenberg J, et al. Long-term recurrence and chronic pain after repair for small umbilical or epigastric hernias: a regional cohort study. Am J Surg 2015;209:725–32.

19. Berger RL, Li LT, Hicks SC, et al. Suture versus preperitoneal polypropylene mesh for elective umbilical hernia repairs. J Surg Res 2014;192:426–31.

20. Christoffersen MW, Olsen BH, Rosenberg J, et al. Randomized clinical trial on the postoperative use of an abdominal binder after laparoscopic umbilical and epigastric hernia repair. Hernia 2015;19:147–53.

21. Erritzoe-Jervild L, Christoffersen MW, Helgstrand F, et al. Long-term complaints after elective repair for small umbilical or epigastric hernias. Hernia 2013;17: 211–5.

Surgical Management of Parastomal Hernias

Jennifer Colvin, MD, Steven Rosenblatt, MD*

KEYWORDS

- Parastomal hernia • Ostomy formation • Fascial repair • Stoma relocation
- Mesh repair

KEY POINTS

- Parastomal hernias are a common complication after ostomy formation that can require surgical repair when they become symptomatic.
- Simple fascial repair is associated with an unacceptably high recurrence rate and should be used in urgent situations as a temporizing measure until a more definitive repair can be performed.
- Stoma relocation also has a high recurrence rate, both at the old and the new ostomy site.
- To help mitigate this situation, prophylactic mesh can and should then be used.
- Operative planning and a thorough understanding of the anatomy of the abdominal wall is of utmost importance, because such repairs can be quite complex.

INTRODUCTION

Parastomal hernias are incisional hernias related to an abdominal wall stoma.[1] The most common complication of stoma creation by far is parastomal herniation, with the incidence ranging from 28.3% for end ileostomy to as high as 48.1% for end colostomy.[2–4] The majority of these defects develop within the first few years after creation; however, the risk for herniation increases over time.[3,4] Risk factors include obesity, chronic corticosteroid use, malnutrition, advanced age, increased intraabdominal pressure, and postoperative wound infection.[3,5,6] The development of parastomal hernias can negatively impact a patient's quality of life and can lead to increased health care costs.[3,7,8] With an estimated 100,000 to 120,000 new stomas created annually in the United States, these hernias are a growing problem that all general surgeons will encounter.[9,10]

PRESENTATION AND DIAGNOSIS

Patients with a parastomal hernia may complain of bulging with coughing or straining and discomfort around the stoma.[8] In addition, patients may have difficulties with

The authors have nothing to disclose.
General Surgery, Cleveland Clinic, 9500 Euclid Avenue, Cleveland, OH 44195, USA
* Corresponding author.
E-mail address: rosenbs@ccf.org

Surg Clin N Am 98 (2018) 577–592
https://doi.org/10.1016/j.suc.2018.01.010
0039-6109/18/© 2018 Elsevier Inc. All rights reserved.

pouching, leading to leakage and skin irritation.[11] If a parastomal hernia is present, it may be possible to palpate a bulge adjacent to the stoma upon Valsava maneuver.[8] However, studies have shown that physical examination alone is often unreliable in diagnosing parastomal hernias.[12] Computed tomography scans of the abdomen are useful because they may be able to detect occult hernias that are missed on physical examination. These radiographic tests are also helpful to delineate the anatomy of the rest of the abdominal wall.[8,13]

MEDICAL MANAGEMENT VERSUS SURGICAL REPAIR

Most patients with asymptomatic parastomal hernias and those with mild symptoms can be managed nonoperatively. Stomal support belts, skin protective sealants, and a flexible appliance are very useful adjuncts in this patient population.[14] It is important that patients have access to wound ostomy nursing care, because this measure has been shown to significantly improve the quality of life in these patients.[15]

Although many parastomal hernias can be managed nonoperatively, approximately 30% of such patients will ultimately require surgical correction.[16] Elective repair can and should be offered to patients with symptoms such as difficulty maintaining a seal on their pouch, significant parastomal pain, and prolapse.[6,8] Emergent surgical management may be required for obstruction, incarceration, or strangulation.[8] Given that the current options for surgical repair still have a high recurrence rate, it is our practice to defer surgical repair unless the patient is having significant pain, obstructive symptoms, skin breakdown, or difficulty pouching.

Current surgical options for these hernias include primary fascial repair, stoma relocation, and mesh repairs, of which there are several options. The decision as to which surgical approach to choose in these patients can be complex. Before proceeding with surgical repair, one must review the patient's comorbidities and ability to tolerate a major operative procedure.[17] The different surgical approaches are discussed in further detail elsewhere in this article.

When planning surgical intervention, it is important to review the patient's previous operative reports, because many such patients have developed recurrences after the initial repair. The etiology of the stoma itself also must be taken into consideration. For example, urostomies may be difficult to relocate and, therefore, surgical repair may require keeping the stoma in situ. Similarly, the type of stoma is important, be it an end or a loop ostomy. Obviously, if the stoma may be reversed at some point, then this is the optimal treatment for parastomal hernias.[6] However, given that many stomas are permanent, this situation is usually not the case.

Preoperative computed tomography scans are crucial for operative planning.[8,18] This study provides essential information regarding the location of the stoma in relation to the defect, the integrity of the abdominal wall musculature, and the size and location of concurrent incisional hernias, which are very common.[18] It is also important to consider the timing of the operation. In cases of elective repair, one should wait a minimum of 3 months, and oftentimes even longer, after a previous intraabdominal surgery.[18]

SURGICAL REPAIR

Appropriate preoperative antibiotics to cover enteric bacteria and appropriate deep vein thrombosis prophylaxis are given. The patient is placed in the supine position and general anesthesia is then induced. A Foley catheter is placed to monitor urine output during the operation. In cases of urostomy hernias, a sterile catheter is used to intubate the stoma, which also can be of assistance in identifying the loop of bowel during adhesiolysis. An adhesive sterile drape is placed over the stoma to avoid contamination of the field, regardless of the approach used.[19,20] The patient is subsequently prepped and draped in the usual sterile fashion.

SIMPLE FASCIAL REPAIR

Simple fascial repair involves a parastomal incision, reduction of the hernia sac, and narrowing of the fascial opening with nonabsorbable sutures.[6] Although this technique avoids a laparotomy, it entails a very high risk of recurrence. One metaanalysis found a recurrence rate of 69.4% for simple fascial repair when approached locally or through a midline laparotomy.[21] Given the unacceptably high recurrence rate, this technique should only be used in patients with small defects, those with contraindications to the use of prosthetic material, or patients who cannot tolerate extensive surgery.[6,8] This technique can also be appropriate as a temporizing measure in urgent situations, to delay intervention until the patient is optimized for a definitive repair.

STOMA RELOCATION

Stoma relocation involves moving the ostomy to a new position and repairing the hernia at the previous site. Recurrences are very common at the new stoma site, with rates as high as 76% documented in some studies.[8] Similarly, this method also is associated with a risk of hernia recurrence as high as 52% at the previous stoma location.[22] This technique can be of some usefulness in cases where the existing stoma location is unsatisfactory.[6] However, the stoma should be repositioned on the contralateral side of the abdomen whenever possible, given the higher recurrence rates when relocated to the ipsilateral side.[23] The use of prophylactic mesh at the new stoma site may also be used, because this technique has been shown to decrease recurrence rates.[24] However, if prophylactic mesh is to be used, it should cover all potential areas of hernia formation: the new stoma site, the previous stoma site, and the midline incision.[17]

If stoma relocation is planned or even just a possibility, care should be taken to place the new stoma in a suitable position. The patient should be examined both in a standing and a sitting position, and coordination with enterostomal nurses for preoperative marking should be done whenever possible.[15] Additionally, the stoma should be placed through the rectus muscle, because this placement has been shown to have a lower recurrence rate compared with placement lateral to the rectus.[25]

MESH SELECTION

The number of available mesh options has skyrocketed over the past decade, which can make this choice much more confusing, regardless of the approach. First and foremost, the type of repair must be taken into consideration when making this decision. Further complicating matters is the concern about placing synthetic mesh in the presence of stomas because of the associated contaminated field and the potential risk of mesh infection. Since its inception, biologic mesh has been increasingly used in such cases owing to the concern for contamination. However, biologic mesh has been shown to be associated with high recurrence rates. One trial examining the use of biologic mesh in contaminated hernia repairs revealed a recurrence rate of 31.3%.[26]

Recent studies however, have called into question the principle of avoiding synthetic mesh in such contaminated cases. Carbonell and colleagues[27] reported favorable surgical site infection and surgical site occurrence rates using lightweight polypropylene synthetic mesh in clean-contaminated and contaminated ventral hernia repairs. Lightweight and medium weight polypropylene meshes have been used in both the open onlay and the retromuscular techniques of parastomal hernia repair in the literature, with favorable outcomes with regard to surgical site infections and recurrence rates.[17,19,20,28–32] Owing to the very real concerns regarding the potential for contamination in the face of an existing stoma, biologic mesh remains a very appropriate consideration at present. However, it is impossible to ignore the high recurrence rates associated with biologic grafts, as well as their significant cost.

Laparoscopy is also a viable alternative in hernia repair. The smaller incisions and lower potential contamination have made this a very reasonable choice. However, this approach raises different concerns for mesh reinforcement. Given the inherent risk of adhesions, erosion, and fistula formation with intraabdominal polypropylene, newer meshes have been developed to minimize these risks of intraperitoneal placement when the laparoscopic approach is used.

Because of the microporous nature of expanded polytetrafluoroethylene (ePTFE), there is less tissue in-growth and, therefore, less risk of adhesions to bowel, which led to the early acceptance of this product for laparoscopic incisional and then parastomal hernia repair. However, a low porosity also results in poor incorporation into the abdominal wall.[33] Additionally, there is a higher risk of mesh infection with ePTFE given the smaller pore size. Such low porosity also contributes to mesh contraction, which is an important consideration, especially when a keyhole is created around the stoma.[33]

To combat the drawbacks of ePTFE, dual-sided barrier-coated composite-type meshes have been developed. With these products, the coated side is placed in contact with the abdominal viscera to minimize bowel adhesions, and the superior surface is placed to optimize tissue incorporation into the abdominal wall.[33] Owing to such benefits, composite mesh is most commonly used when parastomal hernias are repaired with intraperitoneal mesh, be it open or laparoscopic. It is important to note that, although there may be less adhesion formation in the initial postoperative period, there may still be long-term adhesion formation when such coated meshes are used.[34] Similarly, when creating a keyhole in the mesh, shrinkage must also be taken into consideration. Indeed, the smaller pores of heavyweight mesh leads to more shrinkage and, therefore, greater porosity is preferred at present.[33]

Presently, we use a barrier-coated composite mesh for our laparoscopic hernia repairs, which is widely accepted. For open repairs, we are now using medium weight polypropylene mesh placed into the retrorectus space, and mesh infection has not been a frequent complication. Indeed, randomized controlled studies are presently underway comparing biologic and synthetic mesh in such contaminated fields. With time, these trials will help to guide us as to the optimal mesh in the open approach to complex parastomal hernia repairs.

ONLAY MESH REPAIR

The onlay method of repair places the mesh subcutaneously, with fixation to the anterior rectus sheath and aponeurosis of the external oblique muscle.[8] This approach has been found to be a reasonable option associated with low risks of wound (1.9%) and mesh (2.6%) infection.[21] Recurrence rates range from 0% to 20%, with an overall 12-month recurrence rate of 17.2% in one metaanalysis.[19–21,28] Using this technique, it is possible to avoid a formal laparotomy and, therefore, it is advantageous for high-risk patients with small to medium sized hernias.[35] This approach may also be of use in patients with a prohibitive abdomen owing to past surgical history. Still, this procedure does require large skin flaps and the inherent complications associated with a significant postoperative dead space, which puts these patients at greater risk for infection and subsequent mesh infection.[36]

Operative Technique

Using a lateral incision approximately 10 cm away from the stoma, dissection is carried down to the rectus sheath and then continued medially to mobilize the stoma (**Fig. 1**), allowing for the hernia sac to be separated and reduced.[19] The fascial defect is then closed with nonabsorbable suture, maintaining care to avoid narrowing the orifice. Upon completion, the opening should admit approximately 2 fingers.[20] The repair is then reinforced with mesh (**Fig. 2**), which is secured to the surrounding anterior fascia with nonabsorbable suture.[19,21] Indeed, in the existing literature, polypropylene mesh has traditionally been used in the onlay mesh repair.[19,20,29] Occasionally, when it is not possible to reapproximate the defect without excessive tension, although not optimal, the mesh onlay can be placed without fascial closure.[29] As the stoma remains in situ, a slit is created in the mesh to form the keyhole. The tails are then wrapped around the stoma to allow for passage of the bowel.[19,20,28,30] To ensure adequate coverage of the defect laterally, it may help to place the slit medial to the stoma.[20] When the tails are reapproximated, care is taken to avoid constriction of the bowel.[29] Closed suction drains are placed subcutaneously and the wound is closed in 2 layers.[20,29]

OPEN INTRAPERITONEAL MESH REPAIR

Open intraperitoneal mesh repair involves placement of the mesh intraabdominally and fixed posteriorly to the peritoneum.[37] Barrier-coated composite mesh is preferred

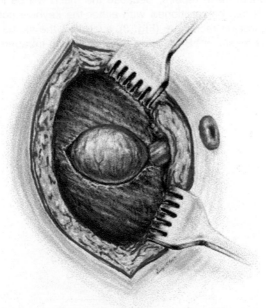

Fig. 1. Hernia sac exposed deep to Scarpa's fascia in preparation for onlay mesh repair. (*From* Franks ME, Hrebinko RL. Technique of parastomal hernia repair using synthetic mesh. Urology 2001;57(3):551–3; with permission.)

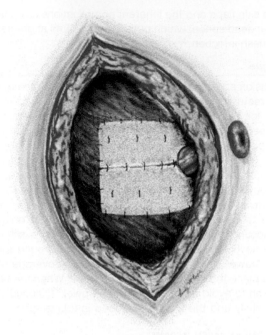

Fig. 2. Onlay mesh sutured in place. (*From* Franks ME, Hrebinko RL. Technique of parastomal hernia repair using synthetic mesh. Urology 2001;57(3):551–3; with permission.)

for the intraperitoneal mesh repairs, because the mesh will be in contact with the viscera. The mesh can be positioned with either the keyhole configuration or with the modified Sugarbaker technique (**Fig. 3**), such that the stoma passes under the lateral edge of the mesh.[37,38] By placing the mesh in an intraperitoneal location via

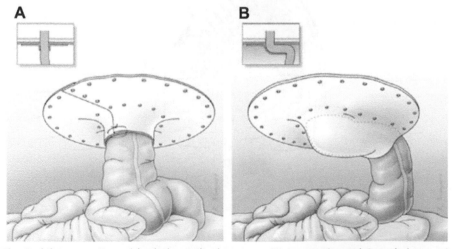

Fig. 3. (*A*) Intraperitoneal keyhole mesh placement. (*B*) Intraperitoneal Sugarbaker mesh placement. (*From* Hansson BME, Slater NJ, van der Velden AS, et al. Surgical techniques for parastomal hernia repair: a systematic review of the literature. Ann Surg 2012;255(4):685–95; with permission.)

a midline incision, it is possible to decrease potential contact with the stoma.[39] Thus, there is theoretically less risk of contamination of the wound and prosthetic material.[38,39] However, this technique places the mesh in contact with the proximal bowel, risking fibrosis, adhesions, and erosion.[38]

It has been shown that, over time, mesh contracts, and subsequently the orifice placed in the mesh for the stoma to pass can enlarge, which may result in higher recurrence rates if the keyhole method is used.[38,40] The modified Sugarbaker technique avoids this problem by lateralizing the bowel, allowing for intact mesh to be used in the repair.[38,39] Sugarbaker's original experience with the technique was excellent, citing low mesh complication rates and no recurrences.[39] However, there are limited data directly comparing the 2 methods of mesh placement in the open technique.

The intraperitoneal keyhole technique has been found to have a mesh infection rate of 2.2% and a wound infection rate of 2.2%.[21] Recurrence rates range between 0.0% and 28.6%, with an overall recurrence rate of 7.2% on metaanalysis.[21,31,41–43] However, all published series had small sample sizes, with the largest study entailing only 16 patients.[31,41–43] In comparison, the intraperitoneal Sugarbaker technique using ePTFE mesh published by Stelzner and colleagues[38] showed a wound infection rate of 5%, no mesh infections, and a recurrence rate of 15% in 20 patients.

Operative Technique: Keyhole

A midline incision is used to enter the abdomen and adhesiolysis is performed to reduce the contents of the hernia sac.[31] If there is a concurrent incisional hernia, its contents should also be dissected free. Adhesiolysis should be continued, so that there are no adhesions to the posterior abdominal wall.[43] At this point, there are 2 options when dealing with the stoma—either it can be taken down and eventually rematured or left in situ. The hernia sac is resected when possible and the parastomal fascial defect is closed posteriorly. The fascial opening at the stoma site should not be overly tight or too loose after reapproximation.[31] The repair is then reinforced with mesh, placing it against the peritoneum so that there is extensive coverage of both the parastomal hernia and the midline incision.[31,43] If the stoma has been taken down, then a small keyhole is created in the mesh through which the stoma is delivered. The bowel is then brought through all layers of the abdominal wall. Care must be maintained to prevent twisting or kinking of the bowel or its mesentery. If the ostomy has remained in place, then a lateral slit is created and wrapped around the stoma.[43] The 2 tails are reapproximated with nonabsorbable suture, which is then run medially to create a keyhole of the appropriate size.[31,43] The mesh is secured circumferentially to the posterior rectus sheath with interrupted transfascial sutures.[43] The abdomen is then closed in layers using the standard technique. Postoperatively, the patient is managed similarly to other laparotomy cases.[31]

Operative Technique: Modified Sugarbaker

The technique used for the open intraperitoneal Sugarbaker repair is initially similar to that described, except for the placement of the mesh. Adhesiolysis, dissection of the hernia sac, and fascial defect approximation are performed as with the open keyhole technique. The bowel—either colon or small intestine—that is immediately proximal to the stoma is then lateralized and fixed to the abdominal wall. The fascial defect and lateralized colon are then covered with mesh, making sure there is an overlap of at least 5 cm in all directions. Using either interrupted or running suture, the mesh is fixed dorsolaterally, allowing the bowel to enter between the mesh and peritoneum without restriction.[38] The remaining 3 edges of the mesh are then secured using transfascial sutures.[38] The abdomen is closed in layers using a standard technique.

RETROMUSCULAR MESH REPAIR

The retromuscular repair involves placement of the mesh posterior to the rectus muscle.[8,21] This approach avoids intraperitoneal placement of mesh and the potential complications of adhesions to the mesh, erosion, or fistula formation.[35] The retromuscular technique is a reasonable consideration if there are concomitant midline hernias, because it allows for wide coverage of multiple defects and can simultaneously address all such defects.[44] This approach is also a good option for multiply recurrent parastomal hernias.[44] This operation is technically challenging, and should not be undertaken by surgeons who are unfamiliar with posterior component separation techniques.[44]

Rosen and colleagues[17] described stoma relocation, posterior component separation, and retrorectus placement of mesh with the new stoma being placed through a keyhole in the mesh. In doing so, the old stoma site is repaired with mesh and the new stoma site and midline are similarly reinforced. In their small series, they reported 1 surgical site infection (8.3%), no mesh infections, and 1 asymptomatic hernia recurrence (8.3%).[17] Similarly, in 1 metaanalysis of such cases, there were no mesh infections and a 4.8% incidence of wound infections using the retromuscular technique.[21] Recurrence rates ranged between 0.0% and 28.6%. However, the pooled recurrence rate was found to be a very reasonable 6.9%.[21,32,45,46]

Pauli and colleagues[44] reported their experience using a transversus abdominis release (TAR) with retromuscular mesh placement using a modified Sugarbaker configuration. In their original series, they reported no stoma-related complications, mesh erosions, or obstructions. However, in a recent study by Tastaldi and colleagues,[47] mesh erosions occurred in 8% of cases and the recurrence rate was not significantly different than the retromuscular keyhole repair.

Operative Technique: Retromuscular Mesh Repair (Keyhole Mesh Placement with and Without Transversus Abdominis Release)

The use of the TAR technique described by Rosen and associates[17] for parastomal hernia repair has been an important development in the treatment of this difficult patient population. The approach allows for optimal wide mesh coverage of all defects. Subsequent closure of the posterior sheath limits the contact between the mesh and the bowel to only a small portion of the stoma as it passes through the abdominal wall.

After entering the abdomen through a generous midline incision, all adhesions to the abdominal wall should be taken down.[8,21] Adhesiolysis should be continued around the stoma to optimize exposure of the involved loop of bowel.[32] The hernia sac is dissected free and reduced as much as possible, whereas the ostomy is left in situ.[48] Just lateral to the linea alba, the posterior sheath is incised and the retrorectus space is developed out to the semilunar line (**Fig. 4**), while taking care to preserve the neurovascular bundles.[17,32,44,48] In such cases, developing the space for optimal mesh underlay may be quite difficult owing to the variable location of stomas through the rectus muscle as well as the size of the parastomal hernia component. Subsequently, a space is created superior and inferior to the ostomy, so that dissection lateral to the stoma can be completed eventually.[45] Just medial to the linea semilunaris, the posterior lamella of the internal oblique is incised and a TAR is performed (**Fig. 5**). Dissection can be performed laterally to the psoas muscle if necessary for optimal mesh overlap. This maneuver allows for the isolation of the stoma as it traverses the abdominal wall, as well as for optimal visualization of the hernia defect on the affected side. Often, a TAR is not necessary on the contralateral side and a simple retrorectus dissection is enough to ultimately reinforce the midline fascial closure.

A

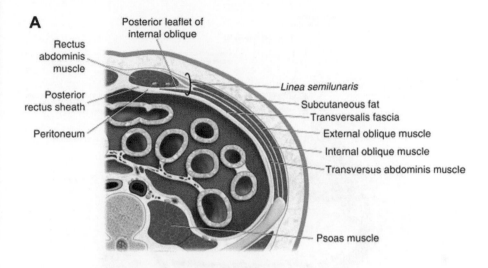

Rectus
abdominis
muscle

Posterior leaflet of
internal oblique

Posterior
rectus sheath

Peritoneum

Linea semilunaris

Subcutaneous fat

Transversalis fascia

External oblique muscle

Internal oblique muscle

Transversus abdominis muscle

Psoas muscle

B

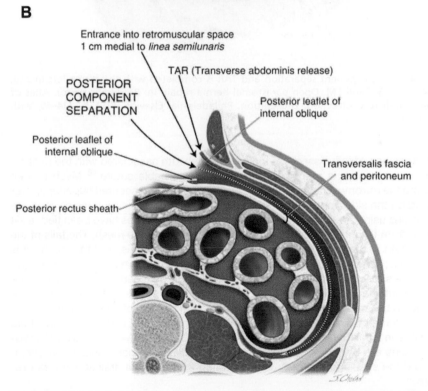

Entrance into retromuscular space
1 cm medial to *linea semilunaris*

TAR (Transverse abdominis release)

POSTERIOR
COMPONENT
SEPARATION

Posterior leaflet of
internal oblique

Posterior leaflet of
internal oblique

Transversalis fascia
and peritoneum

Posterior rectus sheath

Fig. 4. (*A*) Normal abdominal wall anatomy. (*B*) Dissection plane for retromuscular repair. (*From* Winder JS, Pauli EM. Open parastomal hernia repair. In: Rosen MJ, editor. Atlas of abdominal wall reconstruction. 2nd edition. Philadelphia: Elsevier; 2017. p. 124–49; with permission.)

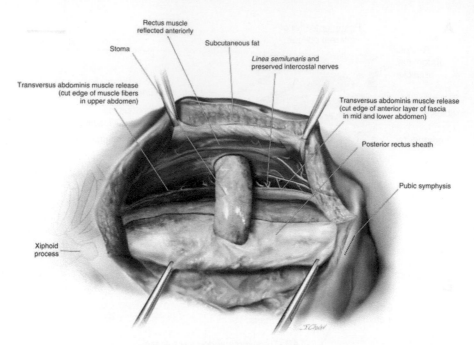

Fig. 5. Posterior component separation and TAR is completed with the stoma left in situ. (*From* Winder JS, Pauli EM. Open parastomal hernia repair. In: Rosen MJ, editor. Atlas of abdominal wall reconstruction. 2nd edition. Philadelphia: Elsevier; 2017. p. 124–49; with permission.)

Upon completion of this dissection, the posterior sheath associated with the midline, as well as the hernia, is reapproximated using absorbable suture.[48] Mesh is then placed into the retromuscular space (**Fig. 6**).[32,45] The mesh is secured superiorly, inferiorly, and on the side opposite the stoma using absorbable suture through separate stab incisions using the suture passing device. Once the sutures have been tied, a slit is created from the site of the ostomy to the lateral edge of the mesh. The tails of the mesh are then secured laterally with further transfascial sutures, and the mesh slit is reapproximated back toward the stoma with a permanent running stitch, being cognizant that the subsequent orifice is neither too tight nor too loose.[32,48] Of course, care must be maintained to prevent twisting or kinking of the stoma or its mesentery. The mesh should be large enough to allow for a minimum of 5 cm of overlap of the fascial defects in all directions.[17] After placement, the mesh should cover any potential old stoma sites in addition to reinforcing the midline and the new stoma site. Closed-suction drains are placed above the mesh. The midline anterior fascia is reapproximated and the skin is closed. The drains are left in place until drainage is less than 30 mL/d.[48]

Retromuscular Mesh Repair with Transversus Abdominis Release and Sugarbaker

Recently described by Pauli, this approach was developed to combine the benefits of the relatively new TAR with the advantages of the Sugarbaker technique.[39] The procedure is the same as described for the retromuscular keyhole repair as described, up until the point of mesh placement. The mesh is not slit nor is a keyhole necessary. The dissection creates a large retromuscular plane where the only structure traversing

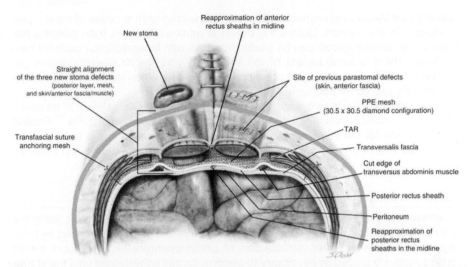

Fig. 6. Retromuscular placement of the mesh, allowing for wide coverage of the parastomal hernia and any abdominal wall defects. TAR, transversus abdominis release. (*From* Winder JS, Pauli EM. Open parastomal hernia repair. In: Rosen MJ, editor. Atlas of abdominal wall reconstruction. 2nd edition. Philadelphia: Elsevier; 2017. p. 124–49; with permission.)

the abdominal wall is the lateralized stoma. This allows for the creation of a large mesh tunnel. The mesh is then positioned with the modified Sugarbaker configuration as described, using a transfascial suture passer to secure the mesh in place with absorbable sutures around the periphery. The parastomal fascial defect is closed primarily and the abdomen is then closed in the midline by suturing the anterior rectus sheaths together.[44] The subcutaneous tissue and skin are closed using a standard technique. Drains are placed as with the retrorectus keyhole technique and remain in place until the output is appropriate.

Just as proposed by Pauli and colleagues,[44] it has been our preference to use medium weight polypropylene mesh for the retromuscular repair. Most papers report using either lightweight or medium weight polypropylene mesh for this technique.[45,46,48] As previously described, given the contamination associated with parastomal hernia repair, there remains continued interest in using biologic mesh.[17]

LAPAROSCOPIC INTRAPERITONEAL MESH REPAIR

Laparoscopic hernia repair involves a minimally invasive approach to the intraperitoneal placement of mesh, with or without approximation of the parastomal fascial defect.[21] The mesh can be placed using either the keyhole or Sugarbaker configuration.

The laparoscopic approach avoids stoma relocation and has fewer wound-related complications owing to the avoidance of a large incision and the potential associated wound morbidity. The minimal access approach also is associated with the added benefits of less postoperative pain, reduced morbidity, shorter duration of stay, and earlier return to work.[49] Laparoscopy allows for the concurrent repair of incisional hernias at the time of operation.[50] Additionally, the published rate of conversion to open is rare, only 3.6% in metaanalysis.[21,50] However, not all parastomal hernias are amenable to laparoscopic repair. Large and incarcerated hernias may be better approached via an open technique.[44] With time, the surgical community has come to accept that fascial approximation is crucial for the long-term success of most types of incisional hernia repairs. Unless the defect is particularly small, then bringing the edges of the fascia together can be problematic. As with laparoscopic incisional hernia repairs, there is some benefit of the so-called hybrid repair whereby the larger defect is reapproximated using an open approach, which is then reinforced with a laparoscopically placed intraperitoneal mesh.

On metaanalysis, the laparoscopic parastomal hernia repair was shown to be associated with a wound infection rate of 3.3% and a mesh infection rate of 2.7%.[21] Pooled recurrence rate for the laparoscopic Sugarbaker technique was found to be significantly lower than the laparoscopic keyhole technique on metaanalysis (11.6% vs 34.6%).[21]

Operative Technique: Laparoscopic Keyhole Technique

Laparoscopically, the abdomen is usually entered contralateral to the stoma, using the preferred approach of the surgeon. However, the entry site may be influenced by prior surgical procedures.[51] After introduction of pneumoperitoneum, additional 5-mm working ports are placed as necessary to perform careful adhesiolysis until the stoma and the abdominal wall are completely dissected free.[50] The ability to visualize potentially occult hernias is an important benefit of the laparoscopic approach. Using the suture passer and small stab incisions, the fascial defects are reapproximated with nonabsorbable suture. As always, care must be maintained to prevent the stoma fascial opening from being either too tight or too loose.[51] Fascial closure may also be attained using a limited overlying incision, with the understanding that this will be reinforced with the hybrid approach as discussed. Usually, a piece of composite mesh is chosen for the repair. In preparation, stay sutures are placed around the periphery of the mesh. A slit is then created in the mesh, and one such suture is placed on each tail. This is then rolled and placed into the abdomen through a trocar and is unfurled. The mesh is then positioned to allow for a 5-cm overlap of the defect,[52] and a keyhole configuration is attained by wrapping the tails around the stoma.[51] These stay sutures are then grasped by the suture passer and sequentially secured. Traditionally, a combination of both tacks and sutures are used to secure the mesh to the posterior abdominal wall.[52] The pneumoperitoneum is then released and the port sites are closed in the usual fashion.

Operative Technique: Laparoscopic Modified Sugarbaker Technique

The technique used for the laparoscopic Sugarbaker repair is initially similar to that listed, again except for the mesh placement. Location of the ports, adhesiolysis, and fascial defect approximation are performed. The bowel proximal to the stoma is lateralized and fixated to the posterior abdominal wall using nonabsorbable suture. Such stitches are placed either extracorporally or intracorporally, based on the surgeon's comfort with the technique. The mesh, obviously without a slit, again is prepared with circumferential stay sutures, before placing it into the abdomen. The mesh is placed and secured intraperitoneally, such that there is adequate overlap of the fascial defect, the stoma, and the lateralized bowel.[50] By placing the mesh in this configuration, a tunnel is created between the abdominal wall and the mesh, through which the lateralized bowel travels.[50] The mesh on either side of the lateralized bowel should be secured first, taking care to avoid making the tunnel overly tight.[52] Similarly, it is important to avoid acute angulation of the bowel as it courses toward the stoma. The repair is then reinforced further with tacks as necessary. The abdomen is desufflated, and the port sites are closed in the standard manner.

ROBOTIC PARASTOMAL HERNIA REPAIR

The use of the robot has become the latest development in the field of abdominal wall reconstruction. The robotic platform may be of benefit in complex parastomal hernia repairs, because it offers articulating instruments with more degrees of freedom. Indeed, over the past few years, this technology has become an area of rapid growth in all aspects of hernia repair—both intraperitoneal and retrorectus. Although there are currently no large published series regarding the use of the robot for parastomal hernia repairs, this approach has been implemented in ventral hernia repairs with increasing popularity. A recent study comparing the laparoscopic and robotic approaches for intraperitoneal mesh placement in incisional hernia repairs showed longer operative times and shorter durations of stay for the robotic group.[53] Such results reinforce the experience of many diverse procedures in many different specialties performed with the robot—specifically whether or not the more rapid recovery justifies the longer case time. Furthermore, in today's climate of cost containment, there remains controversy as to the overall cost of the robot itself, which also needs to be taken into consideration. Clearly, further studies are necessary to determine the quality and efficacy of this platform.

SUMMARY

Parastomal hernias are common complications after ostomy formation that can require surgical repair when they become symptomatic. Operative planning and a thorough understanding of the anatomy of the abdominal wall is of utmost importance, as such repairs can be quite complex.

Simple fascial repair is associated with an unacceptably high recurrence rate and, therefore, should mainly be used in urgent situations as a temporizing measure until a more definitive repair can be performed. Stoma relocation also has a high recurrence rate, both at the old and the new ostomy site. To help mitigate this situation, prophylactic mesh can and should then be used. At this time, the use of mesh—be it synthetic or biologic—clearly is considered to be the standard of care in the repair of parastomal hernias.

Given the lower recurrence rates and acceptable infection risks when compared with biologic reinforcement in incisional hernias associated with contaminated fields, there is literature to support the use of synthetic mesh in such cases. By extrapolating such results, synthetic mesh can be considered a reasonable option in the repair of parastomal hernias, be it placed in the onlay, retromuscular, or intraperitoneal position. However, because of the concern for contamination, biologic mesh remains a popular choice in parastomal hernia repair. Trials are ongoing that will ultimately determine the optimal type of mesh to be used in such complex cases. With these trials, the comparative rates of infection and recurrence, as well as total costs, will have to be carefully considered.

As we have described, there are multiple approaches to repair parastomal hernias with mesh. The open and the laparoscopic mesh repairs are both reasonable options and have shown favorable wound and mesh infection rates. At present, it is difficult to draw conclusions regarding the preferred approach and position of mesh placement based on the available literature, which consists mainly of small retrospective studies. With time, however, controlled trials will eventually assist the surgical community in determining the best technique for these repairs—with the acceptance that all such patients can be very different and a tailored approach to each individual patient is crucial. For this reason, as surgeons, it is and remains imperative that we are comfortable with several of these techniques. Indeed, parastomal hernia repair is a complex case that requires a thorough understanding of all approaches and options in our ultimate quest to find a durable and long-lasting repair for this patient population.

REFERENCES

1. Pearl RK. Parastomal hernias. World J Surg 1989;13(5):569–72.
2. Carlsson E, Fingren J, Hallén A-M, et al. The prevalence of ostomy-related complications 1 year after ostomy surgery: a prospective, descriptive, clinical study. Ostomy Wound Manage 2016;62(10):34–48.
3. Londono-Schimmer EE, Leong AP, Phillips RK. Life table analysis of stomal complications following colostomy. Dis Colon Rectum 1994;37(9):916–20.
4. Glasgow SC, Dharmarajan S. Parastomal hernia: avoidance and treatment in the 21st century. Clin Colon Rectal Surg 2016;29(3):277–84.
5. Israelsson LA. Parastomal hernias. Surg Clin North Am 2008;88(1):113–25, ix.
6. Carne PWG, Robertson GM, Frizelle FA. Parastomal hernia. Br J Surg 2003;90(7): 784–93.
7. Scarpa M, Ruffolo C, Boetto R, et al. Diverting loop ileostomy after restorative proctocolectomy: predictors of poor outcome and poor quality of life. Colorectal Dis 2010;12(9):914–20.
8. Aquina CT, Iannuzzi JC, Probst CP, et al. Parastomal hernia: a growing problem with new solutions. Dig Surg 2014;31(4–5):366–76.
9. Turnbull GB. Ostomy statistics: the $64,000 question. Ostomy Wound Manage 2003;49(6):22–3.
10. Hendren S, Hammond K, Glasgow SC, et al. Clinical practice guidelines for ostomy surgery. Dis Colon Rectum 2015;58(4):375–87.
11. Kald A, Juul KN, Hjortsvang H, et al. Quality of life is impaired in patients with peristomal bulging of a sigmoid colostomy. Scand J Gastroenterol 2008;43(5): 627–33.
12. Gurmu A, Matthiessen P, Nilsson S, et al. The inter-observer reliability is very low at clinical examination of parastomal hernia. Int J Colorectal Dis 2011;26(1): 89–95.
13. Williams JG, Etherington R, Hayward MW, et al. Paraileostomy hernia: a clinical and radiological study. Br J Surg 1990;77(12):1355–7.
14. Kane M, McErlean D, McGrogan M, et al. Clinical protocols for stoma care: 6. Management of parastomal hernia. Nurs Stand 2004;18(19):43–4.
15. Erwin-Toth P, Thompson SJ, Davis JS. Factors impacting the quality of life of people with an ostomy in North America: results from the Dialogue Study. J Wound Ostomy Continence Nurs 2012;39(4):417–22 [quiz: 423–4].
16. Israelsson LA. Preventing and treating parastomal hernia. World J Surg 2005; 29(8):1086–9.
17. Rosen MJ, Reynolds HL, Champagne B, et al. A novel approach for the simultaneous repair of large midline incisional and parastomal hernias with biological mesh and retrorectus reconstruction. Am J Surg 2010;199(3):416–20 [discussion: 420–1].
18. Reynolds HL. Open repair of parastomal hernias. In: Atlas of abdominal wall reconstruction. 1st edition. Philadelphia: Elsevier; 2012. Available at: https://expertconsult.inkling.com/read/rosen-atlas-abdominal-wall-reconstruction-1st/chapter-7/1–introduction. Accessed June 19, 2017.
19. Amin SN, Armitage NC, Abercrombie JF, et al. Lateral repair of parastomal hernia. Ann R Coll Surg Engl 2001;83(3):206–8.

20. Kald A, Landin S, Masreliez C, et al. Mesh repair of parastomal hernias: new aspects of the Onlay technique. Tech Coloproctol 2001;5(3):169–71.
21. Hansson BME, Slater NJ, van der Velden AS, et al. Surgical techniques for parastomal hernia repair: a systematic review of the literature. Ann Surg 2012;255(4): 685–95.
22. Rubin MS, Schoetz DJ, Matthews JB. Parastomal hernia. Is stoma relocation superior to fascial repair? Arch Surg 1994;129(4):413–8 [discussion: 418–9].
23. Allen-Mersh TG, Thomson JP. Surgical treatment of colostomy complications. Br J Surg 1988;75(5):416–8.
24. Stephenson BM, Phillips RK. Parastomal hernia: local resiting and mesh repair. Br J Surg 1995;82(10):1395–6.
25. Sjödahl R, Anderberg B, Bolin T. Parastomal hernia in relation to site of the abdominal stoma. Br J Surg 1988;75(4):339–41.
26. Rosen MJ, Krpata DM, Ermlich B, et al. A 5-year clinical experience with single-staged repairs of infected and contaminated abdominal wall defects utilizing biologic mesh. Ann Surg 2013;257(6):991–6.
27. Carbonell AM, Criss CN, Cobb WS, et al. Outcomes of synthetic mesh in contaminated ventral hernia repairs. J Am Coll Surg 2013;217(6):991–8.
28. Venditti D, Gargiani M, Milito G. Parastomal hernia surgery: personal experience with use of polypropylene mesh. Tech Coloproctol 2001;5(2):85–8.
29. Franks ME, Hrebinko RL. Technique of parastomal hernia repair using synthetic mesh. Urology 2001;57(3):551–3.
30. Ho KMT, Fawcett DP. Parastomal hernia repair using the lateral approach. BJU Int 2004;94(4):598–602.
31. Hofstetter WL, Vukasin P, Ortega AE, et al. New technique for mesh repair of paracolostomy hernias. Dis Colon Rectum 1998;41(8):1054–5.
32. Kasperk R, Klinge U, Schumpelick V. The repair of large parastomal hernias using a midline approach and a prosthetic mesh in the sublay position. Am J Surg 2000;179(3):186–8.
33. Brown CN, Finch JG. Which mesh for hernia repair? Ann R Coll Surg Engl 2010; 92(4):272–8.
34. Schreinemacher MHF, van Barneveld KWY, Dikmans REG, et al. Coated meshes for hernia repair provide comparable intraperitoneal adhesion prevention. Surg Endosc 2013;27(11):4202–9.
35. Hotouras A, Murphy J, Thaha M, et al. The persistent challenge of parastomal herniation: a review of the literature and future developments. Colorectal Dis 2013; 15(5):e202–14.
36. Bröker M, Verdaasdonk E, Karsten T. Components separation technique combined with a double-mesh repair for large midline incisional hernia repair. World J Surg 2011;35(11):2399–402.
37. Al Shakarchi J, Williams JG. Systematic review of open techniques for parastomal hernia repair. Tech Coloproctol 2014;18(5):427–32.
38. Stelzner S, Hellmich G, Ludwig K. Repair of paracolostomy hernias with a prosthetic mesh in the intraperitoneal onlay position: modified Sugarbaker technique. Dis Colon Rectum 2004;47(2):185–91.
39. Sugarbaker PH. Peritoneal approach to prosthetic mesh repair of paraostomy hernias. Ann Surg 1985;201(3):344–6.
40. de Ruiter P, Bijnen AB. Successful local repair of paracolostomy hernia with a newly developed prosthetic device. Int J Colorectal Dis 1992;7(3):132–4.
41. Byers JM, Steinberg JB, Postier RG. Repair of parastomal hernias using polypropylene mesh. Arch Surg 1992;127(10):1246–7.

42. Morris-Stiff G, Hughes LE. The continuing challenge of parastomal hernia: failure of a novel polypropylene mesh repair. Ann R Coll Surg Engl 1998;80(3):184–7.

43. van Sprundel TC, Gerritsen van der Hoop A. Modified technique for parastomal hernia repair in patients with intractable stoma-care problems. Colorectal Dis 2005;7(5):445–9.

44. Pauli EM, Juza RM, Winder JS. How I do it: novel parastomal herniorrhaphy utilizing transversus abdominis release. Hernia 2016;20(4):547–52.

45. Longman RJ, Thomson WH. Mesh repair of parastomal hernias–a safety modification. Colorectal Dis 2005;7(3):292–4.

46. Guzmán-Valdivia G, Guerrero TS, Laurrabaquio HV. Parastomal hernia-repair using mesh and an open technique. World J Surg 2008;32(3):465–70.

47. Tastaldi L, Haskins IN, Perez AJ, et al. Single center experience with the modified retromuscular Sugarbaker technique for parastomal hernia repair. Hernia 2017; 21(6):941–9.

48. Fei YA. modified sublay-keyhole technique for in situ parastomal hernia repair. Surg Today 2012;42(9):842–7.

49. Safadi B. Laparoscopic repair of parastomal hernias: early results. Surg Endosc 2004;18(4):676–80.

50. Hansson BME, Morales-Conde S, Mussack T, et al. The laparoscopic modified Sugarbaker technique is safe and has a low recurrence rate: a multicenter cohort study. Surg Endosc 2013;27(2):494–500.

51. Jani K. Laparoscopic paracolostomy hernia repair: a retrospective case series at a tertiary care center. Surg Laparosc Endosc Percutan Tech 2010;20(6):395–8.

52. Yang X, He K, Hua R, et al. Laparoscopic repair of parastomal hernia. Ann Transl Med 2017;5(3):45.

53. Prabhu AS, Dickens EO, Copper CM, et al. Laparoscopic vs robotic intraperitoneal mesh repair for incisional hernia: an Americas Hernia Society Quality Collaborative analysis. J Am Coll Surg 2017;225(2):285–93.

Flank and Lumbar Hernia Repair

Lucas R. Beffa, MD, Alyssa L. Margiotta, MS, Alfredo M. Carbonell, DO*

KEYWORDS

- Lumbar hernia • Flank hernia • Hernia repair • Robotic • Preperitoneal • Mesh

KEY POINTS

- Lumbar and flank hernias may be either congenital or acquired.
- Large and deforming defects may be best approached open with preperitoneal mesh placement and wide mesh overlap. Smaller defects in those with increased wound morbidity risk are more appropriate for robotic transabdominal preperitoneal repair.
- Surgeons should have a keen understanding of the anatomy of the lateral abdominal wall muscles, the paraspinal and pelvic musculature, and the location of retroperitoneal nerves.
- Although the optimal mesh fixation technique is debatable, wide mesh overlap and potential fixation to bone in addition to percutaneous transfascial sutures is recommended.

INTRODUCTION: NATURE OF THE PROBLEM

Lateral hernias are subclassified into four regions: subcostal (L1), flank (L2), iliac (L3), and lumbar (L4). This article discusses flank hernias that occur lateral to the rectus sheath and lumbar hernias, which are uncommon defects of the posterolateral abdominal wall.[1] Often there is significant overlap with classification, and sometimes these defined anatomic compartments are difficult to differentiate. Although classification of these hernias based on size and location is important to track outcomes, classification also provides a reliable and consistent platform for communication between surgeons and investigators. Nevertheless, the specific location may have little impact on choice of approach or clinical outcomes.

There have been a mere 300 cases of lumbar hernias reported in the literature to date.[2] This is likely because of the rare nature of these defects. Additionally, lumbar hernias are often misdiagnosed as lipomas, fibromas, or muscle strains. The lumbar

Disclosure: Dr. A.M. Carbonell has received teaching honoraria from Intuitive Surgical Corporation. The other authors have nothing to disclose.
Division of Minimal Access and Bariatric Surgery, Greenville Health System, University of South Carolina School of Medicine – Greenville, Greenville, SC, USA
* Corresponding author. Division of Minimal Access and Bariatric Surgery, Greenville Health System, University of South Carolina School of Medicine – Greenville, 701 Grove Road, Greenville, SC 29605.
E-mail address: acarbonell@ghs.org

Surg Clin N Am 98 (2018) 593–605
https://doi.org/10.1016/j.suc.2018.01.009
0039-6109/18/© 2018 Elsevier Inc. All rights reserved.

surgical.theclinics.com

region is defined by the 12th rib superiorly, the erector spinae muscle medially, the iliac crest inferiorly, with the external oblique muscle acting as the lateral border. The anatomic borders of the superior lumbar triangle where a Grynfeltt hernia occurs is defined by the 12th rib, quadratus lumborum, and external oblique. The anatomic borders of the inferior lumbar triangle where Petit hernias occur is defined by the iliac crest, latissimus dorsi, and the external oblique muscle.[3]

These defects may be either congenital or acquired. Congenital lumbar hernias are typically discovered during infancy or early childhood and are associated with other birth defects, such as hydrometrocolpos and anorectal malformations.[4] Congenital lumbar hernias account for approximately 20% of all lumbar hernias, whereas the remaining 80% of lumbar hernias are acquired.[5] Acquired lumbar and flank hernias are either primary (spontaneous) or secondary (trauma or surgery). Primary (spontaneous) flank hernias account for approximately 55% of flank hernias.[6] Conditions that cause increased intra-abdominal pressure, chronic debilitating disease, extreme thinness, or increased aging can result in the formation of a primary flank hernia.[2] Secondary flank hernias make up 25% of flank hernias and usually present after a surgical incision or traumatic event.[7] The most common incisions associated with this type of hernia include flank incisions for nephrectomy or hepatic resections, abdominal aortic aneurysm repair, resection of abdominal wall tumors, iliac bone harvest, and latissimus dorsi flaps used during plastic reconstructive surgery.[8–12] It is theorized that secondary flank hernias arise as a combination of multiple factors. Transection or damage to the nerves that originate laterally from the spine and innervate the abdominal wall is believed to play a major role in the formation of these hernias. This denervation leads to muscular atrophy, creating a weakness or bulging effect in the lumbar triangle or flank that ultimately manifests as a lumbar or flank hernia.[12,13] Surgical incisions are not the sole cause of these secondary flank hernias. Traumatic events, such as avulsion of soft tissues and muscles from their bony attachments, crush injuries, fractures of the iliac crest and pelvis, and incidents that cause sudden increased intra-abdominal pressure, such as high-speed motor vehicle collision with rapid deceleration by seat belt restraint, are also common causes of secondary flank hernias.[7]

As with most hernia surgery, indications for operative repair are based largely on patient symptoms. If there is concern for incarceration or bowel obstruction because of the hernia defect, then repair is mandated either emergently or electively depending on the clinical situation. Patients who present with these hernias usually complain of pain and bulging. If the hernia is interfering with the patient's daily activities, then repair is also recommended. Bulging of the lateral abdominal wall improves with hernia repair. However, the repair rarely results in exact symmetry with the contralateral side. Patients should have this expectation managed preoperatively. The risk of bowel incarceration or a true hernia emergency of lumbar or flank hernias is extremely rare with only a few case reports in the literature. Therefore, repair of these defects if completely asymptomatic is not recommended.

In summary, lateral abdominal wall hernias are a challenge to the general surgeon, with lack of high-quality data to drive operative decision making. The anatomy, location of the defect, cause, and difficulty with mesh placement/fixation because of bony landmarks and neurovascular structures make repair difficult. The risk of incarceration for flank or lumbar hernias is rare (<10%) because of the wide neck of the hernia orifice and location within the abdominal wall itself.[2,14] However, these hernias may become more symptomatic as they grow larger over time and therefore, surgical correction is recommended when a patient presents with a symptomatic hernia.

SURGICAL TECHNIQUE
Preoperative Planning and Patient Selection

Imaging of the abdominal wall is critical in determining the size and location of the defect. Computed tomography scans are an excellent and reliable imaging modality for determining the anatomic relationships within the lumbar area.[15] These defects are approached either open or using a minimally invasive technique. Many of these fascial defects are small and thus amenable to a simple laparoscopic intraperitoneal mesh hernia repair.[16] Our preference, however, is to place mesh extraperitoneal, whether that is performed open or robotic. Patients with large hernia defects (>15 cm), significant herniated visceral mass, thin atrophic skin, or large dystrophic scars are approached open in our practice, because this allows for proper management of the skin and soft tissue. We reserve robotic preperitoneal repair for smaller defects in patients with a high risk of wound complications, such as the obese, active smokers, and patients with poorly controlled diabetes. In our opinion, the robotic approach confers the benefit of extraperitoneal mesh placement, similar to open surgery, with a minimally invasive approach and its attendant low wound morbidity.

Preparation and Patient Positioning

The patient is placed in a lateral decubitus position using a bean bag, ensuring the midline remains exposed for adequate transfascial suture fixation. If a robotic approach is chosen, we prefer a semilateral decubitus position to gain better trocar access to the abdominal cavity.

Surgical Procedure (Open Technique)

The open surgical technique is as follows:

  Step one: The patient is positioned in the lateral decubitus position using a bean bag for stabilization of the torso. The bed is flexed to widen the space between the costal margin and iliac crest (**Fig. 1**).

  Step two: The surgical incision is made through the previous incision, or directly over the defect if no previous surgical interventions have been performed.

  Step three: Dissection is carried down to the hernia sac, and the hernia sac is circumferentially dissected free from the surrounding fascial edges or bony structures depending on location of the hernia. The hernia sac is typically entered, although not necessarily in all cases. Lysis of adhesions is carried out until the

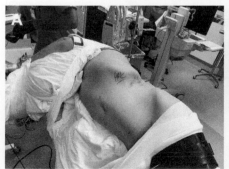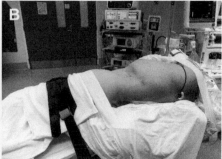

Fig. 1. (*A*) Lateral decubitus positioning of patient with the help of a bean bag. (*B*) Posterior view of lateral decubitus position.

bowel or omentum falls back into the abdominal cavity, thus protecting the viscera during preperitoneal dissection. Once the visceral contents are safely freed, the hernia defect is then measured.

Step four: The preperitoneal plane is developed starting at the junction of the fascial edge and hernia sac (**Figs. 2** and **3**). During large or loss of domain flank hernia repairs, it may be beneficial to keep one side (or both sides) of the hernia sac attached to the peritoneum. This provides valuable tissue coverage when closing the visceral sac. This plane is developed out for a minimum of 5 cm in all directions of the hernia defect edge. This dissection typically includes exposing the psoas muscle and tendon posteriorly, iliac crest inferiorly, underneath costal margin to expose diaphragmatic muscle fibers, and medially to the border of the rectus muscle.

Step five: The peritoneum is then inspected for any holes created during dissection, and those larger than 1 cm are reapproximated with absorbable suture. Next, the peritoneum is closed with a running, slowly absorbable suture. The bed is then unflexed, which allows for more accurate measurement of the preperitoneal pocket (**Fig. 4**). A mid-weight, macroporous, uncoated polypropylene mesh is selected and shaped to the appropriate size of this pocket (**Fig. 5**).

Step six: The mesh is fixated in place. If choosing to fixate to the iliac crest, permanent bone anchors with permanent suture may be placed on the inner table of the iliac crest. If fixating to the costal margin, ensure that mesh extends beyond the ribs and covers the exposed diaphragmatic fibers. Multiple slowly absorbable sutures are used to suture directly through the cartilaginous edge of the rib (**Fig. 6**). Posteriorly, the mesh is fixated to the psoas tendon with slowly absorbable suture. Medially, the mesh is fixated using transfascial, slowly absorbable sutures. A closed suction drain is then placed directly on top of the mesh, and brought through the skin medially.

Step seven: The hernia defect is then closed with a slowly absorbable suture using a small stitch technique (**Fig. 7**). Redundant and attenuated muscle is excised to eliminate lateral bulging after repair. Alternatively, the muscles are first closed and the closure imbricated to minimize laxity (**Figs. 8** and **9**).

Step eight: If a skin flap was created for muscular plication, a closed suction drain is placed on top of the fascia in the subcutaneous space. Skin is reapproximated in two layers with absorbable sutures and skin glue (**Fig. 10**).

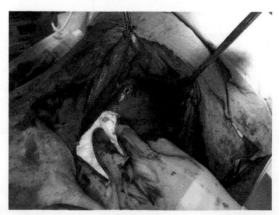

Fig. 2. Preperitoneal plane being developed. Fascial edges grasped with Allis clamps.

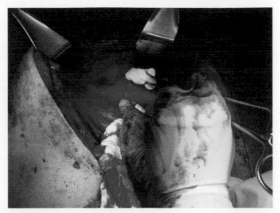

Fig. 3. Preperitoneal pocket being developed bluntly. Transversus abdominis muscle being retracted.

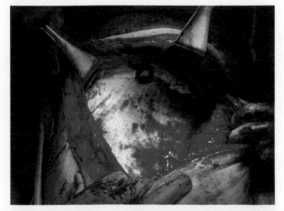

Fig. 4. Completed preperitoneal dissection. Pocket for mesh is demonstrated by the sponge.

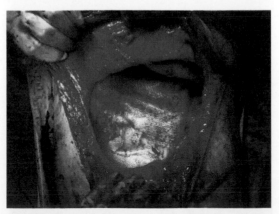

Fig. 5. Uncoated polypropylene mesh placed into the preperitoneal plane with mesh overlap under the costal margin.

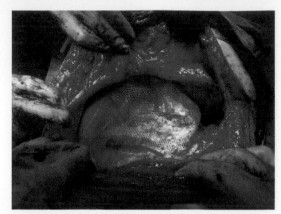

Fig. 6. Mesh is sewn directly to the costal margin with multiple interrupted slowly absorbable sutures.

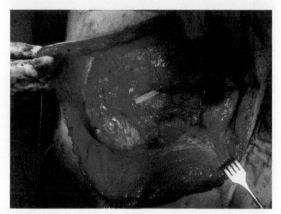

Fig. 7. Skin flaps raised to demonstrate attenuated oblique musculature.

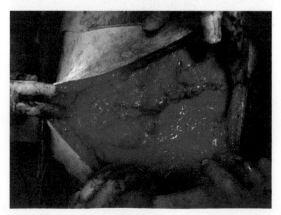

Fig. 8. Attenuated oblique musculature closed.

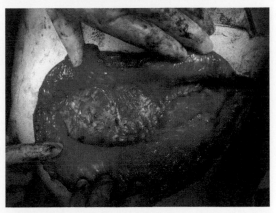

Fig. 9. Initial oblique muscle closure now imbricated.

Surgical Procedure (Robotic Preperitoneal Technique)

The robotic preperitoneal surgical technique is as follows:

Step one: The patient is positioned lateral and flexed on a bean bag, similar to the open approach. Entry into the abdominal cavity is gained by any technique preferred by the surgeon; we prefer an optical trocar entry.

Step two: A 12-mm camera port and two 8-mm ports are placed along or just off the midline. An assistant 12-mm trocar is placed low in the abdomen (**Fig. 11**). The robot is then docked in the standard fashion.

Step three: Much like the laparoscopic transabdominal preperitoneal approach to inguinal hernias, the peritoneum is incised vertically at least 5 cm medial to the most proximal border of the defect to ensure space for adequate mesh overlap (**Fig. 12**). If the peritoneum immediately under the rectus muscle is exceedingly thin and the peritoneal flap cannot be started, an alternative is to use the retromuscular plane initially and then access the preperitoneal plane. To do this, incise the posterior rectus sheath vertically. A retromuscular dissection is carried out

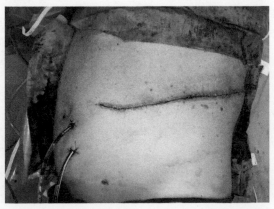

Fig. 10. Skin closed. One drain retromuscular and second subcutaneous.

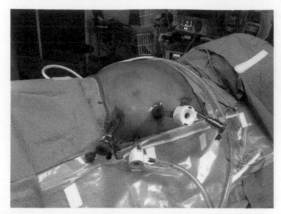

Fig. 11. Robotic trocar positioning before robotic docking.

dorsal to the rectus muscle and once the lateral edge of the rectus sheath is reached, the sheath is incised dorsally, entering the preperitoneal plane. The preperitoneal dissection can then commence from there.

Step four: Dissection is carried out in the preperitoneal plane. Once the hernia sac is reached, it is reduced from the hernia defect and dissection continues lateral to the hernia defect. If the hernia sac cannot be easily reduced, it is left in situ, understanding this creates a large defect in the peritoneum that requires later closure. It is important to ensure the preperitoneal dissection is carried out for 5 cm from the edge of the defect in all directions. The preperitoneal pocket is subsequently measured (**Fig. 13**).

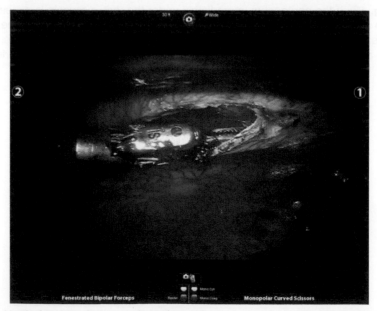

Fig. 12. Vertical incision being made in the peritoneum, medial to the hernia defect.

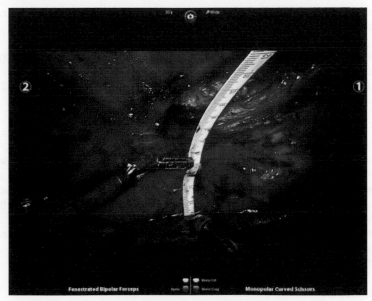

Fig. 13. Completely dissected preperitoneal pocket being measured.

Step five: The hernia defect is reapproximated horizontally using a slowly absorbable barbed suture (**Fig. 14**). If the hernia sac was left in situ, every few fascial suture bites should also incorporate a bite of the hernia sac. This imbricates the hernia sac and decreases the size of the resulting seroma.

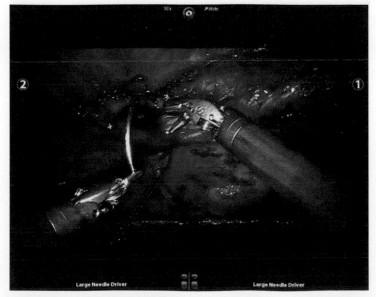

Fig. 14. Suture closure of the hernia defect.

Step six: Next an appropriately sized mid-weight, macroporous polypropylene mesh is trimmed to size and placed into the preperitoneal pocket with at least 5 cm overlap in all directions.

Step seven: The mesh is fixated at its corners and along the edges using either absorbable suture or a fixation device (**Fig. 15**).

Step eight: The peritoneal flap is closed with a slowly absorbable barbed suture (**Fig. 16**).

Postoperative Care

The patient is placed on an enhanced recovery pathway, which focuses on minimizing narcotic use. Patients are instructed to ambulate the same day of surgery. There are no diet restrictions and patients are discharged when their pain is controlled. If a drain is used, it is typically removed immediately before discharge, regardless of output volume. The patient is not given any lifting restrictions after surgery. They are instructed to gradually increase their activity, returning to normal duties once they are no longer taking narcotic medicine. Most flank hernia repair patients take 2 to 3 weeks to return to work, and most are back to baseline activity levels after approximately 6 weeks.

CLINICAL RESULTS

Flank and lumbar hernias are rarely reported in the literature, with only case series, retrospective reviews, and case reports to guide the general surgeon in decision making and counseling patients on outcomes. There are no randomized trials on the subject to provide strong recommendations regarding these difficult hernias. Given this paucity of evidence, optimal techniques and approaches remain elusive. Clinical results for open and laparoscopic repairs differ in many ways, not only in technique, but also in recurrence rates, wound complications, length of stay, and other

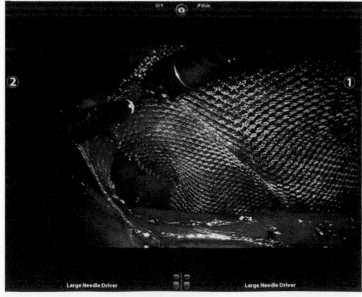

Fig. 15. Mesh being fixated with a tacking device.

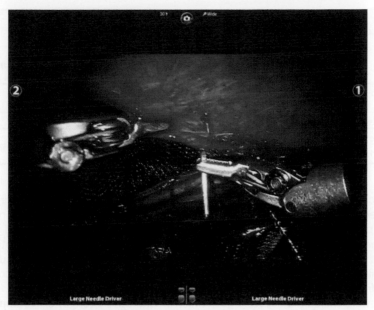

Fig. 16. Closure of the peritoneal flap.

outcomes. Furthermore, there are no published reports on the robotic approach to flank and lumbar hernias, and thus we review the outcomes of open and traditional laparoscopic intraperitoneal onlay mesh repairs.

Studies that enrolled a minimum of three patients undergoing flank and lumbar hernia repairs were reviewed and outcomes summarized in **Tables 1** and **2**. Open flank hernia repairs required a longer length of stay (5.1–15 days[17–21]) when compared with laparoscopic repairs (2–3.1 days[17,22,23]). Postoperative analgesic consumption was higher with open repairs when compared with laparoscopic repairs,[17,20,21] although the mesh fixation technique for laparoscopic repair varied between studies. Carbonell and colleagues[20] reported transfascial fixation every 4 cm to 6 cm along the abdominal wall portion of the hernia and then the use of bone anchors every 1.5 cm to 2 cm along the inner table of the iliac crest with no hernia recurrences. The wound and complication rate ranged from 0% to 40%, with the

Table 1
Open preperitoneal repairs of flank and lumbar hernias

Author, Year of Study	Number of Patients	Length of Hospital Stay (d)	Postoperative Analgesic Consumption (d)	Complication Rate (%)	Recurrence Rate (%)
Moreno-Egea et al,[17] 2013	20	5.1	15.9	40	15.9
Phillips et al,[18] 2012	16	6.3	—	19	0
Veyrie et al,[19] 2013	61	7	—	18	4.9
Fei & Li,[24] 2010	23	—	—	13	13
Carbonell et al,[20] 2005	10	5.2	0	0	0
Petersen et al,[21] 2002	4	15	0	0	0

Table 2
Laparoscopic intraperitoneal mesh onlay repairs of flank and lumbar hernias

Author, Year of Study	Number of Patients	Length of Hospital Stay (d)	Postoperative Analgesic Consumption (d)	Complication Rate (%)	Recurrence Rate (%)
Moreno-Egea et al,[17] 2013	35	2.5	6.8	37	2.9
Edwards et al,[22] 2009	27	3.1	—	3.7	0
Yavuz, et al,[25] 2009	7	8.1	—	0	0
Shekarriz et al,[23] 2001	3	2	—	0	0

overall complication rate being lower in laparoscopic flank hernia repair when compared with an open approach. However, the different complications that were reported in each study were inconsistent. Complications reported varied widely between studies, which spanned the clinical spectrum from asymptomatic seromas to ureteral and bowel injuries. Open repairs had a higher hernia recurrence rate, which ranged from 0% to 15.9%, whereas laparoscopic repair recurrences ranged from 0% to 2.9%.[17–24]

There were multiple disadvantages, which weaken the strength of recommendations that can be made regarding clinical outcomes when comparing these studies. The number of patients enrolled in each trial is small; mesh size used for repair is not reported in every study; and length of follow-up varied widely, with some being only 3 months. The type of flank hernia being repaired (traumatic or incisional), hernia location, and mesh fixation were inconsistent. Additionally, none of these trials were randomized to eliminate selection bias and provide strong, clear evidence. These confounding factors erode conclusions that can be drawn from the current literature available on flank and lumber hernias. Despite these downsides, some conclusions can still be extracted. Laparoscopic flank hernia repairs seem to have a shorter length of stay, lower rate of overall complications, and possibly a lower recurrence rates when compared with open repairs.

SUMMARY

Lumbar and flank hernias are rare and continue to prove challenging to address for the general surgeon. Their unique location, anatomic borders, and proximity to major neurovascular structures add to their complexity. Patients should be counseled adequately in the preoperative period about outcomes and expectations following repair. A preperitoneal-based repair with transfascial and bone anchor mesh fixation provides a durable repair. The traditional laparoscopic approach is associated with a shorter length of stay, less postoperative pain analgesic consumption, and a lower complication rate. There are some limitations to these studies, and prospective, randomized trials are needed in this subject. Although there are currently no published reports of robotic transabdominal preperitoneal hernia repair for flank and lumbar hernias, this approach provides the benefits of both the open and minimally invasive approach and may ultimately replace the laparoscopic technique.

REFERENCES

1. Muysoms F, Miserez M, Berrevoet F, et al. Classification of primary and incisional abdominal wall hernias. Hernia 2009;13(4):407–14.

2. Moreno-Egea A, Baena EG, Calle MC, et al. Controversies in the current management of lumbar hernias. Arch Surg 2007;142(1):82–8.
3. Cavallaro G, Sadighi A, Paparelli C, et al. Anatomical and surgical considerations on lumbar hernias. Am Surg 2009;75(12):1238–41.
4. Wakhlu A, Wakhlu AK. Congenital lumbar hernia. Pediatr Surg Int 2000;16(1–2): 146–8.
5. Stamatiou D, Skandalakis JE, Skandalakis LJ, et al. Lumbar hernia: surgical anatomy, embryology, and technique of repair. Am Surg 2009;75(3):202–7.
6. Swartz WT. Lumbar hernias. J Ky State Med Assoc 1954;52(9):673–8.
7. Burt BM, Afifi HY, Wantz GE, et al. Traumatic lumbar hernia: report of cases and comprehensive review of the literature. J Trauma 2004;57(6):1361–70.
8. Kretchmer HL. Hernia of the kidney. J Urol 1951;65(6):944–9.
9. Soto Delgado M, Garcia Urena MA, Velasco Garcia M, et al. Lumbar eventration as complication of the lumbotomy in the flank: review of our series. Actas Urol Esp 2002;26(5):345–50 [in Spanish].
10. Moon HK, Dowden RV. Lumbar hernia after latissimus dorsi flap. Plast Reconstr Surg 1985;75(3):417–9.
11. Mickel TJ, Barton FE Jr, Rohrich RJ, et al. Management and prevention of lumbar herniation following a latissimus dorsi flap. Plast Reconstr Surg 1999;103(5):1473–5.
12. Fulham SB. Lumbar hernia. J R Coll Surg Edinb 1985;30(5):315–7.
13. Orcutt TW. Hernia of the superior lumbar triangle. Ann Surg 1971;173(2):294–7.
14. Teo K, Burns E, Garcea G, et al. Incarcerated small bowel within a spontaneous lumbar hernia. Hernia 2010;14(5):539–41.
15. Baker ME, Weinerth JL, Andriani RT, et al. Lumbar hernia: diagnosis by CT. AJR Am J Roentgenol 1987;148(3):565–7.
16. Heniford BT, Iannitti DA, Gagner M. Laparoscopic inferior and superior lumbar hernia repair. Arch Surg 1997;132(10):1141–4.
17. Moreno-Egea A, Alcaraz AC, Cuervo MC. Surgical options in lumbar hernia: laparoscopic versus open repair. A long-term prospective study. Surg Innov 2013; 20(4):331–44.
18. Phillips MS, Krpata DM, Blatnik JA, et al. Retromuscular preperitoneal repair of flank hernias. J Gastrointest Surg 2012;16(8):1548–53.
19. Veyrie N, Poghosyan T, Corigliano N, et al. Lateral incisional hernia repair by the retromuscular approach with polyester standard mesh: topographic considerations and long-term follow-up of 61 consecutive patients. World J Surg 2013; 37(3):538–44.
20. Carbonell AM, Kercher KW, Sigmon L, et al. A novel technique of lumbar hernia repair using bone anchor fixation. Hernia 2005;9(1):22–5.
21. Petersen S, Schuster F, Steinbach F, et al. Sublay prosthetic repair for incisional hernia of the flank. J Urol 2002;168(6):2461–3.
22. Edwards C, Geiger T, Bartow K, et al. Laparoscopic transperitoneal repair of flank hernias: a retrospective review of 27 patients. Surg Endosc 2009;23(12):2692–6.
23. Shekarriz B, Graziottin TM, Gholami S, et al. Transperitoneal preperitoneal laparoscopic lumbar incisional herniorrhaphy. J Urol 2001;166(4):1267–9.
24. Fei Y, Li L. Comparison of two repairing procedures for abdominal wall reconstruction in patients with flank hernia. Zhongguo Xiu Fu Chong Jian Wai Ke Za Zhi 2010;24(12):1506–9 [in Chinese].
25. Yavuz N, Ersoy YE, Demirkesen O, et al. Laparoscopic incisional lumbar hernia repair. Hernia 2009;13(3):281–6.

Inguinal Hernia
Mastering the Anatomy

Heidi J. Miller, MD, MPH

KEYWORDS

- Inguinal herniorrhaphy • Lichtenstein • TAPP • Anatomy • Bassini • Inguinodynia

KEY POINTS

- Success of inguinal herniorrhaphy is defined by low recurrence and complication rates and relies on the surgeon's knowledge and understanding of groin anatomy and physiology.
- Open tension-free mesh repair remains the most common and gold standard repair of inguinal hernias, building on knowledge and understanding of groin anatomy developed throughout history.
- A standardized dissection of the myopectineal orifice, following anatomic landmarks, allows for identification of all possible groin hernias and adequate mesh coverage of defects.

INTRODUCTION

Inguinal hernias are a common problem that affect a large number of people around the globe. This leads to a surgical disease of significant scope, with 20 million inguinal hernia repairs completed annually worldwide, and in the United States more than 800,000 are completed by 18,000 surgeons across the country.[1] The success of an inguinal hernia repair is defined by the permanence of the operation while creating the fewest complications at minimal cost and allowing patients an early return to activity. This success relies and depends on the surgeon's knowledge and understanding of groin anatomy and physiology. This article reviews relevant anatomy to inguinal hernia repair as well as technical steps to common repair techniques as they relate to this anatomy.

GENERAL ANATOMY AND IMPORTANT STRUCTURES AND LANDMARKS

- External landmarks of the abdominal wall are used for all approaches to gain access to the correct area of the groin for hernia repair. For open approaches, the

The author has nothing to disclose.
Department of Surgery, MSC 10 5610, University of New Mexico, Albuquerque, NM 87131, USA
E-mail address: hjmillermd@gmail.com

initial incision is based on external landmarks, and for minimally invasive approaches, the use of external landmarks helps guide dissection and prevent complications. Take note of the anterior superior iliac spine (ASIS), the pubic tubercle, and the inguinal ligament (**Fig. 1**).

- Layers of the abdominal wall
  - From superficial to deep, the layers of the abdominal wall in the inguinal region are skin, subcutaneous tissue, Scarpa and Camper fascias, external oblique (EO) fascia and muscle, internal oblique (IO) fascia and muscle, transversus abdominis muscle (TAM), transversalis fascia (TAF), preperitoneal fat, and peritoneum. Medially the rectus abdominis muscle is encased by the anterior rectus sheath (ARS) throughout and the posterior rectus sheath above the

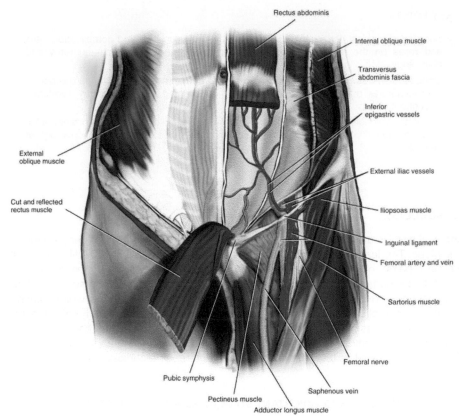

Fig. 1. The inferior epigastric vessels are important landmarks on the anterior abdominal wall, particularly because of their risk for injury during laparoscopic trocar entry. The artery arises from the lower medial aspect of the external iliac artery. The vein flows into the external iliac vein just cranial to the inguinal ligament. The femoral nerve emerges from within the substance of the psoas major muscle to be exposed directly under the tough inguinal ligament. This view shows the upper portion of the adductor longus, as well as the pectineus muscle. The latter overlies the obturator foramen (canal) and the obturator externus muscle, through which penetrate the obturator nerve plus the obturator vessels (not shown). Note also that the saphenous and femoral veins cross above the pectineus muscle. (*From* Baggish MS. Basic pelvic anatomy. In: Baggish MS, Karram MM, editors. Atlas of pelvic anatomy and gynecologic surgery. 4th edition. Philadelphia: Elsevier; 2016. p. 5–58; with permission.)

arcuate line (**Fig. 2** shows cross-section of the layers and **Fig. 3** shows the layers in relation to the inguinal region).

- ○ The TAF is the innermost fascial layer of the abdominal wall muscles. It has 2 laminal layers, the more superficial of which is vascular; the deeper layer is an avascular plane that makes a beneficial dissection plane into the preperitoneal space (**Fig. 4** shows the separation of these layers during a laparoscopic dissection).
- Myopectineal orifice (MPO) (**Fig. 5** shows anterior and posterior views of the MPO and **Fig. 6** is a laparoscopic view of the dissected MPO)
  - ○ The MPO was first described by Dr Henri Fruchaud in 1956 as a distinct area of weakness in the pelvic region and is believed to have become weakened during the evolutionary process as humans became bipedal, stood, and stretched this area that already contained natural openings and areas of weakness.[2]
  - ○ The MPO is bordered by the conjoined tendon superiorly and Cooper ligament inferiorly. The medial border is the rectus abdominus muscle and rectus sheath, and the lateral border is the iliopsoas muscle. The MPO is divided by the inguinal ligament, which runs diagonally from the ASIS to the pubic tubercle. The suprainguinal space of the MPO contains the internal inguinal ring, through which the spermatic cord penetrates the abdominal wall to course through the inguinal canal and into the scrotum. This is the site of an indirect inguinal hernia, which is a pathologic opening or weakness in the TAF, allowing the peritoneum and its contents to bulge through the internal ring alongside the spermatic cord or round ligament.

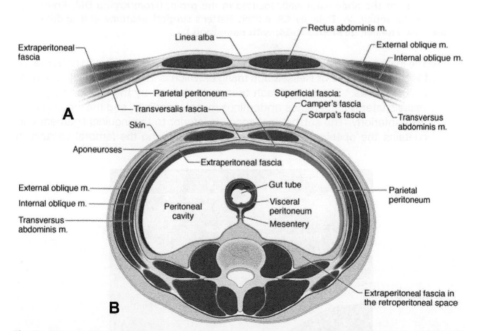

Fig. 2. Cross-section representation of the layers and musculature and the abdominal wall. A, focus on the anterior abdominal wall below the arcuate line. B, above the arcuate line. m, muscle. (*From* Morton DA, Foreman KB, Albertine KH. The big picture: gross anatomy. New York: The McGraw-Hill Companies, Inc; 2011. Available at: www.accessmedicine.com; with permission.)

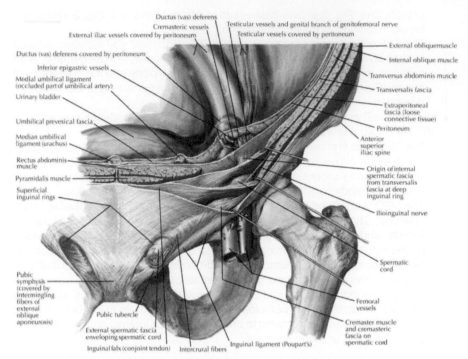

Fig. 3. Layers of the abdominal wall, focused in the groin. (*From* Krpata DM, Rosen MJ. Open inguinal repair. In: Delaney CP, editor. Netter's surgical anatomy and approaches. Philadelphia: Elsevier; 2014. p. 341–54; with permission.)

- o The inferior epigastric vessels run medial to this and create the third border of the medial triangle or Hesselbach triangle, which is the area of development of direct hernias.[3] The Hesselbach triangle is defined by the inferior epigastric vessels laterally, the rectus abdominus muscle medially, and the inguinal ligament inferiorly. The subinguinal space is inferior to the inguinal ligament and contains the opening for the femoral canal, allowing the femoral vessels to

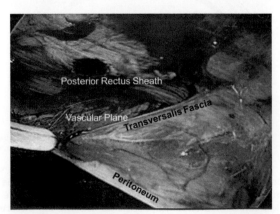

Fig. 4. Laparoscopic photo of dissection planes between the posterior rectus sheath, TAF, and peritoneum.

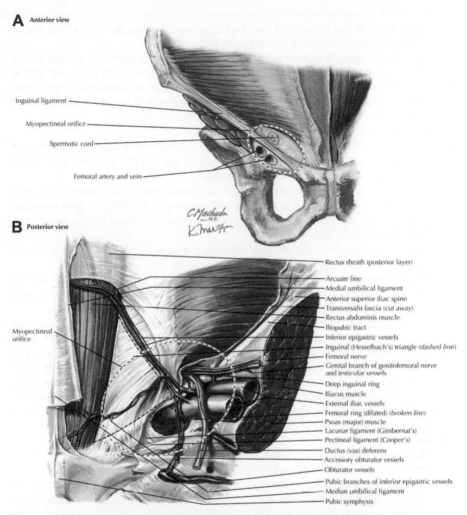

A Anterior view

Inguinal ligament

Myopectineal orifice

Spermatic cord

Femoral artery and vein

B Posterior view

Rectus sheath (posterior layer)
Arcuate line
Medial umbilical ligament
Anterior superior iliac spine
Transversalis fascia (cut away)
Rectus abdominis muscle
Iliopubic tract
Inferior epigastric vessels
Inguinal (Hesselbach's) triangle (dashed line)
Femoral nerve
Genital branch of genitofemoral nerve and testicular vessels
Deep inguinal ring
Iliacus muscle
External iliac vessels
Femoral ring (dilated) (broken line)
Psoas (major) muscle
Lacunar ligament (Gimbernat's)
Pectineal ligament (Cooper's)
Ductus (vas) deferens
Accessory obturator vessels
Obturator vessels
Pubic branches of inferior epigastric vessels
Median umbilical ligament
Pubic symphysis

Myopectineal orifice

Fig. 5. Anterior and posterior views of myopectineal orifice. (*From* Elliott HL, Novitsky YW. Laparoscopic inguinal hernia repair. In: Delaney CP, editor. Netter's surgical anatomy and approaches. Philadelphia: Elsevier; 2014. p. 357; with permission.)

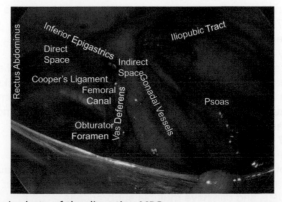

Fig. 6. Laparoscopic photo of the dissection MPO.

pass through the abdominal wall and allowing for weakness in the TAF, especially in women, due to a wider pelvic shape.
  ○ The entire MPO is vulnerable to the development of hernias because of the normal anatomic gaps in the tissue to allow structures to pass out of the abdomen into the lower extremities or pelvis as well as the aponeurotic nature of the area, whereas the rest of the abdominal wall is covered with layers of thick muscle.
- Iliopubic tract (IPT)
  ○ The IPT is a thickening of the TAF that fans out laterally in the transversalis and iliac fasciae. Medially it attaches posterior to the Cooper ligament and it runs parallel and deep to the inguinal ligament.
  ○ The IPT is an important landmark for the preperitoneal approach to inguinal hernia repair, because it is the posterior divider of the MPO. It also provides the superior border of the triangle of pain, providing clues for the prevention of postoperative inguinodynia.
  ○ The IPT is used in tissue reconstruction of the floor of the inguinal canal, especially in the Shouldice procedure.
- Conjoint tendon: fusion of the medial fibers of the IO aponeurosis (IOA) and the transversus abdominis fascia, which then turns inferiorly to insert into the crest of the pubis and the Cooper ligament[4]
- Inguinal ligament: fibrous band made of thickened folds of the EOA that extends from the ASIS to the pubic tubercle; fibers of the inguinal ligament that pass laterally and attach to the pectin pubis form the Cooper ligament (pectineal ligament)
- Inguinal canal: the passage that transmits structures from the pelvis to the perineum, formed by fetal migration of the gonad; it is approximately 4 cm long and connects the deep inguinal ring (opening in the TAF superior to the inguinal ligament and lateral to the inferior epigastric arteries) to the superficial inguinal ring (V-shaped opening in the EOA, superior-medial to the pubic tubercle).
- Nerves[1,5]
  ○ Nerves of the inguinal region arise from the lumbar plexus; they innervate abdominal muscles and supply sensation to the skin and peritoneum. Inguinodynia is a common complication in inguinal hernia repair, and it becomes of greater concern as techniques continue to be refined, implant technology improves, and recurrence rates become very low. Injury or entrapment can cause pain, and transection can lead to pain or numbness. It is often difficult to differentiate somatic and neuropathic pain.
  ○ The risk of chronic inguinodynia increases with the presence of preoperative pain, younger age, open surgery, neurolysis, postoperative complications, and high 7-day postoperative pain score.
  ○ The incidence of severe chronic pain affecting quality of life, daily activities, and ability to work has been found to be 0.5% to 6%.
  ○ Both acute and chronic postoperative pain should be treated early with multimodal pharmacologic management. Diagnostic nerve blocks, exclusion of meshoma or recurrence, and further work-up should be completed prior to consideration of surgical intervention, which should not be undertaken earlier than 1 year after original surgery.
  ○ See **Fig. 7** for a representation of the sensory dermatomes.
    ▪ Lateral femoral cutaneous nerve (LFCN)
      • Root leaves L2/3 and enters the abdomen medial and caudal to the ASIS and runs in the lateral fringe of the psoas muscle, either below or along the IPT, and can have multiple subbranches.

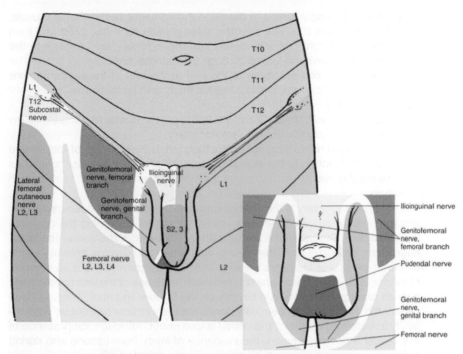

Fig. 7. Lower extremity anatomy: proximal innervation (peripheral nerves labeled on right side of the body, dermatomes on the left). n, nerve. (*From* Brown DL. Lower extremity block anatomy. In: Farag E, Mounir-Soliman L, Brown DL, editors. Brown's atlas of regional anesthesia. 5th edition. Philadelphia: Elsevier; 2017. p. 89–96; with permission.)

- The LFCN supplies sensation to the upper lateral thigh
- Genitofemoral nerve (GFM)
  - Arises from first and second lumbar nerves. Located centrally on the psoas medial to the iliohypogastric nerve (IHN) and ilioinguinal nerve (IIN). The genital branch of the GFM perforates the abdominal wall at the IPT near and lateral to the internal inguinal ring. It runs within the cremasteric fascia with the external genital vessels. The femoral branch of the GFM passes under the inguinal ligament to follow the external iliac artery. Each branch has been found to have as many as 3 subbranches.
  - The genital branch of the GFM supplies sensation to labia majora or the cremasteric reflex.
  - The femoral branch of the GFM supplies the skin over the femoral triangle, anterior medial thigh.
- Iliohypogastric nerve (IHN)
  - Can share a root with the IIN, leaving from T12/L1 and emerging in the lateral edge of the psoas muscle, crossing the quadratus lumborum muscle (QLM). The IHN enters the TAM at the iliac crest and branches and then enters the IO above and in front of the ASIS. It then runs deep to the EO just above the inguinal canal and penetrates the EO within 1 cm to 2 cm cranial to the external ring.
  - The IHN provides the sensory innervation of the suprapubic region
- Ilioinguinal nerve (IIN)

- Leaves L1 and courses of the QLM then anterior to the iliacus muscle. The IIN enters the TAM near the anterior end of the iliac crest and then passes through IOM and moves into the inguinal canal anterior to the spermatic cord and leaves through the external ring.
  - The IIN supplies sensation to the skin at the root of the penis, anterior third of the scrotum, anterior medial thigh, and labia majora
  - Femoral nerve
    - Root emerges from L2/3/4 lateral to the psoas muscle and travels below the IPT laterally toward the femoral artery.
    - The femoral nerve supplies motor function to the muscles of the leg and sensory function to the skin of the inner thigh via the anterior cutaneous femoral nerve
- Vasculature
  - The external iliac artery is the arterial supply to the groin. The deep circumflex iliac and inferior epigastric arteries branch off before becoming the common femoral artery. The internal spermatic artery arises from the aorta. The obturator artery branches from the internal iliac artery and passes anteroinferiorly on the lateral wall of the pelvis. In up to 80% of pubic rami, there is an aberrant obturator artery that has an anastomosis with branches of the iliac or epigastric arteries forming a ring that run directly on the Cooper ligament. This has been named the *corona mortis* because significant hemorrhage can occur, with difficulty in obtaining control if the vessel is torn or cut. Although the presence of this vessel is not uncommon, the incidence of injury from tacking and during minimally invasive surgical (MIS) repair is rarely reported.[6–8]
  - There are multiple venous plexi for drainage of the groin, including the panpiniform plexus. These also can be clinically significant when injured and are intertwined with fatty tissues in the spermatic cord and preperitoneal space of Retzius. It is injury or thrombosis of the panpiniform plexus that leads to testicular atrophy after hernia repair.[9]

OPEN TISSUE REPAIR

Tissue repairs require in-depth understanding of the muscular and fascial anatomy of the groin. At least 1 technique should be in a surgeon's arsenal for patients who present but are not candidates for mesh repair. The Bassini-Halsted repair was the gold standard inguinal hernia repair for half a century. Bassini studied 262 repairs with no mortality between 1885 and 1890, with a 1-year recurrence rate of less than 3%.[10] McVay[11] did a thorough study of groin anatomy and suggested additional steps in the repair of inguinal hernias, recognizing Cooper ligament as a source of strength for tissue closures. He also evaluated 580 of his repairs and showed a similar recurrence rate but with significant decrease in the rate after he started using Cooper ligament for the posterior reconstruction.[12]

- Bassini repair[10]
  - A 5 cm to 6 cm groin incision is made from the pubic tubercle laterally in the Langer lines
  - Expose the EO aponeurosis (EOA) and incise into the external ring.
  - Identify and protect the IIN.
  - Raise flaps of the EOA for approximately 3 cm to 4 cm above inguinal floor.
  - Encircle the spermatic cord or round ligament, identify the hernia sac in the anteriomedial location, dissect the sac away from the other tissues, and reduce the contents of the sac into the abdomen.

- ○ Suture ligate the hernia sac, if necessary the round ligament may be ligated and transected.
- ○ Assess and open the floor of the inguinal canal.
- ○ Identify and assess the mobility of the conjoint tendon.
- ○ Identify and clear the shelving edge of the inguinal ligament.
- ○ Make a relaxing incision of the IOA or ARS for any tension.
- ○ Suture the conjoined tendon to the shelving edge with interrupted permanent sutures. It is possible to close the internal ring completely in women; it may be closed tightly around the spermatic cord with enough space to pass a hemostat or Kelly clamp. This may require an additional stitch lateral to internal ring if the space is large.
- ○ Close the EOA, scarpa's fascia and skin in layers.
- McVay repair[11] (**Fig. 8**)
  - ○ Follow steps 1-6 of the Bassini repair, as described above.
  - ○ Assess the floor of the canal, incise the TAF as well as any weak or attenuated fascia, and identify the ipsilateral Cooper ligament.
  - ○ Make a relaxing incision in the ARS.
  - ○ Suture the conjoint tendon to the ipsilateral Cooper ligament with interrupted permanent suture from the pubic tubercle to the femoral vein.
  - ○ The key transition suture includes a bite each of the Cooper ligament, conjoint tendon, femoral sheath, and the shelving edge of the inguinal ligament.
  - ○ The internal ring is then reduced in size with lateral sutures as necessary.
  - ○ Close the EOA, scarpa's fascia and skin in layers.
- Nerves most commonly injured during open repair are the IIN, IHN, and g-GFN, most commonly during dissection. Neurectomy during open repair does not reduce the incidence of chronic induinodynia. International guidelines recommend identification of all 3 nerves, thus reducing the risk to less than 1%.[5]

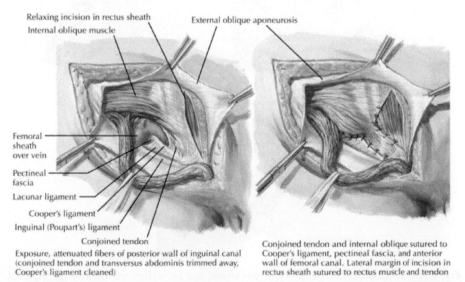

Fig. 8. McVay repair. (*From* Krpata DM, Rosen MJ. Open inguinal repair. In: Delaney CP, editor. Netter's surgical anatomy and approaches. Philadelphia: Elsevier; 2014. p. 341–54; with permission.)

OPEN TENSION-FREE MESH REPAIR

The Lichtenstein hernioplasty has become the new gold standard inguinal hernia repair. It can be done under local or general anesthesia, is easy to learn and reproduce, can be completed quickly, and has low recurrence and complication rates.

- Lichtenstein repair[13] (**Fig. 9**)
  - ○ A 5-cm to 6-cm groin incision is made from the pubic tubercle laterally within the Langer lines.
  - ○ Open the EOA and raise flaps approximately 3-4 cm above the inguinal floor, taking care to avoid any underlying nerves.
    - ▪ Visualize the iliohypogastric and ilioinguinal nerves.
  - ○ Separate the spermatic cord and cremaster muscle from the floor of the inguinal canal and the pubic bone.
    - ▪ The IIN, external spermatic vessels and the genital branch of the GFN shoudl be included with the cord structures.
  - ○ Incise the cremasteric sheath in order to identify an indirect hernia sac, then dissect the sac free of the cord structures and invert in the abdomen without ligation of the cord.
    - ▪ A large direct hernia sac can be inverted with absorpbable sutures.
    - ▪ Large scrotal sacs can be transected if they are difficult to dissect out. The proximal section should be suture ligated, and the distal section kept open.

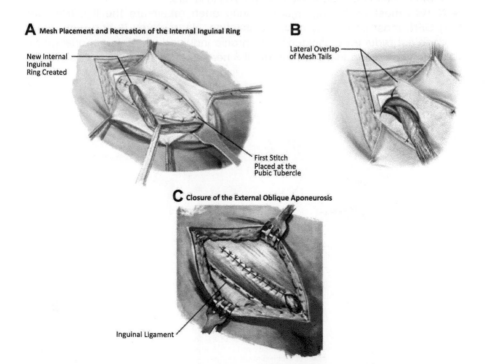

A Mesh Placement and Recreation of the Internal Inguinal Ring

New Internal Inguinal Ring Created

B

Lateral Overlap of Mesh Tails

First Stitch Placed at the Pubic Tubercle

C Closure of the External Oblique Aponeurosis

Inguinal Ligament

Fig. 9. Lichtenstein repair. (*A, B*) Mesh placement and recreation of the internal inguinal ring. (*C*) Closure of the EOA to recreate the external inguinal ring. (*From* Krpata DM, Rosen MJ. Open inguinal repair. In: Delaney CP, editor. Netter's surgical anatomy and approaches. Philadelphia: Elsevier; 2014. p. 341–54; with permission.)

- Place a large 7 cm × 15 cm mesh that overlaps the pubic tubercle by 1.5 cm - 2cm. Suture the mesh to the ARS superior to the pubic tubercle, avoiding the periosteum.
- Continue to suture along the border of the mesh to the shelving edge.
  - A femoral hernia can be repaired by opening the posterior wall to expose the Cooper ligament, reduction of the hernia sac, and placing a suture between the mesh and Cooper ligament.
- Slit the mesh laterally and position the cord structures between the two tails.
- Fixate the mesh to the conjoint tendon with 2 interrupted sutures, including the ARS and IOA.
- Fixate the 2 mesh tails to the inguinal ligament and recreate the internal ring, leaving 5 cm or more of mesh overlap lateral to the internal ring.
- Close the EOA, scarpa's fascia and skin in layers.

MINIMALLY INVASIVE REPAIR

Laparoscopic inguinal hernioplasty was first described in the early 1990s and can be completed from multiple approaches, including transabdominal preperiotoneal (TAPP), totally extraperitoneal (TEP), or robotic TAPP. Laparoscopy in comparison with open inguinal hernioplasty has been shown to have longer operative times, increased cost, and longer learning curve but has the benefit of decreased immediate postoperative pain and earlier return to work.[14–17] Technical errors have been found, however, to be the cause for recurrences and chronic pain, including insufficient mesh coverage and inadequate dissection of the MPO.[18] To reduce recurrence rates and chronic pain complications, a recent description of a critical view of the MPO has been published.[19] (see **Fig. 6**). Additional anatomic landmarks for MIS repair help identify potential downfalls or danger zones of the dissection. The first is the triangle of doom (**Fig. 10**), which contains the external iliac vessels and femoral nerve and is outlined by the vas deferens, gonadal vessels, and peritoneal reflection. The triangle of pain (**Fig. 11**) contains at least the LFCN, FN, and f-GFN and possibly other nerves, described previously, and is defined by the gonadal vessels medially, the IPT superiorly, and the peritoneal reflection laterally.

- TAPP inguinal hernia repair
  - Laparoscopic access is acquired by the surgeon's approach of choice. Insufflation is achieved and 3 ports are placed. Port placement is usually at the

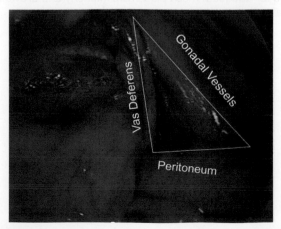

Fig. 10. Triangle of Doom.

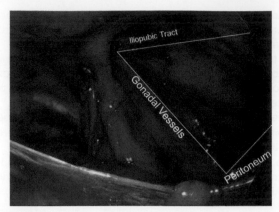

Fig. 11. Triangle of Pain.

umbilicus, with bilateral ports placed approximately 10 cm lateral to the midline and slightly cranial to the middle port (**Fig. 12**).
- The working space of Retzius is accessed via creation of a peritoneal flap. By incising the peritoneum above the imaginary line between bilateral ASIS, nerve injury during closure can be avoided.
- The dissection of the flap follows the preperitoneal space, separating the TAF in the deep, avascular plane. This leaves the inferior epigastric vessels protected by the TAF and leads the dissection directly into preperiotoneal space of Retzius.
- The medial dissection in the preperitoneal space at the midline leads into the space of Retzius and to the pubic symphysis. This space is dissected across the midline to expose the bilateral pubic tubercles and Cooper ligaments.
- The dissection is continued laterally from the midline to expose the Hesselbach triangle in order to visualize a direct defect, if present. If a direct defect is identified the dissection should definitely be taken across the midline to expose the contralateral Cooper ligament and allow adequate space for medial mesh overlap.
- Further posterior dissection drops the bladder away from the Cooper ligament, and allows for adequate mesh placement inferiorly and allows for inspection of the obturator foramen.

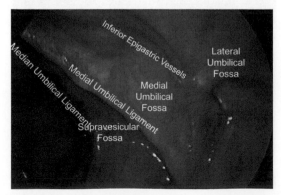

Fig. 12. Internal pelvic landmarks.

- ○ Dissection between Cooper ligament and the iliac vein allows for visualization of the femoral orifice to evaluate for a femoral hernia.
- ○ Lateral dissection of the peritoneal flap is undertaken, following the preperitoneal space, and sweeping the peritoneum inferiorly and laterally beyond the ASIS. Care should be taken in the triangle of pain to avoid contact with nerves or the body of the psoas muscle.
- ○ The indirect sac is then dissected off of the cord structures, until they are parietalized. This dissection is not complete until the cord structures lie flat and are free of movement with the flap is pulled upward. The psoas muscle and iliac vessels should also be visualized during this step.
- ○ The cord structures should be inspected as they leave the abdomen in order to identify cord lipomas, usually found lateral to the cord elements. These should be dissected out and can be used to cover the inferior border of the mesh within the flap.
- ○ Place mesh to completely overlap the MPO, securing as deemed necessary to avoid mesh slippage or folding (**Fig. 13**). Most 10-cm × 15-cm meshes are adequate for coverage, although a larger mesh may at times be needed.[19] Fixation with tacks or sutures should be avoided below the IPT, along the psoas, or caudal to the ASIS line to avoid injury to nerves. LFCN and IIN are the most commonly injured nerves during MIS repair, either injured during lateral dissection or impinged with tacks if exposed medially to the ASIS. Fibrin glue has been found to provide adequate mesh fixation with possible decrease in postoperative chronic pain.[20]
- ○ Closure of the peritoneal flap is undertaken, with suture, glue, or tacking, ensuring that no penetrating fixation is placed inferior to the ASIS line.
- • TEP inguinal hernia repair
- ○ A skin incision is made near the umbilicus, allowing access to either side of the linea alba and dissection down to the ARS. The ARS is incised and the rectus muscle dissected bluntly, and a port is placed anterior to the posterior rectus sheath.
- ○ Access to the preperitoneal space is gained through blunt dissection, which can be achieved with the aid of a balloon dissector. Following the posterior rectus sheath inferiorly, the arcuate line is traversed. The TAF must be penetrated to enter the true preperitoneal space and access the space of Retzius.

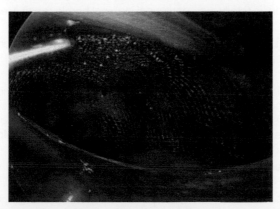

Fig. 13. Laparoscopic mesh overlapping the entire MPO.

○ Working ports are placed, frequently along the midline as the dissection takes place. Insufflation of the preperitoneal space is achieved.

○ The dissection proceeds in a similar fashion as a TAPP repair, and is described in steps 4 to 11 above under TAPP inguinal hernia repair.

TAPP and TEP have been studied closely, and both have been found safe and successful approaches to inguinal hernia repair. Some studies have shown increased risk of bowel injury with TAPP and increased vascular injury with TEP. Any noted difference in outcomes or complications, however, is likely more related to the type of hernia repaired than the technique used.[21] The rate of chronic postoperative pain is doubled, however, with the use of more than 10 tacks during a TAPP repair.[22]

SUMMARY

Inguinal hernia repair is one of the most commonly performed surgeries in the United States and around the world. Because of this, the complexity of both the anatomy and the repair technique is often overlooked. An understanding of inguinal anatomy, however, allows the surgeon to develop a full arsenal of approaches to this problem, providing options for patient and surgeon depending on the situation.

REFERENCES

1. Chen DC, Hiatt JR, Amid PK. Operative management of refractory neuropathic inguinodynia by a laparoscopic retroperitoneal approach. JAMA Surg 2013; 148(10):962.

2. Stoppa R. Henri Fruchaud (1894-1960), man of courage, anatomist and surgeon. Hist Sci Med 1997;31(3–4):281–6.

3. Agarwal AK, Mukherjee R. Franz Kaspar Hasselbach (1759-1816). Indian J Surg 2008;70(2):96–8.

4. Moore K, Dalley A. Clinically Oriented Anatomy, 4th Addition. Philadelphia: Lippincott Williams & Wilkins; 1999.

5. Reinpold W, Schroeder AD, Schroeder M, et al. Retroperitoneal anatomy of the iliohypogastric, ilioinguinal, genitofemoral, and lateral femoral cutaneous nerve: consequences for prevention and treatment of chronic inguinodynia. Hernia 2015;19(4):539–48.

6. Ates M, Kinaci E, Kose E, et al. Corona mortis: in vivo anatomical knowledge and the risk of injury in totally extraperitoneal inguinal hernia repair. Hernia 2016;20(5): 659–65.

7. Darmanis S, Lewis A, Mansoor A, et al. Corona mortis: an anatomical study with clinical implications in approaches to the pelvis and acetabulum. Clin Anat 2007; 20(4):433–9.

8. Hong HX, Pan ZJ, Chen X, et al. An anatomical study of corona mortis and its clinical significance. Chin J Traumatol 2004;7(3):165–9. Available at: https://extranet. uj.edu.pl/,DanaInfo=apps.webofknowledge.com+full_record.do?product=UA& search_mode=AdvancedSearch&qid=3&SID=V1zmk7es8ETMpgnXF6E&page =1&doc=21&cacheurlFromRightClick=no.

9. Wantz GE. Testicular atrophy and chronic residual neuralgia as risks of inguinal hernioplasty. Surg Clin North Am 1993;73(3):571–81.

10. Banks SB, Cotlar AM. Classic groin hernia repair...lest we forget. Curr Surg 2005; 62(2):249–52.

11. McVay CB. An anatomic error in current methods of inguinal herniorrhaphy. Ann Surg 1941;113(6):1111–2. Available at: http://www.ncbi.nlm.nih.gov/pubmed/17857829.
12. MCVay CB, Chapp JD. Inguinal and femoral hernioplasty- the evaluation of a basic concept. Ann Surg 1968;148(4):499–510.
13. Amid PK. Lichtenstein tension-free hernioplasty: Its inception, evolution, and principles. Hernia 2004;8(1):1–7.
14. Kark AE, Kurzer MN, Belsham PA. Three thousand one hundred seventy-five primary inguinal hernia repairs: advantages of ambulatory open mesh repair using anesthesia. J Am Coll Surg 1998;186(4):447–56.
15. Peitsch WKJ. A modified laparoscopic hernioplasty (TAPP) is the standard procedure for inguinal and femoral hernias: a retrospective 17-year analysis with 1,123 hernia repairs. Surg Endosc 2014;28(2):671–82.
16. Novitsky YW, Czerniach DR, Kercher KW, et al. Advantages of laparoscopic transabdominal preperitoneal herniorrhaphy in the evaluation and management of inguinal hernias. Am J Surg 2007;193(4):466–70.
17. Matsutani T, Nomura T, Hagiwara N, et al. Laparoscopic transabdominal preperitoneal inguinal hernia repair using memory-ring mesh: a pilot study. Surg Res Pract 2016;2016:9407357.
18. Phillips EH, Rosenthal R, Fallas M, et al. Reasons for early recurrence following laparoscopic hernioplasty. Surg Endosc 1995;9(2):140–5. Available at: http://www.ncbi.nlm.nih.gov/entrez/query.fcgi?cmd=Retrieve&db=PubMed&dopt=Citation&list_uids=7597581.
19. Daes J, Felix E. Critical view of the myopectineal orifice. Ann Surg 2017;266(1):e1–2.
20. Topart P, Vandenbroucke F, Lozac'h P. Tisseel vs tack staples as mesh fixation in totally extraperitoneal laparoscopic repair of groin hernias: a retrospective analysis. Surg Endosc 2005;19(5):724–7.
21. Köckerling F, Bittner R, Jacob DA, et al. TEP versus TAPP: comparison of the perioperative outcome in 17,587 patients with a primary unilateral inguinal hernia. Surg Endosc Other Interv Tech 2015;29(12):3750–60.
22. Belyansky I, Tsirline VB, Klima DA, et al. Prospective, comparative study of postoperative quality of life in TEP, TAPP, and modified lichtenstein repairs. Ann Surg 2011;254(5):709–15.

Inguinal Hernia
Four Open Approaches

Shirin Towfigh, MD

KEYWORDS

• Inguinal hernia • Lichtenstein • Shouldice • Bassini • McVay • Mesh

KEY POINTS

• Open inguinal hernia repair options should be tailored to the needs and risk factors of each patient.
• Knowledge of the complex inguinal anatomy is the key to reduce complications and improve outcomes.
• Open anterior mesh repair is the most common approach for inguinal hernia repairs, with the best outcomes for most patients.
• Open anterior tissue repair is an option for inguinal hernia repair, especially for small hernias.
• Femoral hernias must be evaluated for intraoperatively among women.

INTRODUCTION

Inguinal hernias are among the most common hernias repaired throughout the world. They are more commonly diagnosed among men, at a rate 10 or more times higher than women.[1] That said, the existence of inguinal hernias in women should not be discounted, because they can occur and often present differently than in males. For example, men tend to present primarily with a bulging mass in the groin, at times with associated pain. Women tend to present with groin pain radiating to their upper inner thigh, vagina, or around to their lower back, and may not demonstrate a bulging mass in the groin.[2] Also, femoral hernias are at least 3 times more common among women. These hernias can present insidiously, as with intestinal obstruction. Symptoms may include groin pain radiating down the anterior mid thigh. Examination can be nondiagnostic.

Surgical techniques for inguinal hernias are plentiful, first introduced in ancient Egypt. The open approach is the most commonly performed technique. This approach may involve either a pure tissue repair (suture repair) or the addition of a mesh implant. In the United States and Europe, the mesh repair is most commonly performed.

The most common and well-studied mesh repair is the Lichtenstein technique. This technique involves an onlay patch of mesh. Other techniques include the Gilbert bilayer

Disclosure Statement: The author has nothing to disclose.
Beverly Hills Hernia Center, 450 North Roxbury Drive #224, Beverly Hills, CA 90210, USA
E-mail address: DrTowfigh@BeverlyHillsHerniaCenter.com

repair, the plug technique, and the open retroperitoneal mesh repair. Variations to the open retroperitoneal mesh repair have been described by many (Stoppa, Nyhus, Wantz, Kugel). It is also the basis behind the transinguinal preperitoneal and transrectus sheath preperitoneal techniques. Modern guidelines do not recommend any plug type repair, owing to the high volume of mesh used and its risks for erosion and chronic pain.[3]

Tissue repairs involve suturing of the defect in a manner to reduce recurrence and chronic pain. Common tissue repairs that have been well-studied include the Shouldice, Bassini, and McVay repairs. The retroperitoneal Nyhus-Condon repair is also useful. The tissue repair remains a valuable approach for those with 1 or more of the following factors: low risk for hernia recurrence, small indirect inguinal hernia, not a candidate for mesh repair (eg, contaminated field), high risk for mesh-related complications such as chronic pain (eg, chronic pain syndrome, fibromyalgia),[4] and/or prefers not to have mesh implantation.[5] In the past, a tissue repair was considered optimal for women, because they tend to have small hernias, and it was believed that they were less likely to have an underlying collagen disorder. With improvements in population studies looking at outcomes among women, it is evident that women have more hernia recurrences and/or chronic pain, with tissue repairs and anterior mesh repairs. This is partially due to the rate of missed femoral hernias, noted to be the diagnosis in 50% of hernia recurrences in women.[6] Although femoral hernias can be repaired via tissue repair, the outcomes are poor, with a high risk for recurrence and chronic pain. Modern guidelines now recommend a laparoscopic approach if the expertise is available, or open preperitoneal mesh repair, for women.[3]

SURGICAL TECHNIQUE
Preoperative Planning

For elective hernia repairs, planning is directed at reducing perioperative complications and improving outcomes. Any modifiable risk factors for a poor outcome should be addressed, which includes treating chronic constipation and a chronic cough. If there are signs of prostatism, such as nocturia, or straining to improve slow urinary stream and completely empty the bladder, it should be optimally treated either medically or surgically. In many situations, these risk factors are primary contributors to worsening symptoms or enlargement of the inguinal hernia.

Nicotine use has been linked to poor healing and hernia recurrence.[7] Cessation is preferred, especially if the hernia repair is complex, giant, and/or multiply recurrent. Patients taking antiplatelet or antithrombotic medications are at greater than average risk for critical bleeding or hematoma after hernia repair. Thus, repair should be performed at a time when it is considered medically safe to be off these medications or bridged with a short-acting reversible medication, such as heparin or enoxaparin. Operating while the patient is on aspirin, if necessary for cardioprotection, is typically safe, although with increased risk of ecchymosis and clinically nonsignificant hematoma.[8]

The planned technique for hernia repair should be tailored to the patient's needs. For example, an open tissue repair may be preferred in a yoga instructor with a small inguinal hernia. An open mesh repair may be recommended for an elderly patient with a scrotal component to his hernia. Laparoscopic options with mesh should also be discussed, especially for patients with recurrence from an open repair, bilateral inguinal hernias, many athletes, women, and those with femoral hernias.

Preparation and Patient Positioning

For all open repairs, the patient is placed supine, with both arms laid out and padded. Consider removing any pillows from under the knees, because that may narrow the working space and risk a tighter than intended repair. Clipping hairs in the operative field may help with patient comfort from tape removal; there are conflicting studies whether this reduces surgical site infection.[9,10] Surgical preparation of the sterile field may include prepping the genitalia. This practice is most helpful if the surgeon needs to manipulate the spermatic cord or the testicle, for example, to help in the anatomy of the operation. When draping, reduce the total surface area of exposed skin to reduce the risk of surgical site infection (**Fig. 1**).

The use of Foley catheterization is often not necessary for open approaches. The bladder is typically not in the way of the operation and the surgical duration is low. This configuration may contribute to the reduced risk of postoperative urinary retention seen with open versus laparoscopic inguinal hernia repairs (1.1% vs 7.9%).[11] Intravenous fluids should be restricted to less than 750 mL, with goal of 400 mL, to reduce the risk of postoperative urinary retention.[11] Most open hernia repairs can be performed under local anesthesia with sedation. This measure can also reduce the risk of postoperative urinary retention. The larger, scrotal hernias are more likely to require muscle relaxation under general anesthesia.

Elective inguinal hernia repairs are considered clean operations. That said, surgical site infection risks have been reported from 0% to 18%. Most operations in low-risk populations can be safely performed without the need for antibiotic prophylaxis, with a 2% to 3% surgical site infection risk. The addition of antibiotics has reduced this risk to 1% to 2%, which was statistically insignificant. Antibiotic prophylaxis is recommended when implanting mesh, with bilateral open inguinal hernia repairs, recurrent inguinal hernias, other high-risk populations (eg, diabetic, immunosuppressed), and in high-risk environments.[3]

Suture choice is variable. In general, permanent monofilament sutures are preferred, of the size 2-0. The traditional Shouldice repair is performed with a steel suture. For some mesh repairs, a sutureless repair or the judicious use of absorbable suture has been advocated by some.[12]

Mesh choice depends on the technique chosen (eg, onlay, sublay, bilayer, plug). Common choices include polypropylene, polyester, expanded polytetrafluoroethyl, and polyvinylidene difluoride, although the biomaterials industry is evolving with the introduction of synthetic resorbable and hybrid mesh. Outcomes based on the weight of the mesh (eg, heavyweight, lightweight) have been studied, with conflicting results.[3] It seems use of lightweight mesh (<40 g/m^2) is associated with improved shorter term recovery and pain, with no long-term differences as compared with heavyweight mesh (>90 g/m^2). Some studies show concern for an increase in the recurrence rate with lightweight mesh.[13] Mesh weight alone should not be a criterion to determine outcome, because the mesh material, pore size, configuration, and size also contribute to overall outcome. Mesh size should be at least 3 × 6 inches, to reduce recurrence risk.

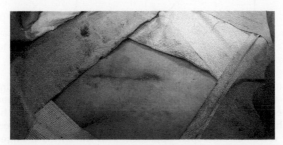

Fig. 1. Drape patient to minimize skin exposure. Setup for a left inguinal hernia repair.

Surgical Approach

Step 1: incision

The choice of incision depends on the operation (**Fig. 2**).

- For most anterior inguinal hernias, a 4-cm incision in the groin is adequate.
- Follow Langer's line, along the ilioinguinal ligament.
- If a patient has a prior incision, for example, Pfannenstiel or abdominoplasty, you can choose to use that, understanding that it may require extension or may be too cephalad.
- For an open retroperitoneal approach, make the incision 2 fingerbreadths cephalad to the inguinal ligament.
- Use self-retaining retractors (eg, Weitlaner or wound protector) and prevent over-retraction of wound to reduce postoperative pain, edema, and ecchymoses.

Step 2: exposure of the hernia

- Incise the external oblique aponeurosis, starting at external ring, along its fibers.
- Be careful to prevent injury to underlying ilioinguinal nerve. Consider a wheal of local anesthetic to lift the aponeurosis off the muscle and nerve.
- In males: Use a Penrose to circle the spermatic cord and hernia sac.
- Be careful to include and preserve the genital branch of the genitofemoral nerve. The best technique is to stay close to the pubic tubercle when encircling the cord.

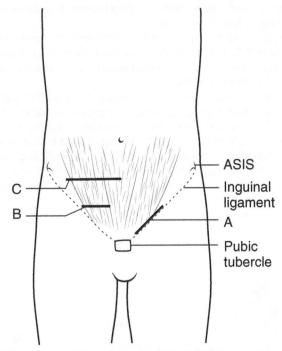

Fig. 2. Groin incision options. ASIS, anterior superior iliac spine. *A*, inguinal incision along Langer's line, directly over inguinal ligament, which follows a line between ASIS and pubic tubercle. *B*, transverse incision for inguinal approach. This may sometimes be close to a Pfannenstiel incision that can be extended laterally for better cosmetic outcome. *C*, low transverse incision for retromuscular open approach. This incision is 2 fingerbreadths above the inguinal ligament and extends the width of the rectus muscle.

- In females: Carefully dissect off the round ligament and hernia sac off the underlying muscle.
- In females: One can choose to sacrifice the round ligament. Be careful to identify and not injure the genital branch of the genitofemoral nerve in this process.

Step 3: handling of the nerves

- Identify all 3 nerves: Ilioinguinal, iliohypogastric, and genital branch of the genitofemoral nerve (**Fig. 3**).[3,13]
- Preservation of the nerves, without skeletonization or dissection, is the best option to reduce risk of postoperative neuropathic pain.
- If the nerve is injured or at risk for injury (eg, densely adherent to hernia sac), consider high transection of the nerve and burial of the nerve end into the internal oblique muscle to reduce the risk of neuroma.
- Preplanned neurectomy is not recommended.

Step 4: reduction of the hernia sac

- Perform high dissection of all hernia sacs, that is, completely return all peritoneum and its contents to the abdomen.
- Ligation of the hernia sac may contribute to acute postoperative pain. For large or redundant sacs, ligation may help to reduce recurrence rates.[3]
- For indirect inguinal hernias, carefully dissect the peritoneum and its contents off the spermatic cord or round ligament, identifying nerves and the vas deferens in the process.
- In females, if the round ligament is transected, use that as a handle to adequately reduce the peritoneum en masse with the round ligament (**Fig. 4**).

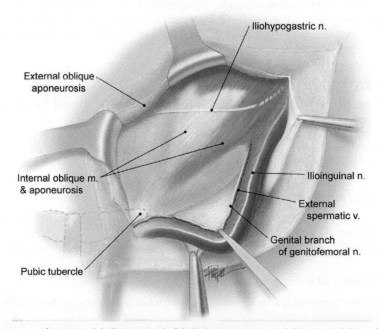

Fig. 3. Preserved nerves: (a) ilioinguinal, (b) iliohypogastric, and (c) genital branch of the genitofemoral nerve (n.). v., vein. (*Courtesy of* D. Chen, MD, Santa Monica, CA.)

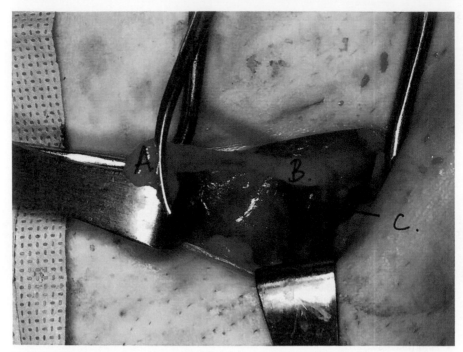

Fig. 4. Transected left round ligament (A), with associated indirect inguinal hernia fat content (B) seen through internal ring (C).

- For large scrotal hernias, consider transection of the sac. Leave the distal peritoneum deep within the scrotum. This step will reduce hematoma and seroma risks. Consider marsupialization of the distal sac via opening it up along its anterior surface.

Step 5: handling of lipomas

- Fat within the inguinal canal can cause pain. This fat should be reduced or excised.
- Spermatic cord fat is normal and should be left alone. This fat is distinct from cord lipomas, which should be excised, because they may cause pain or feeling of a mass or swelling in the groin or scrotum.

Step 6: ruling out femoral hernia

- In women, assess the femoral space transinguinally. This examination can be performed via a finger through the internal ring.
- If a femoral hernia is noted, it should be included as part of the hernia repair.

Step 7: handling of a direct inguinal hernia

- Once the contents are reduced, consider primarily closing the direct defect, using absorbable suture.[13]
- This measure allows for reduced bridging of the repair, and improved outcome.
- The same technique can be used for a blown out pelvic floor.

Step 8: repair of hernia

Mesh repair: Lichtenstein onlay (**Fig. 5**)
- Inferiorly, flat mesh is secured to the inguinal ligament with a running suture starting at the pubic tubercle and stopping at the level of the internal ring (**Fig. 5B**).
- Too lateral of a suture placement can entrap the genitofemoral nerve branches and/or the lateral femorocutaneous nerve.
- Superiorly, the mesh is secured to the rectus abdominis and conjoint tendon using interrupted sutures (**Fig. 5C**).
- The iliohypogastric nerve is at risk for suture entrapment with this step. Some advocate the use of absorbable suture to reduce the risk of permanent entrapment and pain.
- In males, the mesh is slit laterally to medially, with the lower tail being approximately one-third of the width of the upper tail. This measure recreates the internal ring.
- The spermatic cord is placed within this slit. In the Amid modification of this technique, a single stitch is used to secure the 2 tails to the shelving edge of the inguinal ligament. This allows for a tunneling of the spermatic cord, with a lesser perceived risk of cord entrapment (**Fig. 5D**).
- In females, if the round ligament is sacrificed, no mesh slitting is necessary.
- The tails are laid flat under the external oblique aponeurosis laterally. No fixation is necessary.
- The external oblique aponeurosis is reapproximated with absorbable suture.
- Alternatives to fixation
   - Glue fixation has been reported, with a single suture used to fix the tails together and possibly another suture to fix the mesh medially to the pubic tubercle.

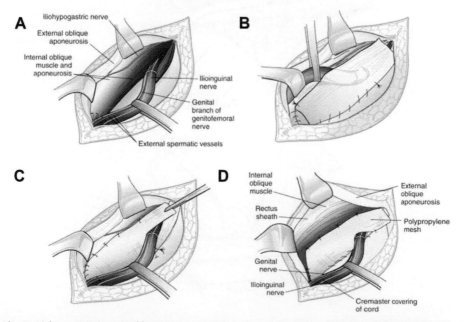

Fig. 5. Lichtenstein inguinal hernia repair with onlay mesh. (*From* Malangoni MA, Rosen MJ. Hernias. In: Townsend CM Jr, Beauchamp RD, Mark EB, et al, editors. Sabiston textbook of surgery [Chapter 44]. 20th edition. Philadelphia: Elsevier; 2017. p. 1100; with permission.)

○ Self-fixating mesh is available, requiring at most 1 suture to close the tail around the mesh.
○ There is no strong evidence to show superiority of 1 fixation option over another.[14]

Gilbert bilayer (**Figs. 6** and **7**)

- Similar to the Lichtenstein onlay repair, this technique includes a posterior sublay mesh repair as well.
- A wide posterior dissection is made bluntly to accommodate for the posterior mesh portion.
- Be careful to prevent vascular injury with this blunt dissection. Vessels at risk include the inferior epigastric vessels, femoral vessels, and obturator branches.
- The bridge between the 2 mesh layers is placed through the indirect or direct defect.
- The posterior layer must have adequate space preperitoneally to accommodate for flat placement of the mesh. This step is important, because this portion of the mesh is at risk for folding and causing pain or recurrence.

Kugel, Stoppa, Nyhus, and transrectus sheath preperitoneal sublay (**Figs. 8** and **9**)

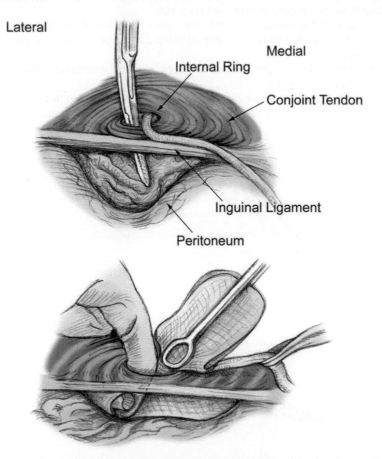

Fig. 6. Bilayer hernia repair. (Image reproduced with permission from Medscape Drugs & Diseases (https://emedicine.medscape.com/), Open Inguinal Hernia Repair, 2018, available at: https://emedicine.medscape.com/article/1534281-overview.)

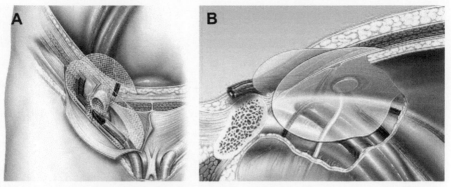

Fig. 7. (*A*) Prolene hernia system anterior view. (*B*) Prolene hernia system posterior view. (*Courtesy of* Ethicon, Inc, Somerville, NJ; with permission).

- Similar in concept to the laparoscopic repair, a mesh is used to cover the myopectineal orifice in the preperitoneal space.
- A low transverse 5-cm incision is made 2 fingerbreadths cephalad to the inguinal ligament and pubic tubercle. Alternatively, a low midline incision can be made; this technique is preferred for giant or bilateral hernias.

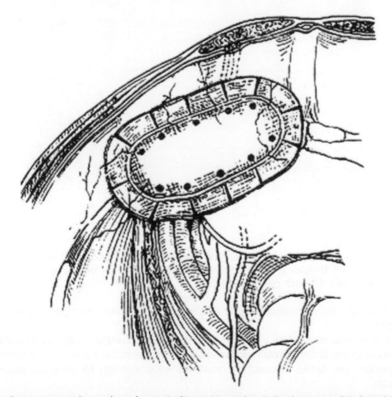

Fig. 8. Open retroperitoneal mesh repair. (*From* Natarajan B, Burjonrappa SC, Cemaj S, et al. Basic features of groin hernia and its repair. In: Yeo CJ, editor. Shackelford's surgery of the alimentary tract. 7th edition. Philadelphia: Elsevier; 2013. p. 579; with permission.)

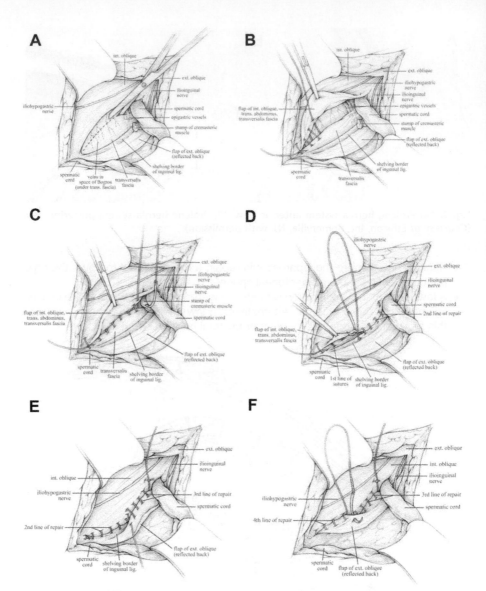

Fig. 9. Shouldice technique tissue repair. ext., exterior; int., interior; lig., ligament; trans., transversalis. (*From* Shouldice EB. The Shouldice repair for groin hernias. Surg Clin North Am 2003;83(5):1163–87; with permission.)

- Muscle-sparing dissection is made, accessing the retromuscular preperitoneal space.
- The preperitoneal space is developed bluntly and widely, reducing all contents to expose the entire myopectineal space, from the pubic tubercle to the anterior superior iliac spine. Dissection must be wide enough to accommodate the mesh.
- Be careful not to injure the deep inferior epigastric vessels in this process.
- Mesh placement should be flat and with appropriate coverage and overlap with the pubic tubercle and Cooper's ligament.

- The mesh is sutured to the rectus abdominis insertion onto the pubic tubercle medially. Additional sutures may be placed to Cooper's ligament inferior to the femoral space and superiorly to the rectus abdominis.
- An alternative approach is the transinguinal preperitoneal approach. This approach involves placement of retroperitoneal mesh via an inguinal incision and may require opening the pelvic floor.

Tissue repair: The Shouldice technique (**Fig. 9**)

- The incision and hernia dissection is similar to the mesh repair (as described).
- Instead of mesh implantation, the pelvic floor is opened widely.
- Start at the internal ring and transversely open the transversalis fascia toward the pubic tubercle (**Fig. 9A**).
- Bluntly dissect the retroperitoneal tissue, including the hernia sac, peritoneum, and any retroperitoneal fat, off the posterior wall of the pelvic floor.
- Identify the pelvic floor anatomy in preparation for the suture repair.
  - ○ Inferior flap: transversalis fascia edge, shelving edge of inguinal ligament, external oblique aponeurosis.
  - ○ Superior flap: transversus abdominis, internal oblique.
- Classically, the cremasteric muscle and genital nerve branch are resected.
- There are 4 layers of suture with this technique.
  - ○ Layer 1: Start medially. Suture transversalis fascia edge of inferior flap to underside of transversus abdominis muscle of superior flap. Include the proximal stump of the cremasteric muscle surrounding the spermatic cord at the internal ring (**Fig. 9B, C**).
  - ○ Layer 2: Reverse with the same suture, now sewing laterally to medially. Sew the shelving edge of the inguinal ligament inferiorly to the transversus abdominis superiorly **Fig. 9D**.
  - ○ Layer 3: Start laterally at the internal ring. Suture the external oblique aponeurosis, just anterior to shelving edge, and inferiorly to partial thickness of the internal oblique. Continue medially to include the anterior rectus fascia overlying the pubic tubercle (**Fig. 9E**).
  - ○ Layer 4: Reverse with the same suture, now sewing medially to laterally. Sew another layer of external oblique aponeurosis inferiorly to the internal oblique superiorly (**Fig. 9F**).
- If the cremasteric muscle was resected, then pulley up the distal cremasteric muscle around the spermatic cord and sew it to the anterior rectus fascia, to prevent low-lying testicle.

Bassini (**Fig. 10**)

- This is similar to the Shouldice repair, but with only a single layer of sutures and traditionally with interrupted sutures (as discussed).
- The pelvic floor is widely opened. Modern modifications skip this step, with varied results.
- Classically, the cremasteric muscle is resected, but the genital nerve branch is preserved.
- Sutures are placed to approximate the superior flap to the inferior flap, that is, the internal oblique and transversus abdominis superiorly to the transversalis fascia and shelving edge of the inguinal ligament inferiorly.
- A relaxing incision may be necessary superolaterally to reduce tension on this repair.
- Modifications of this technique separate this single row of sutures into 2 separate rows, as in layers 2 and 4 of the Shouldice technique.

McVay (**Fig. 11**)

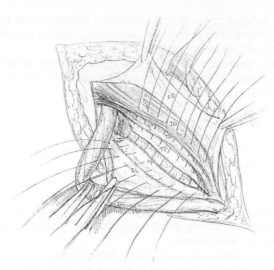

Fig. 10. Bassini tissue repair. (*From* Lao OB, Fitzgibbons RJ Jr, Cusick RA. Pediatric inguinal hernias, hydroceles, and undescended testicles. Surg Clin North Am 2012;92(3):487–504; with permission.)

- This is similar to the Bassini repair, but repairs femoral hernias at the same setting (as discussed).
- The pelvic floor is widely opened.
- The cremasteric muscle and genitofemoral nerves are preserved.
- Also known as the Cooper's ligament repair, sutures are placed to approximate the superior flap to the inferior flap laterally and to Cooper's ligament medially.
- The inferior flap transition from Cooper's ligament to transversalis fascia and shelving edge of inguinal ligament begins at the level of the femoral vein.

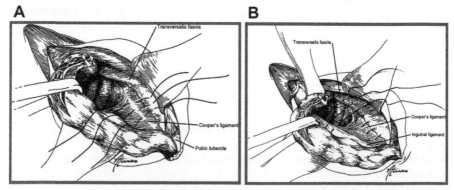

Fig. 11. McVay tissue repair for right femoral hernia. (*A*) Interrupted sutures from transversalis fascia to Cooper's ligament, medial to the external iliac vessels, closing the femoral space. (*B*) Interrupted sutures transitioning from transversalis fascia to inguinal ligament, lateral to the external iliac vessels. (*From* Gore DC. Inguinal herniorrhaphy (McVay; Cooper's ligament repair). In: Townsend CM, Evers BM, editors. Atlas of General Surgical Techniques. Philadelphia: Elsevier; 2010. p. 802–810; with permission.)

- A relaxing incision may be necessary superolaterally to reduce tension on this repair.

Nyhus iliopubic tract repair (**Fig. 12**)

- This approach is similar to the open retroperitoneal mesh repair (as discussed).
- This technique is best applied to incarcerated or strangulated hernias, because it allows for a nonmesh repair extraperitoneally after addressing the at-risk hernia contents intraperitoneally via the same incision.
- A 5-cm, low transverse incision is made 2 fingerbreadths cephalad to the inguinal ligament.
- Once the hernia is reduced and the peritoneum is dissected widely off the posterior wall of the pelvic floor, the repair can be performed.
- Using interrupted sutures, the transversalis arch is approximated to the iliopubic tract.

Immediate postoperative care

Postoperatively, the patient should be monitored for pain control and urination. Ice packs over the incision can help with pain, edema, and ecchymosis. Narcotics should be minimized and fluids should be restricted to reduce the risk of urinary retention.[11] Antiinflammatory medications have a much more significant impact than narcotics on pain control for hernia repairs, because much of the pain is inflammatory in nature.[15] Most patients should not require significant pain medication for longer than 3 to 7 days.

REHABILITATION AND RECOVERY

Postoperative recovery can vary among patients. In general, as long as pain is contained, patient activity need not be restricted. In fact, there is no evidence that restricting patient activity offers any advantage in terms of hernia recurrence or outcome.[3] This includes return to work and most exercises.

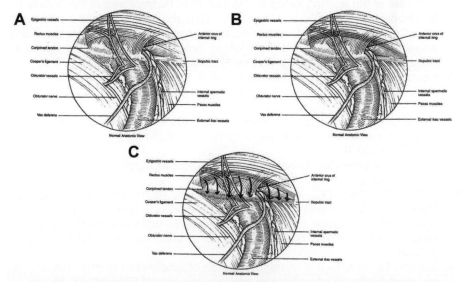

Fig. 12. Nyhus preperitoneal open iliopubic tract repair. (*A*) Preperitoneal anatomy. (*B, C*) The transversalis arch (*pink*) and il is sutured down to the iliopubic tract (*blue*) with interrupted sutures (*arrows*). (*Adapted from* Essential Surgical Procedures. In: Inguinal and femoral hernia – laparoscopic repair. Elsevier Inc; 2016. p. e68–84; with permission.)

SUMMARY

Open inguinal hernia approaches are varied. The best studied approaches are reviewed herein. The common factor among them is the imperative anatomy knowledge of the surgeon. This knowledge is key to improved outcomes. A tailored approach is best to determine which open technique, if any, is most appropriate for the patient. Although the anterior mesh approach is the most commonly applied, there is support in using the posterior approach or a tissue repair for subsets of patients, such as women.

REFERENCES

1. Kingsnorth A, LeBlanc K. Hernias: inguinal and incisional. Lancet 2003;362: 1561–71.
2. Towfigh S. Obscure groin pain in women. In: Campanelli G, editor. Inguinal hernia surgery. Milan (Italy): Springer-Verlag; 2017. p. 181–6.
3. The HerniaSurge Group. International guidelines for groin hernia management. Hernia 2018;22(1):1–165.
4. Towfigh S. Foreign body reaction, fibromyalgia, and autoimmune disorders. In: Jacob BP, Chen DC, Ramshaw B, et al, editors. The SAGES manual of groin pain. New York: Springer-Verlag; 2016. p. 429–34.
5. Neumayer L, Towfigh S. Inguinal hernia. In: Cameron JL, Cameron AM, editors. Current surgical therapy. 11th Edition. New York: Elsevier; 2013.
6. Nilsson H, Holmberg H, Nordin P. Groin hernia repair in women – a nationwide register study. Am J Surg 2017. [Epub ahead of print].
7. Junge K, Rosch R, Klinge U, et al. Risk factors related to recurrence in inguinal hernia repair: a retrospective analysis. Hernia 2006;10(4):309–15.
8. Korte W, Cattaneo M, Chassot PG, et al. Peri-operative management of antiplatelet therapy in patients with coronary artery disease: joint position paper by members of the working group on Perioperative Haemostasis of the Society on Thrombosis and Haemostasis Research (GTH), the Working Group on Perioperative Coagulation of the Austrian Society for Anesthesiology, Resuscitation and Intensive Care (OGARI) and the Working Group Thrombosis of the European Society for Cardiology (ESC). Thromb Haemost 2011;105:743–9.
9. Kowalski TJ, Kothari SN, Mathiason MA, et al. Impact of hair removal on surgical site infection rates: a prospective randomized noninferiority trial. J Am Coll Surg 2016;223(5):704–11.
10. Lefebvre A, Saliou P, Lucet JC, et al. Preoperative hair removal and surgical site infections: network meta-analysis of randomized controlled trials. J Hosp Infect 2015;91(2):100–8.
11. Kowalik U, Plante MKK. Urinary retention in surgical patients. Surg Clin North Am 2016;96:453–67.
12. O'Neill SM, Chen DC, Amid PK. Groin hernia repair: open techniques. In: Novitsky Y, editor. Hernia surgery. Cham (Switzerland): Springer; 2016.
13. Simons MP, Aufenacker T, Bay-Nielsen M, et al. European Hernia Society guidelines on the treatment of inguinal hernia in adult patients. Hernia 2009;13: 343–403.
14. Sanders DL, Waydia S. A systematic review of randomized control trials assessing mesh fixation in open inguinal hernia repair. Hernia 2014;18:165–76.
15. Bjurstrom MF, Nicol AL, Amid PK, et al. Pain control following inguinal herniorrhaphy: current perspectives. J Pain Res 2014;7:277–90.

Minimally Invasive Approaches to Inguinal Hernias

Charlotte M. Horne, MD, Ajita S. Prabhu, MD

KEYWORDS

- Inguinal hernia • Minimally invasive repair • Transabdominal preperitoneal approach
- Total extraperitoneal approach • Robotic inguinal hernia repairs

KEY POINTS

- Both the transabdominal preperitoneal approach and the total extraperitoneal approach to inguinal hernias provide an effective means of repairing inguinal hernias.
- The robotic platform can be used and may help to decrease immediate postoperative pain; however, as this is a fairly new technique, more research will help further determine long-term outcomes.
- In all methods of fixation, we ensure adequate fixation medially with tacks placed on Cooper's ligament.
- Awareness of the nerves and vessels helps to guide dissection as well as prevent inadvertent injury during mesh fixation.

INTRODUCTION

Inguinal hernia repair is one of the most commonly performed operations by a general surgeon.[1] Historically, repair was conducted via an open approach; however, since the description of minimally invasive techniques two decades ago, there has been a shift to a laparoscopic approach. Initial pitfalls of the laparoscopic approaches included high recurrence rates, as mesh reinforcement was not routine, as well as postoperative pain due to tack placement. Now minimally invasive inguinal hernia repair is associated with minimal morbidity, mortality, and low recurrence rates. Laparoscopic repair has been associated with decreased postoperative pain, earlier return to work, and improved cosmetic outcomes when compared with an open apporach.[2] Despite this, there is no definitive evidence that suggests superiority to an open approach. The two main minimally invasive approaches are a transabdominal preperitoneal approach (TAPP) or a

The author has nothing to disclose.
The Cleveland Clinic, Department of General Surgery, 9500 Euclid Avenue, Cleveland, OH 44113, USA
E-mail address: HORNEC@ccf.org

total extraperitoneal approach (TEP). Extensive comparison of these 2 techniques has been conducted, and there is yet to be definitive evidence to support a superior approach.[3] We feel both techniques to be equally effective when performed by an experienced surgeon and choice of approach is at the discretion of the operating surgeon.

Advantages of a minimally invasive approach include the ability to address bilateral hernias through the same incisions, as well as, in the setting of recurrent inguinal hernia repair, these approaches can allow for dissection in virgin tissue planes. The most challenging part of these procedures is appropriate identification of inguinal anatomy. It is important to identify major neurovascular structures early and be cognizant about their location through to the completion of the operation. Knowledge of the anatomy also can guide dissection in a safe manner and limit postoperative morbidity.

TRANSABDOMINAL PREPERITONEAL REPAIR
Patient Selection

Although most inguinal hernias can be approached from an intraperitoneal approach, some relative contraindications include multiple previous abdominal operations as well as the inability to tolerate general anesthesia. Recurrent and bilateral inguinal hernias may benefit from a laparoscopic approach. We routinely give our patients prophylactic heparin and preoperative antibiotic prophylaxis before incision. A Foley is placed preoperatively and removed at completion of the operation to minimize urinary retention postoperatively.

Patient Positioning and Port Placement

Patients are placed in the supine position. Access is gained at the umbilicus using a Hassan technique. Once access is gained and the abdomen is insufflated, two 5-mm ports are placed slightly cephalad to the level of the umbilicus just lateral to the rectus sheath bilaterally under direct visualization. If adhesiolysis is required, we recommend that this be done sharply if possible.

The preferred dissection plane is the preperitoneal plane, which can be identified by the presence of the transversalis muscle fibers superiorly. Recognizing entry into the pretransversalis plane, which can be identified by the recuts muscle superiorly, is essential, as transition to the preperitoneal plane must be done lateral to the inferior epigastric vessels for proper mesh placement.

Initial Dissection

Initial dissection begins at the medial umbilical fold. An incision is made in the peritoneum just lateral to the fold using scissors with cautery. This incision is should be made as close as possible to the umbilicus to create a space to accommodate an appropriate-sized piece of mesh. Next, further lateral dissection lengthens the peritoneal flap. When carrying out the dissection laterally, it is important to maintain the plane high on the abdominal wall. Creation of the peritoneal flap is complete when the flap is lateral to the inferior epigastric vessels and the anterior superior iliac spine (ASIS) has been reached (**Fig. 1**).

After the peritoneal flap is created, dissection is begun at the medial aspect to identity the pubic tubercle and Cooper ligament. This is successfully completed bluntly due to the lack of significant structures medial to the inferior epigastric vessels. Once the pubis has been reached, further dissection is completed medial to the epigastric vessels, to fully expose the Cooper ligament.

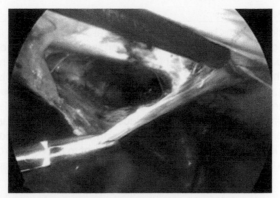

Fig. 1. Dissection is started just lateral to the medial umbilical fold. One grasper is used to pull the incised peritoneal flap to assist in dissection. (*From* Rosen MJ. Transabdominal preperitoneal inguinal hernia repair. In: Atlas of abdominal wall reconstruction. 2nd edition. Elsevier; 2017. p. 418; with permission.)

Lateral Dissection

Next, attention is turned to the lateral aspect (**Fig. 2**). This should occur immediately on the peritoneal flap to maintain hemostasis. Working laterally to medially, dissection is carried toward the inferior epigastric muscles. To facilitate dissection, appropriate tension must be maintained on the peritoneal flap. Filmy adhesions are pushed gently to develop the lateral plane. The lateral extent of dissection is reached when the curve of the abdominal wall begins to take a downward trajectory. It is in this dissection plane the testicular vessels and vas deferens will be encountered. The peritoneum can be bluntly dissected off the spermatic cord. It is imperative that the structures of the spermatic cord are identified and fully mobilized to conclude the lateral dissection. This can be checked by pulling on the peritoneal flap and ensuring that the cord structures do not move with it. In women, we routinely divide the round ligament, to facilitate further dissection.

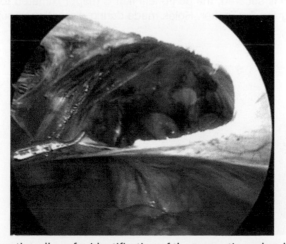

Fig. 2. Lateral dissection allows for identification of the spermatic cord and vas deferens. All moves should occur in a medial to lateral fashion to avoid injury to the inferior epigastric vessels. (*From* Rosen MJ. Transabdominal preperitoneal inguinal hernia repair. In: Atlas of abdominal wall reconstruction. 2nd edition. Elsevier; 2017. p. 420; with permission.)

Hernia Reduction

After the spermatic cord has been identified, the presence of a direct, indirect, or combined hernia defect can be determined. Direct hernias can be reduced by retraction of the hernia with countertraction against the transversalis fascia. To confirm the entirety of the hernia sac has been reduced, the Cooper ligament should be visualized from its medial aspect to the epigastric vessels. Indirect hernias are reduced best by, first, mobilizing the cord structures off the hernia sac. Next, by applying lateral retraction, the indirect hernia can be successfully reduced. Often, if you are unable to reduce the hernia, further dissection of the hernia sac off the spermatic cord needs to be completed. Cord lipomas should be resected if present to prevent perception of recurrence. This should be done with cautery, as often there is a blood vessel supplying the lipoma.

Mesh Selection and Fixation

We routinely use a 12 × 15-cm piece of heavyweight polypropylene mesh to ensure adequate coverage of the hernia defect. Although anatomically shaped meshes can be used, we find that these are more expensive and do not provide superior results. We choose to use a heavyweight mesh, as this has been shown to be equivalent to lightweight mesh in terms of recurrence and postoperative pain.[4] Maintaining a high lateral dissection during the creation of the peritoneal flap creates a space that accommodates this size of mesh. As the most likely location for recurrence is at the medial aspect, we ensure adequate fixation of the mesh by placing 2 ProTacks directly on the pubis and Cooper ligament and another tack placed high and medial (**Fig. 3**). The mesh is secured laterally by another tack placed lateral to the epigastric vessels above the iliopubic tract. Placing the tack here avoids the impaling nerves. Controversy exists as to the optimal securement of the mesh, with current methods including tackers, glue, and sutures. It is our opinion that appropriate placement of tacks with awareness to location of the pathways of the nerves, can help minimize chronic pain postoperatively.

After the mesh is secured, the peritoneal flap is reapproximated to the abdominal wall, again using the ProTacker. Holes made during dissection should be closed at this point.

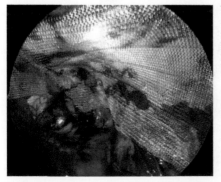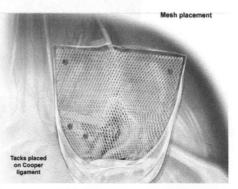

Fig. 3. Two tacks are placed on the Cooper ligament, with 2 other tacks placed high medially and high laterally. *Left panel* indicates intra-operative appearance. *Right panel* is a pictorial reference. (*From* Rosen MJ. Transabdominal preperitoneal inguinal hernia repair. In: Atlas of abdominal wall reconstruction. 2nd edition. Elsevier; 2017. p. 428; with permission.)

Laparoscopic ports are removed under direct visualization and the fascia at the umbilical port is closed using a figure of 8 stitch. The Foley catheter is removed at completion of the operation. Patients are discharged the day of surgery after they have voided. Patients are not routinely given lifting restrictions postoperatively and are counseled to increase their activity as they are able to tolerate.

Pearls and Pitfalls

- Maintaining the peritoneal dissection high on the abdominal wall during creation of the peritoneal flap laterally helps to provide a space large enough to accommodate an appropriate-sized piece of mesh.
- Moves should be carried out in a lateral to medial dissection when clearing the Cooper ligament and medial to lateral fashion during lateral dissection to prevent injury to the inferior epigastric vessels.
- Large indirect hernia sacs can be ligated and incompletely reduced if complete reduction causes significant risk to the contents of the spermatic cord. This puts these patients at higher risk for postoperative seroma and this should be carefully monitored.
- Counter pressure should be applied on the abdominal wall while tacks are being placed to ensure tacks are not inadvertently placed below the iliopubic tract, which may result in a nerve injury.

LAPAROSCOPIC TOTALLY EXTRAPERITONEAL HERNIA REPAIRS
Preoperative Planning

Like TAPP hernia repairs, a TEP approach can be used in most inguinal hernia repairs. Relative contraindications to this approach include previous surgery in the retroperitoneum, certain types of previous inguinal hernia repair, significant history of prior lower abdominal surgery, and inability to tolerate general anesthesia. It is also imperative that operative notes from previous hernia repairs are obtained, as this may dictate the most appropriate way to approach the hernia. Use of a previous patch and plug or hernia system can result in a technically difficult TEP and these may benefit from an open repair.

In-depth knowledge of inguinal anatomy is essential for a safe, effective, and efficient repair. Principal spaces that will be developed are the space of Retzius medially and the space of Bogros laterally. Once these spaces have been identified and dissected, the myopectineal orifice is identified and the hernia defect can be appreciated.

Patient Positioning

The patients undergo induction of general anesthesia, first-generation cephalosporins are given 1 hour before incision, unless patient allergies dictate otherwise, and a Foley catheter is placed perioperatively. We routinely place a Foley to limit postoperative urinary retention and facilitate identification of a bladder injury; however, it is reasonable to have the patient void just before the operation. Patients are placed in the supine position with arms tucked at the side. The operating surgeon stands on the side contralateral to the hernia, with the assistant on the opposite side of the patient.

Incision and Initial Dissection

A 10-mm incision is made just lateral to the umbilicus on the side opposite of the hernia. In the setting of bilateral hernia repair, the incision should be made opposite the side of the larger hernia. This allows for improved visualization as well as an increased amount of space to work in. The anterior fascia is identified and divided either sharply or with cautery, the rectus muscles are retracted laterally, and the posterior sheath is exposed. We routinely use a 10-mm dissecting balloon trocar to develop our preperitoneal space; however, initial blunt dissection with the camera is feasible and can result in moderate cost savings. The balloon trocar is directed toward the pubis and subsequently inflated under direct visualization. The balloon should be inflated completely if possible. The dissecting trocar is then exchanged for a 10-mm trocar.

To create the preperitoneal space without the dissecting balloon, the plane is first gently developed with finger dissection. We next continue the dissection at the midline to the pubis with a blunt laparoscopic probe. The trocar is then inserted in the preperitoneal plane and insufflated, which assists in further dissection of this space. To complete the dissection, the laparoscopic camera can be used to create enough space so subsequent ports can be placed. Care must be taken to avoid inadvertent injury to the peritoneum, as this will result in insufflation of the abdominal cavity and make visualization and subsequent dissection more difficult.

We then place two 5-mm trocars under direct visualization. Care must be taken to ensure that the inferior-most trocar is at least 2 cm above the pubic symphysis to ensure for adequate range of motion. The superior 5-mm trocar should be placed as close to the 10-mm port as possible to increase the space between the 2 working trocars to facilitate dissection as well as surgeon ergonomics.

As with an intra-abdominal approach, inguinal anatomy can again prove challenging for even the experienced surgeon. Careful attention to location of the inferior epigastric and iliac vessels is essential to ensure safe dissection. We start our initial dissection by clearing off the Cooper ligament (**Fig. 4**). This is a safe place to begin the dissection because of the lack of important neurovascular structures. The Cooper ligament is exposed using a laparoscopic Kittner through the superior port with dissection directed inferiorly to maintain the adequate plane.

Lateral Dissection

Next, we turn our attention laterally to expose the transversalis muscle. This dissection will develop the space of Bogros, which is the lateral continuation of the space of Retzius. Developing this plane allows for access into the myopectineal orifice and

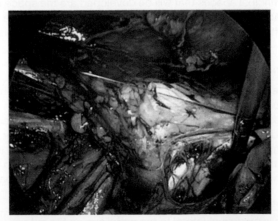

Fig. 4. Medial dissection begins with identification of the Cooper ligament (*bottom right*) and dissection directly on top of the ligament. Care must be taken here to avoid the corona mortis. (*From* Rosen MJ. Transabdominal preperitoneal inguinal hernia repair. In: Atlas of abdominal wall reconstruction. 2nd edition. Elsevier; 2017. p. 439; with permission.)

further delineation of the hernia defect. To develop this space, we use laparoscopic Kittners, with one applying gentle superior retraction against the transversalis fascia and the other used to push the peritoneum inferiorly. Care must be taken to ensure dissection is not carried out in a plane to cephalad, as this will develop a plane superior to the transversalis fascia. The lateral extent of dissection is often encountered when it becomes no longer technically feasible to progress more laterally due to the limits of the instruments.

After lateral dissection is complete, dissection is turned medially toward the internal ring. It is essential that the operator is cognizant of the iliac vessels, as these can be closely associated with the cord structures. Upward traction against the abdominal wall can facilitate entry into the preperitoneal plane. Dissection should be carried down to the internal ring, to allow for full exposure of the spermatic cord.

Dissection of the Spermatic Cord

The next step is to create a window around the spermatic cord. We do this by first identifying the vas deferens. Once the vas deferens is identified, this is retracted superiorly. Attachments are bluntly dissected until all the contents of the cord have been identified. During this dissection, work should occur in a superior manner, as the contents of the triangle of doom lie inferiorly. Constant upward retraction on the abdominal wall and epigastric vessels facilitates dissection of structures off the spermatic cord (**Fig. 5**). After the spermatic cord is identified, determination of the presence of direct, indirect, or combination of both is present.

If a direct hernia is encountered, reduction can be facilitated by applying retraction inferiorly while the other hand bluntly dissects attachments off the hernia sac. The goal of the retraction and dissection should be to identify the distal-most portion or top of the hernia sac. Once this has been identified, it can be held in one hand, with careful inferiorly directed tension, while the other hand dissects the hernia free of surrounding adhesions. The hernia has been completely reduced when the full extent of the direct defect can be visualized.

Mesh Selection and Placement

We routinely use a 4 × 6-inch heavyweight polypropylene mesh, although a lightweight mesh is another feasible option. Preshaped meshes can be used; however, we do not routinely use these because of their cost.

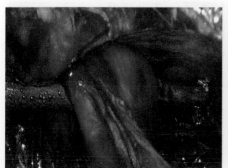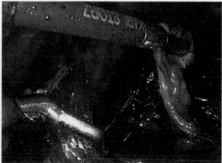

Fig. 5. First the hernia sac and cord structures are identified and isolated (*left*). Next, the cord structures are dissected off the hernia sac (*right*). Upward retraction against the abdominal wall can facilitate this dissection.

To facilitate the placement of the mesh, the medial aspect can be marked so it can be easily identified. The mesh is then rolled and placed through the 10-mm port into the preperitoneal space. The mesh is subsequently positioned at the pubis and is tacked using a ProTacker to the Cooper ligament (**Fig. 6**). We routinely anchor the mesh medially first, as this facilitates unrolling of the mesh in a narrow space. It is imperative that appropriate midline coverage is achieved, as this is the most common location of recurrence. Next, the mesh is unrolled laterally, and the superior aspect is anchored to the superior aspect of the abdominal wall.

As with TAPP, other types of methods to secure the mesh in place have been investigated. These include absorbable tacks, glue, or even no fixation. We routinely use titanium tacks, as there is some evidence to suggest that this is associated with decreased chronic pain.[5]

We do not routinely explore both groins at the time of the index operation, because if there is no concern for a contralateral hernia and they are asymptomatic, potential operative exploration could result in postoperative morbidity. We do routinely explore the contralateral groin if there is concern for a hernia on preoperative examination or a large defect is noted intraoperatively.

After the mesh is anchored and hemostasis is achieved, the abdomen is desufflated under direct visualization. This ensures that the mesh lays smoothly in the space. The fascia is closed with a figure of 8 0-vicryl suture, the Foley is removed, and the patient is awakened from general anesthesia. Patients are routinely discharged on the same day after voiding in the post anesthesia care unit (PACU).

Pearls and Pitfalls

- As space is limited in the TEP, careful placement of ports to facilitate ease of dissection is key. To achieve optimal space between the 2 working ports, we place our inferior port first and then, using a finder, place the superior port as close to the 10-mm port as possible without impaling the balloon of the balloon port. Placement of the inferior port must be 2 cm above the pubis. If this port is placed too inferiorly, dissection will be limited by the pubis.
- When placing the ports, especially with placement of the preperitoneal dissecting port, care must be taken to avoid penetrating the peritoneum, as insufflation of the abdomen can make further dissection and visualization more difficult.

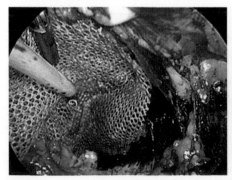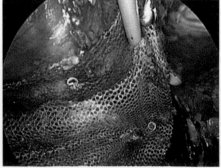

Fig. 6. Two tacks are placed on the Cooper ligament (*left*) and then the mesh is unrolled and tacked laterally (*right*). Palpation on the abdominal wall while tacking ensures tacks are placed about the iliopubic tract.

- The corona mortis often can be encountered during the dissection of the Cooper ligament. Gentle dissection here with early identification of this vein and control can prevent inadvertent vascular injury.
- Tacks should be placed superior to the iliopubic tract to avoid injury to nerve structures. This can be ensured by palpation against the abdominal wall when the tacks are fired.
- Early recognition of the inferior epigastric allows for prevention of an inadvertent avulsion of these vessels. Once identified, they can be retracted superiorly throughout the lateral dissection to aid in visualization and prevent vascular injury.

ROBOTIC TRANSABDOMINAL PREPERITONEAL INGUINAL HERNIA REPAIR
Introduction

As chronic groin pain remains the Achilles' heel of the inguinal hernia repair, different fixation techniques, including glue, various types of tacks, and suturing the mesh in place present possible solutions to this problem. As intracorporeal suturing proves to be technically challenging due to the limited range of motion of the trocars in a laparoscopic transabdominal approach to hernia repair, use of the robotic platform in these situations can help to overcome these ergonomic restrictions. Robotic inguinal hernia repair presents a reasonable option to inguinal hernia repairs, and there are some data to suggest improvement in immediate postoperative pain when compared with a standard laparoscopic approach.[6]

Patient Selection

Like laparoscopic transabdominal and TEP approaches, relative contraindications to a robotic approach include an extensive intra-abdominal surgical history, previous pelvic radiation, and a history of surgery in the retroperitoneum. We routinely obtain all previous operative reports, as certain hernia repairs can lead to increased technical difficulty of the repair. Also, patients must be healthy enough to tolerate general anesthesia for the duration of the operation.

Patient Positioning and Port Placement

Patients are placed supine on the operating table with arms tucked at their side. The operative area is clipped and appropriate preoperative antibiotics are given before incision. A vertical skin incision, large enough to accommodate a 12-mm balloon port, is made 4 cm cephalad to the umbilicus. Dissection is carried down to the linea alba, which is divided, and the abdomen is entered under direct visualization. We then secure the anterior fascia using 0-vicryl sutures. A 12 mm balloon port is then inserted. The abdomen is insufflated to 15 mm Hg and a brief inspection of the abdominal cavity is completed. Next, two 8-mm ports are placed at the same level as the initial 12-mm port, approximately 4 cm cephalad to the umbilicus, under direct visualization. We ensure that there is approximately 8 cm between the ports, as this facilitates full range of motion of the robotic arms. The patient is placed in mild reverse Trendelenburg and the robot is docked. The robot is docked from above the patient, so in the setting of bilateral hernia repairs, undocking and redocking are not required.

To facilitate progression through the operation, the mesh and required sutures are placed in the abdomen through the 12 mm port before docking the robot. As the SI robotic platform requires the camera to be removed and redocked when material is entered through the 12-mm port, we prefer to place the required materials before starting our dissection to minimize operative time. These are placed out of the surgical field but in a place where they can be easily retrieved, such as in the pelvis.

OPERATIVE STEPS
Creation of the Peritoneal Flap

As in the TAPP, we start our dissection by first identifying the medial umbilical ligament, the peritoneum is incised, and the peritoneal flap is created. We dissect in a medial to lateral fashion, ensuring to stay high on the abdominal wall to create a space large enough to incorporate the mesh. The lateral extent of the flap is reached when the position cephalad but corresponding to the ASIS is encountered. The correct dissection plane is the preperitoneal plane. To facilitate dissection in this place, superior traction on the abdominal wall allows for appropriate tension to maintain this plane.

After the peritoneal flap is created, we start our dissection medially at the Cooper ligament. Care must be taken when dissecting here to avoid the corona mortis. Dissection is carried out in a medial to lateral fashion. Medial retraction on the peritoneal flap creates the appropriate tension to facilitate further dissection out laterally. Filmy adhesions are bluntly dissected off the peritoneal flap and dissection is completed once the peritoneum is visualized taking a downward curve toward the retroperitoneum (**Figs. 7** and **8**).

Identification of Cord Structures and Hernia Reduction

Next, we identify the spermatic cord as well as its relation to the hernia sac. In the setting of an indirect hernia, the contents of the cord are carefully dissected bluntly off the hernia sac and the hernia sac is reduced in its entirety. We are careful not to skeletonize the cord but do take down the peritoneal attachments bluntly to ensure there is enough mobility at the base of the peritoneum to hold the mesh. The spermatic cord structures are adequately dissected when they are not tethered to the underlying peritoneum. This can be tested by pulling on the peritoneal flap and ensuring that the cord structures do not move. Direct hernias are most easily reduced by appropriate upward retraction on the transversalis fascia and then downward countertraction on the hernia sac (**Fig. 9**).

Mesh Choice and Placement

Once an adequate peritoneal flap has been created, and the sac has been reduced, the mesh can now be appropriately positioned and secured. As with the laparoscopic TAPP repairs, we use a 12 × 15-cm piece of heavyweight mesh because it is both cost-effective and provides a durable repair. The mesh is secured at midline to the Cooper ligament using a 0-Surgilon interrupted suture. Interrupted sutures are then placed high medially and high laterally for further securement. Care must be taken to avoid the deep inferior epigastric vessels and the iliopubic tract when suturing at the medial and lateral aspects, respectively. The mesh is then inspected to ensure it is secured with appropriate tension and enough medial coverage. Next, the peritoneal

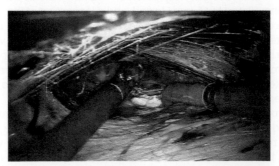

Fig. 7. Medial dissection is carried immediately inferiorly to identify and clear off the Cooper ligament, as seen here in the center.

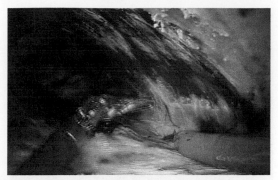

Fig. 8. The peritoneal flap is retracted medial and filmy adhesions are pushed superiorly for the lateral dissection of the peritoneal flap. We can identify we are in the preperitoneal plane by the transverse running muscles of the transversus abdominus.

flap is closed in a lateral to medial running fashion using a 3 to 0 absorbable V-Loc suture. Tears in the peritoneum are fixed at this time as well (**Figs. 10** and **11**).

On completion of closure of the peritoneal flap, all needles are removed under direct visualization, the 8-mm ports are removed under direct visualization, the abdomen is desufflated, and the anterior fascia is closed in a figure of 8 fashion with an 0-Vicryl suture (**Fig. 12**).

At completion of the case, the Foley catheter is removed, and patients are discharged the same day, after voiding in the PACU. Patients are not given any lifting restrictions postoperatively and are normally limited from heavy activity due to pain.

Pearls and Pitfalls

- To facilitate suturing of the mesh in place, trocars should be placed 4 cm above the level of the umbilicus. Optimal distance between trocars is 8 cm.
- We decrease the number of moves by placing all required mesh and sutures in the abdomen before starting our dissection. These can be easily retrieved when needed.
- Care must be taken to ensure to identify the inferior epigastrics when placing the superior medial anchoring stitch to avoid impaling the epigastrics.
- Lateral anchoring sutures must be placed above the iliopubic tract, in order to avoid injuries to the nerves. The iliopubic tract is the lateral border of the triangle of pain.

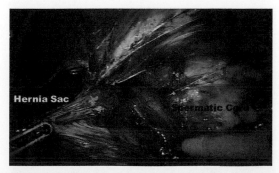

Fig. 9. Medial retraction on the hernia sac facilitates dissection off the cord structures. This is completed bluntly. As you can see, this is an indirect hernia, as it lies lateral to the epigastric vessels, which can be seen superiorly.

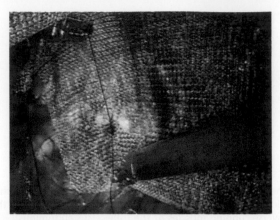

Fig. 10. Medial anchoring of the mesh to the Cooper ligament.

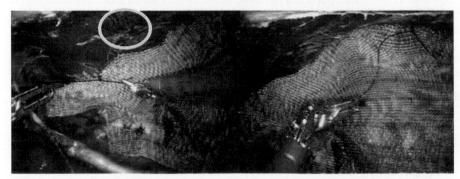

Fig. 11. Superior medial and superior lateral fixation of the mesh. Care must be taken to avoid the inferior epigastric vessels (*circled*) when placing the medial fixation suture.

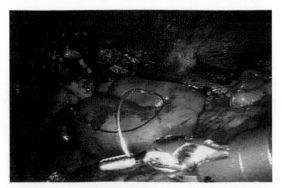

Fig. 12. The peritoneal flap is closed using a running V-Loc suture. Holes made in the peritoneum are also closed at this time.

SUMMARY

Both the TAPP and TEP approaches to inguinal hernias provide an effective means of repairing inguinal hernias. The robotic platform can be used and may help to decrease immediate postoperative pain; however, as this is a fairly new technique, more research will help further determine long-term outcomes. In general, less is more when it comes to anchoring the mesh. In all methods of fixation, we ensure adequate fixation medially with tacks placed on the Cooper ligament. Subsequent tacks are used sparingly, only to ensure mesh lies flat. In general, the biggest pitfall to these operations is inadequate identification of important neurovascular structures. Awareness of the nerves and vessels helps to guide dissection as well as prevent inadvertent injury during mesh fixation.

REFERENCES

1. Barbaro A, Kanhere H, Bessell J, et al. Laparoscopic extraperitoneal repair versus open inguinal hernia repair: 20-year follow up of a randomized controlled trial. Hernia 2017;21:723–7.
2. Neumayer L, Giobbie-Hurder A, Jonasson O, et al. Open mesh versus laparoscopic mesh repair of inguinal hernia. N Engl J Med 2004;350:1819–27.
3. Köckerling F, Bittner R, Jacob DA, et al. TEP versus TAPP: comparison of the perioperative outcome in 17,587 patients with a primary unilateral inguinal hernia. Surg Endosc 2015;29:3750–60.
4. Koning G, de Vries J, Borm G, et al. Health status one year after transinguinal hernia repair and Lichtenstein's method: an analysis alongside a randomized clinical study. Hernia 2013;17:299–306.
5. Belyansky I, Tsirline V, Klima D, et al. Prospective, comparative study of postoperative quality of life in TEP, TAPP and modified Lichetenstein repairs. Ann Surg 2011;254:709–15.
6. Waite K, Herman M, Doyle P. Comparison of robotic versus laparoscopic transabdominal preperitoneal (TAPP) inguinal hernia. J Robot Surg 2016;10:239–44.

Approach to the Patient with Chronic Groin Pain

Q. Lina Hu, MD, David C. Chen, MD*

KEYWORDS

- Chronic pain • Inguinodynia • Chronic postoperative inguinal pain • Inguinal hernia
- Neurectomy

KEY POINTS

- Chronic postoperative inguinal pain has become a primary outcome parameter after elective inguinal hernia repair; hernia recurrence rates have decreased owing to tension-free mesh-based repairs.
- A thorough and systematic preoperative workup is imperative to identifying the most likely cause(s) of pain.
- A multidisciplinary approach to pain management is important, using a combination of behavioral, topical, pharmacologic, and interventional modalities.
- Triple neurectomy is the most widely accepted and effective surgical treatment of neuropathic inguinal pain refractory to conservative measures.
- Hernia recurrence, meshoma, and postherniorrhaphy orchialgia may be addressed in the same operation for triple neurectomy using an open, laparoscopic, or hybrid approach.

INTRODUCTION

Chronic postherniorrhaphy inguinal pain is a potential cause of postoperative morbidity after inguinal hernia repair. For the most part, inguinal hernia repair is a routine procedure with a short period of convalescence and minimal long-term complications.[1] However, given that more than 20 million patients worldwide undergo inguinal hernia surgery annually, any, even rare, long-term complication can be of significant impact.[2] The hernia recurrence rate, which had historically been the most important outcome parameter, has decreased dramatically with the advent of tension-free techniques and the routine use of prosthetic mesh material.[2] Chronic pain, however, remains a persistent challenge and is emerging as arguably the most patient-centered outcome affecting patient productivity, employment, and quality of life.

Chronic postoperative pain is defined as pain that develops after a surgical procedure lasting more than 2 months, excluding other causes of pain.[3] For pain after hernia

Disclosure Statement: The authors have nothing to disclose.
Department of Surgery, University of California at Los Angeles, 757 Westwood Plaza, Los Angeles, CA 90095, USA
* Corresponding author. Lichtenstein Amid Hernia Clinic at UCLA, 1304 15th Street, Suite 102, Santa Monica, CA 90404.
E-mail address: dcchen@mednet.ucla.edu

Surg Clin N Am 98 (2018) 651–665
https://doi.org/10.1016/j.suc.2018.02.002
0039-6109/18/© 2018 Elsevier Inc. All rights reserved.

surgical.theclinics.com

repair, the definition for chronicity is extended to 3 to 6 months to allow postoperative mesh-related inflammatory processes to subside. The reported incidence of postherniorrhaphy pain varies according to the literature owing differing definitions, endpoints, and methodologies from 0% to 63%, but the estimated risk of moderate to severe chronic pain is 10% to 12%, with a smaller percentage (0.5%–6.0%) affecting activities of daily life or employment.[4–7]

PATHOPHYSIOLOGY

The pathophysiology underlying the development of inguinodynia is complex and variable depending on the specific types of pain, including somatic, neuropathic, nociceptive (inflammatory nonneuropathic) and visceral pain. Somatic pain, sometimes referred to as periostitis pubis, is localized to the pubic tubercle and is typically caused by damage to the periosteum of the pubic tubercle from a deep medial anchoring suture.[8] Neuropathic pain is thought to arise from injury to the inguinal nerves resulting in pain in the sensory distribution of the affected nerves. Most commonly, the involved nerves include the ilioinguinal nerve, iliohypogastric nerve, and genital branch of the genitofemoral nerve. With laparoscopic approaches, the femoral branch of the genitofemoral nerve or the lateral femoral cutaneous nerve may also be involved. Rarely, the femoral nerve may be injured with lateral fixation with open repairs or overdissection and penetrating fixation with laparoscopic techniques, leading to motor deficits. The nerve injury can occur intraoperatively or postoperatively, and the mechanisms include indirect or direct structural damage and entrapment injuries, caused by suture or fixation devices, folded mesh or meshoma, or perineural inflammation and scarring.[7,9] Nociceptive pain is the result of tissue injury and the local inflammatory reaction, and is mediated by endogenous inflammatory mediators acting on nociceptors.[9,10] Finally, visceral pain is experienced with intestinal or spermatic cord or other periurethral structure involvement.[7,9] It is, however, important to note that these pain classifications are not discrete categories but exist on a spectrum with extensive overlap, making diagnosis and management a challenging clinical dilemma (**Table 1**).

RISK FACTORS

Young age, female gender, and high preoperative and postoperative pain levels have been identified as risk factors for the development of chronic pain after inguinal hernia repair.[11] One study showed that the results from preoperative pain tests may predict 4% to 54% of the variance in postoperative pain experience and may be helpful in the preoperative stratification of patients into low- and high-risk groups.[12] Psychological and social factors such as depression have been well-demonstrated to contribute to chronic postoperative pain, but have not been well-studied in chronic postherniorrhaphy pain.[13] Genetic research has also identified potential genetic polymorphisms that may contribute to an individual's susceptibility to the generation and experience of pain.[10]

The development of chronic pain is independent of surgical technique. Although there is evidence to suggest that laparoscopic approaches may result in less postoperative pain, the incidence of significant pain equilibrates over time.[5,7,9] Regardless of the specific technique, the careful identification and protection of the inguinal nerves is of utmost importance, and evidence suggests that chronic pain can be reduced to less than 1% with proper handling of the nerves.[6] In terms of the type of mesh material, lightweight mesh in open repairs has been shown to be associated with a lower risk of chronic pain compared with heavy-weight mesh, possibly owing to greater biocompatibility and elasticity.[14] The evidence for mesh fixation techniques is mixed, with some showing potentially decreased pain with glue fixation and others showing a

Table 1
Types of pain, causes, and symptoms

Type of Pain	Potential Causes	Symptoms
Somatic	• Damage to periosteum of pubic tubercle, usually from a deep medial anchoring suture	• Localized to pubic tubercle as area of maximal tenderness
Neuropathic	• Intraoperative or postoperative injury to inguinal nerves	• Pain in the sensory distribution of the inguinal nerves • "Sharp, stabbing, burning, throbbing, shooting, and prickling" • Radiating to scrotum, labium, or upper thigh • Associated with hypoesthesia, hyperesthesia, paresthesia, allodynia, and hyperalgesia • Trigger point with positive Tinel sign • Worse with ambulation, twisting/stretching of upper body, stooping/sitting, hyperextension of hip, and sexual intercourse • Improves with lying down or flexion of hip and thigh
Nociceptive	• Tissue injury and local inflammatory reaction, mediated by endogenous inflammatory mediators acting on nociceptors	• Deep, dull, constant ache • "Gnawing, tender, pounding, pulling" • Localized over the entirety of the groin area or prosthetic • No specific trigger point or radiating component
Visceral	• Injury or involvement of intestinal content, spermatic cord, or other periurethral structures	• Sexual dysfunction/ejaculatory pain • Located at superficial ring or testicular/labial region • Gastrointestinal complaints

Data from Refs.[4,5,7,21,25,35]

similar risk between self-gripping and sutured mesh.[15,16] However, it is reasonable to assert that avoiding excessive application of sutures and tacks is advisable and that atraumatic fixation decreases the potential mechanisms for nerve injury.

With regard to the type of anesthesia, infiltration of anesthesia in the operative field in open repairs has been shown to result in early postoperative pain relief, fewer complications, lower cost, and early recovery and discharge.[17,18] Regional anesthesia is not recommended owing to the greater risk for urinary retention and other rare, but severe, complications inherent to invasive anesthetic technique without documented benefits compared with other forms of anesthesia.[18] General anesthesia may be used in conjunction with local anesthetic, but there are insufficient data to draw firm conclusions.[18]

Finally, although the evidence is mixed, postoperative complications and the need for reoperation have been identified as risk factors predictive of residual pain after hernia surgery.[11,19]

RELEVANT ANATOMY

The neuroanatomy of the groin is complex and highly variable from the retroperitoneal lumbar plexus to the terminal branches exiting through the inguinal canal.[20] An in-depth knowledge of and familiarity with the neuroanatomy of the inguinal region are essential to avoiding nerve injury (**Fig. 1**). The 3 nerves most often implicated are the ilioinguinal nerve, iliohypogastric nerve, and genital branch of the genitofemoral nerve, although the femoral branch of genitofemoral nerve and the lateral femoral cutaneous nerve may also be involved when a laparoscopic or open preperitoneal approach is used.

The ilioinguinal nerve typically enters the inguinal canal medial to the anterior superior iliac spine and travels on the anterior surface of the spermatic cord through the canal. It is covered by an investing fascia derived from the transversalis fascia and the transversus abdominis and internal oblique muscles, which protects the nerve from direct contact with the mesh. Contrary to prior teaching, dissection of the ilioinguinal nerve from the cord is not recommended because disruption of the investing fascia increases the risk of perineural scarring or entrapment by the implanted mesh.

The iliohypogastric nerve enters the inguinal canal medial to the ilioinguinal nerve and travels between the layers of the internal and external oblique muscles, exiting at the cleavage plane between the muscles at the conjoint tendon. It is similarly covered by the investing fascia as it travels over the internal oblique muscle. Approximately 5% of patients do not have a visible iliohypogastric nerve in the inguinal canal because it may run a subaponeurotic course below the internal oblique aponeurosis.[21] This variation is important to note intraoperatively so as to avoid passing suture or fixation material through the internal oblique aponeurosis in the anticipated course of this nerve.

The genital branch of genitofemoral nerve enters the deep inguinal ring and traverses the inguinal canal within the spermatic cord. It is most easily identified by its proximity to the external spermatic vein, which appears as a blue line immediately adjacent to the nerve. Care must be taken when isolating the cord from the inguinal floor to visualize the nerve and maintain its position with the other cord structures. This nerve is covered by the deep cremasteric fascia, which similarly should be kept intact to avoid perineural scarring or contact between the nerve and mesh.

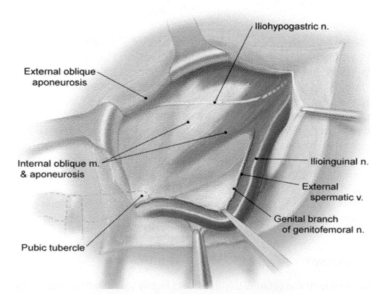

Fig. 1. Inguinal nerve anatomy, anterior view. n., nerve; v., vein.

In addition to the anterior nerves, in the preperitoneal space, the genital and femoral branches of the genitofemoral nerve and the lateral femoral cutaneous nerve may also be encountered (**Fig. 2**). The genitofemoral trunk exits from the lumbar plexus from the nerve roots of L1. The nerve exits the psoas in the retroperitoneum and travels on its anterior surface. The nerve then divides into a genital and a femoral branch, at which point its course becomes more variable. The genital branch usually travels medially to the iliac vessels toward the internal ring and the femoral branch passes lateral under the iliopubic tract toward the anterior thigh. The ilioinguinal and iliohypogastric nerves are not visible in the preperitoneal field, but are at risk of injury with penetrating fixation through the transversalis fascia as they traverse the inguinal canal superficial to the operative field. The lateral femoral cutaneous nerve exits at L3 and passes over the iliacus muscle lateral to the psoas muscle, traveling to the lateral thigh. The femoral nerve trunk traverses in the retroperitoneal space posterolateral to the psoas, and avoidance of lateral fixation especially below the iliopubic tract is essential.

SYMPTOMATOLOGY

The signs and symptoms of chronic postherniorrhaphy pain reflect the variable and overlapping nature of its causes. Somatic pain is usually localized to the pubic tubercle as the area of maximal tenderness. Patients suffering from neuropathic pain often describe pain in the sensory distribution of the inguinal nerves, which can be constant or intermittent, and can be localized or radiating to the scrotum or femoral triangle. The pain is often described as sharp, stabbing, burning, throbbing, shooting, and prickling, and can be associated with other negative sensory phenomena, including reduced sensation (hypoesthesia), increased sensation (hyperesthesia), a burning sensation (paresthesia), pain to a nonpainful stimulus (allodynia), or increased pain response to a painful stimulus (hyperalgesia).[8] Occasionally, a trigger point will reproduce the neuropathic pain symptoms upon palpation. Neuropathic pain is often aggravated by ambulation, stooping or sitting, hyperextension of the hip, or sexual intercourse.[7] Nonneuropathic or nociceptive pain is typically deep, dull, and constant, and may be localized over the entirety of the groin area or the prosthetic. It may be exacerbated by strenuous exercise or position, especially if mesh is involved.[9] Visceral pain is generally related to sexual dysfunction or ejaculatory pain in the region of the superficial ring or the testicular/labial region.[9] It may also manifest as gastrointestinal

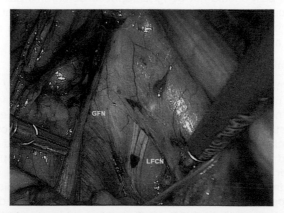

Fig. 2. Preperitoneal neuroanatomy (genitofemoral [GFN] and lateral femoral cutaneous [LFCN] nerves).

complaints if obstruction, adhesions, infection, fistula, or inflammation affect the adjacent viscera.

DIAGNOSIS

The evaluation of a patient with inguinodynia should characterize the type and potential cause of pain. Despite the inclination to suspect chronic postherniorrhaphy pain as the most logical cause, it is crucial to consider the vast breadth of differential diagnoses, including but not limited to surgical, neurologic, infectious, urologic, or gynecologic causes.

A detailed history and review of original operative report can help to determine the likely potential causes and which nerves are at risk based on mechanism and anatomy. Tinel's test can be used to reproduce neuropathic pain by tapping medial to the anterior superior iliac spine or over the area of maximum tenderness. Dermatosensory mapping is a readily available, simple examination that helps to standardize descriptions of neuropathic pain and identify potential nerve involvement. However, owing to overlapping sensory innervations, peripheral communication, and common routes of origin, it is often difficult to distinguish between individual inguinal nerves involved in neuralgic pain.[22,23] In addition to a thorough history and physical examination, the administration of validated pain, function, and quality-of-life instruments may help to delineate the type and severity of pain.

Ultrasound examination is a common initial modality to detect recurrence or meshoma.[24] If ultrasound findings are nondiagnostic, cross-sectional computed tomography scan or MRI of the abdominal wall may be helpful in excluding these pathologies and other differential diagnoses.[25] MRI is currently considered the best valid diagnostic imaging tool for differentiating causes of uncertain inguinal pain, but interpretation is radiologist dependent.[26] Diagnostic and therapeutic local anesthetic block can help to identify ilioinguinal, iliohypogastric, and/or genitofemoral neuralgia. When the results of nerve blocks are equivocal, needle electromyogram and magnetic resonance neurography may provide additional information.[27–29]

TREATMENT

Most patients with postoperative inguinodynia will experience symptom improvement with time, requiring only expectant management and conservative measures. However, postoperative pain should not be ignored, because chronic pain develops from persistence of acute pain and may not be reversible once centralization occurs. The management of chronic postherniorrhaphy pain is complex and a multimodal and multidisciplinary approach is advised (**Box 1**).

Noninterventional Pain Management

In terms of pharmacologic treatment, nonsteroidal antiinflammatory drugs and steroids have been used with some degree of success, especially in inflammatory nociceptive pain and nerve entrapment secondary to inflammation and edema. However, it is usually not sustainable to use these medications in the long term owing to side effects. First-line pharmacologic treatment for chronic pain includes γ-aminobutyric acid analogs and antidepressants such as selective serotonin-norepinephrine reuptake inhibitors or tricyclic antidepressants. Opioids and tramadol are considered second-line treatment alternatives, but may be used during episodic exacerbations of severe neuropathic pain or during titration of other first-line medications. In the case of failure of, or contraindication to, first- and second-line treatments, a few other medications can be considered, including selective serotonin reuptake inhibitors,

---

Box 1
Nonsurgical treatment options

Pharmacologic

First line
γ-Aminobutyric acid analogs (gabapentin, pregabalin)
Selective serotonin-norepinephrine reuptake inhibitors
Tricyclic antidepressants

Second line
Opioids
Tramadol

Third line
Other medications
Selective serotonin reuptake inhibitors
Bupropion
Cannabinoids
Anticonvulsants
Dextromethorphan
Memantine
Clonidine or mexiletine

Topical

Lidocaine

Capsaicin

Nonpharmacologic

Physiotherapy

Acupuncture

Mind–body therapy

Interventional

Inguinal nerve blocks

Neuroablation techniques

Neuromodulation techniques

Data from Refs.[30–35]

---

bupropion, cannabinoids, anticonvulsants, dextromethorphan, memantine, clonidine, or mexiletine. However, data regarding their efficacy in the treatment of neuropathic pain are meager or conflicting.

There are no specific studies evaluating nonpharmacologic treatment such as physiotherapy, acupuncture, and mind–body therapies, but these techniques have been shown to improve pain after surgery and other chronic pain conditions.[30] Given the relatively small anatomic area of inguinodynia, topical medications such as lidocaine or capsaicin patches can sometimes be used. However, they usually do not absorb far enough to treat the underlying condition. Thus, based on the high cost of repeated applications and scarce evidence, topical medications are recommended to be used only as adjunctive treatment or when the patient's comorbidities complicate use of the first-line alternatives.[31–34]

Interventional Pain Management

Nerve blocks of the inguinal nerves can be both diagnostic and therapeutic. They may be used preoperatively to select for patients who may respond favorably to surgical neurectomy. Historically, these nerve blocks were performed using only anatomic landmarks as guidance for needle placement. However, recent advances in ultrasound imaging have allowed for nerve blocks under direct visualization, which have reduced the risk of intraperitoneal needle placement and small volume injections. Neuroablative techniques, such as chemical neurolysis, cryoablation, and pulsed radiofrequency ablation, can be used when nerve blocks provided significant but temporary pain relief.[26] Finally, neuromodulation techniques, either peripheral nerve field stimulation, spinal cord stimulation, or dorsal root ganglion stimulation may be considered when other modalities such as pharmacologic, interventional, and surgical measures have failed.[35] Multiple case reports or case series have shown promising results; however, stringent and careful patient selection is critical.

Surgical Pain Management

Patients with chronic pain refractory to pharmacologic and interventional treatment modalities may be considered for surgical intervention. However, it is important to note that the failure of conservative measures in and of itself is not an indication for surgery. In general, surgical treatment is not recommended until at least 6 months to 1 year after the initial hernia repair.[6,36]

Successful operative outcomes depend on choosing patients with potentially remediable causes of pain, such as recurrence, meshoma, foreign body sensation, neuropathic pain, or orchialgia.[36] A systematic and thorough preoperative evaluation to identify the specific etiologies of pain is imperative. Overt or occult hernia recurrence is important to rule out and should be addressed when identified. Meshoma identified clinically or radiographically may improve with meshectomy. Neuropathic pain isolated to the inguinal distribution, not present before the initial operation, and responsive to diagnostic nerve blocks, has the highest likelihood to improve with surgery. Finally, coexisting orchialgia can potentially be addressed with neurectomy of autonomic nerves investing the vas deferens.

The goal of remedial surgery is to simultaneously address all likely causes to prevent subsequent risk and difficulty of reoperation while balancing this against the potential morbidity of surgery. Isolated selective inguinal nerve neurolysis or neurectomy, removal of mesh and fixation material, and revision of the prior herniorrhaphy are common but, in general, less effective options of treatment owing to ultrastructural changes of the nerve fibers, anatomic variations and cross-innervation of the inguinal nerves, and coexisting causes of pain.[6]

Triple neurectomy of the ilioinguinal, iliohypogastric, and genitofemoral nerves, pioneered in our institute in 1995, is currently a universally accepted surgical treatment for neuropathic pain refractory to conservative measures and is arguably the most effective option.[6] Operative neurectomy in conjunction with removal of meshoma, when present, provides effective relief in the majority of patients with refractory inguinodynia.[6]

Risks of surgery

Operative remediation of inguinodynia is not a benign intervention, and it is critical to discuss the potential benefits, risks, and consequences of surgery to appropriately manage patient expectations. In addition to the usual operative risks, specific considerations include permanent numbness, deafferentation hypersensitivity, inability to access or identify 3 inguinal nerves, abdominal wall laxity from partial denervation of the oblique muscles with retroperitoneal neurectomy, numbness in the labia in females that can interfere with sexual sensation, and testicular atrophy and loss of a cremasteric reflex in male patients. Risks related to reoperation in a scarred field include bleeding, disruption of the prior hernia repair, vascular injury, and testicular loss.

Finally, there is the potential for ongoing pain and disability despite successful neurectomy owing to the nociceptive component of pain, neuroplasticity, afferent hypersensitivity, and centralization of pain.

Surgical Technique

Open triple neurectomy and groin exploration

Triple neurectomy involves resecting segments of the ilioinguinal nerve, iliohypogastric nerve, and genital branch of the genitofemoral nerve from a point proximal to the original surgical field to the most distal accessible point, and can be performed through an open or laparoscopic approach. In the open technique, the standard inguinal incision is used for surgical exposure, which may be the same incision as the original repair. Extending the incision more cephalad and lateral facilitates the exposure of the proximal portions of the ilioinguinal and iliohypogastric nerves and allows for access to the inguinal canal proximal to the scarred mesh and operative field.

The ilioinguinal nerve can be identified lateral to the internal ring, between the ring and the anterior superior iliac spine. The iliohypogastric nerve is identified within the anatomic cleavage plane between the external and internal oblique aponeurosis. It is then traced proximally within the fibers of the internal oblique muscle to a point proximal to the field of the original hernia repair (**Fig. 3**). If the nerve has a subaponeurotic course, the internal oblique aponeurosis is split to visualize the hidden portion. The inguinal segment of the genital branch of the genitofemoral nerve can be identified adjacent to the external spermatic vein along the cord or within the internal ring through the lateral crus of the ring. The nerves should be resected proximal to the field of original hernia repair. The cut ends of all 3 nerves should be ligated to avoid neuroma formation and buried into the muscle to protect the nerve stump from future scarring of the operative field.

The disadvantages of the open anterior approach are its complexity and technical difficulty operating within a scarred surgical field, placing the spermatic cord and vascular structures at greater risk of compromise. However, the advantage of this technique is that it allows for the possibility of a single stage for triple neurectomy as well as surgical correction for other coexisting causes of pain, such as recurrence or meshoma (**Fig. 4**). Occasionally, testicular pain owing to postherniorrhaphy orchialgia accompanies inguinodynia and must be distinguished from the scrotal pain

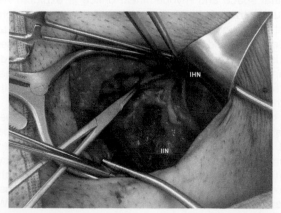

Fig. 3. Open inguinal neurectomy and mesh removal. IHN, iliohypogastric nerves IIN, ilioinguinal nerve.

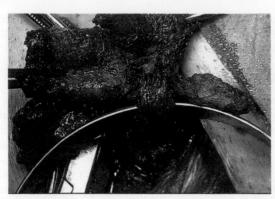

Fig. 4. Open meshectomy with cord preservation.

seen in genital neuralgia in inguinodynia. If true orchialgia exists, triple neurectomy alone is insufficient to alleviate pain. Postherniorrhaphy orchialgia is likely caused by neuropathy of the paravasal nerve fibers originating from the deep pelvic plexus and the autonomic fibers that accompany the cord structures, and may be treated with segmental resection of the lamina propria of the vas deferens. This procedure has been successful, but these results are less predictable and consistent.[19]

Endoscopic groin exploration

In the recent decades, preperitoneal repairs of inguinal hernia have become ubiquitous. However, inguinodynia that arises after these repairs poses a more complex challenge because the repairs can cross both the anterior and posterior planes. Nerve, vas deferens, and spermatic cord injuries associated with these operations are often too proximal to be addressed from an open anterior approach. In these situations, an endoscopic approach, either retroperitoneal or transabdominal, offers a desirable alternative.

The first step of endoscopic groin exploration is diagnostic laparoscopy, because it allows for the assessment of the presence of recurrent hernias, interstitial hernias, mesh migration, and intraabdominal adhesions that could be potentially contributing to the patient's symptoms. If any offending tacks or fixation devices are identified, they can be removed from the intraperitoneal space without violating the preperitoneal space.

The preperitoneal space and myopectineal orifice is explored next and can be approached through a transabdominal or totally extraperitoneal approach. The myopectineal orifice should be assessed for recurrence, retained lipoma, and mesh migration. The peritoneal flap should be separated from the mesh and preserved if possible.

If a recurrence is identified and the mesh is otherwise flat, a larger dissection space may be created and additional mesh can be placed, leaving the original mesh in place. Alternatively, the recurrence may be addressed with an anterior modified Lichtenstein repair, avoiding the preperitoneal plane altogether.

If a meshoma is identified after an initial repair by isolated preperitoneal laparoscopic mesh (total extraperitoneal, transabdominal preperitoneal), open preperitoneal mesh placement (transinguinal preperitoneal technique, Kugel, transrectus sheath extraperitoneal procedure), or plug technique, the mesh removal may sometimes be accomplished entirely through a laparoscopic approach (**Fig. 5**). Meshoma is typically scarred, fixated, or contracted around the epigastric and iliac vessels or the cord structures and can sometimes be adherent to the bladder as well. When separation from these structures is difficult, it is often prudent to leave a small cuff of mesh behind to minimize injuries. Meshoma pain is usually related to the amount of mesh present,

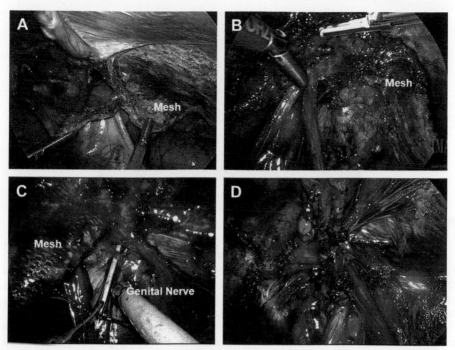

Fig. 5. (*A*) Superior approach to mesh and the myopectineal orifice. (*B*) Inferior approach to mesh and the myopectineal orifice. (*C*) Simultaneous genital neurectomy. (*D*) Preperitoneal mesh removed with small rim of mesh left on cord structures.

its 3-dimensional configuration, and bulk. Reduction in the mass of meshoma can potentially be sufficient to alleviate symptoms.

Neurectomy of the genitofemoral and lateral femoral cutaneous nerves may be performed to address the neuropathic pain component of the patient's symptoms. The genital and femoral branches of the genitofemoral nerve may be identified over the psoas and iliac vessels as they pass toward the internal ring and iliopubic tract. The lateral femoral cutaneous nerve can be identified lateral to the psoas passing over the iliacus muscle toward the lateral thigh. Neurectomy of these 2 nerves may be safely and effectively performed with minimal morbidity in this location (see **Fig. 5C**).

As in the open technique, neurectomy in of itself will not address orchialgia. Laparoscopic paravasal neurectomy may be accomplished by taking the autonomic nerve fibers in the tissue between the skeletonized vas and spermatic vessels proximal to the injury and scarring (**Fig. 6**).

Endoscopic retroperitoneal triple neurectomy
As in the open technique, the goal of laparoscopic triple neurectomy is to resect the ilioinguinal nerve, iliohypogastric nerve, and genital branch of the genitofemoral nerve. The retroperitoneal approach is advantageous over the open approach because it allows nerve resection proximal to any potential sites of neuropathy and the neuroanatomy of the inguinal nerves is less variable in this region. However, resecting the main trunks of these nerves also increases the distribution of numbness and may cause some oblique muscle denervation and bulging. The patient should be placed in the lateral decubitus position and the table flexed to open the space between the iliac crest and costal margin.

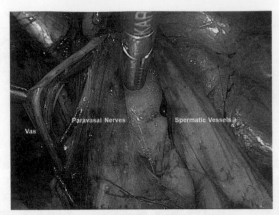

Fig. 6. Paravasal autonomic nerves enveloping the vas deferens.

The lumbar plexus should be defined before any neurectomy is performed. The iliohypogastric and ilioinguinal nerves frequently share a common trunk and can be seen overlying the quadratus muscle at L1 (**Fig. 7**A). They can be resected over the quadratus muscle. We recommend placing a clip proximally and distally to close the neurilemma and to identify the location in case future blocks are needed.

The dissection is then continued toward the groin where the genitofemoral nerve trunk can be identified running over the psoas muscle (see **Fig. 7**B). It is resected over the psoas in the same fashion. If in the preoperative evaluation the dermatomal

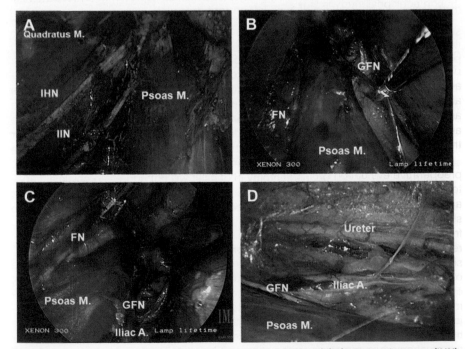

Fig. 7. (A) Cephalad view of retroperitoneal ilioinguinal (IIN) and iliohypogastric nerves (IHN). (B) Caudal view with genitofemoral nerve (GFN) isolated. (C) Lateral view with femoral nerve (FN) identified. (D) View of GFN with iliac and ureter. A., artery; M., muscle.

distribution of the femoral branch of the genitofemoral nerve is not affected, the separate femoral trunk should be identified and preserved if possible.

The lateral femoral cutaneous nerve originates at L3 and is identified lateral to the psoas, crossing the iliacus muscle below the iliac crest. This may be sacrificed with isolated lateral femoral cutaneous nerve neuropathies seen with penetrating fixation and overdissection. The femoral nerve can also be found lateral and deep to the psoas muscle, but does not require specific dissection (see **Fig. 7**C). Of note, the ureter and iliac vessels should be identified medial to the psoas and protected (see **Fig. 7**D).

CLINICAL OUTCOMES

Triple neurectomy was first described by our institute in 1995. Our experience has included more than 800 patients using an open approach and 90 cases using a laparoscopic retroperitoneal approach. Since 2004, we have incorporated resection of the intramuscular segment of the iliohypogastric nerve as described in this article. With this technique, we are now able to achieve satisfactory resolution of postherniorrhaphy inguinodynia in more than 95% of patient whose original repair did not enter the preperitoneal space. Before this modification, only the extramuscular portion of the nerve was resected with an associated success of 85%.[21]

In patients with inguinodynia after preperitoneal mesh repairs, we have performed open extended triple neurectomy including main trunk of the genitofemoral nerve with a greater than 90% success rate in this highly selected cohort. In patients with coexisting orchialgia, we have additionally combined paravasal neurectomy with neurectomy. In our experience with 24 patients, orchialgia was resolved in 83% of patients. These limited series demonstrate safety and efficacy for both procedures, though additional study is indicated before they become standard practice.

SUMMARY

Chronic postherniorrhaphy pain is a significant problem with consequences affecting patient productivity, employment, and quality of life. Currently, there is no universally accepted definition, etiology, classification, or surgical management and best available recommendations are derived from case reports, case series, expert opinion, and expert consensus. In-depth knowledge of the inguinal neuroanatomy is crucial, and meticulous identification, preservation, and pragmatic neurectomy can prevent this disabling complication.

In approaching a patient with chronic inguinodynia, a systematic and thorough preoperative evaluation is crucial to identify the etiologies and types of pain. Owing to the complex nature of chronic pain, a multimodal and multidisciplinary treatment approach is necessary. Pharmacologic and interventional modalities have been shown to be efficacious in the management of pain. Patients with chronic pain refractory to conservative measures after 6 months to 1 year after the initial hernia repair may be considered for surgical intervention. Operative remediation aims to simultaneously address all likely causes to prevent subsequent risk and difficulty of reoperation. Triple neurectomy remains the most definitive and accepted remedial operation performed and when performed in conjunction with the removal of meshoma or paravasal neurectomy, when indicated, provides effective relief in majority of patients with refractory inguinodynia. Outcomes are highly dependent on patient selection, and a logical plan of care must be tailored for each patient based on the mechanism, symptoms, anatomy, and technical considerations. Prevention is by far the most important and effective means of preventing inguinodynia and improving patient outcomes.

REFERENCES

1. Bay-Nielsen M, Thomsen H, Andersen FH, et al. Convalescence after inguinal herniorrhaphy. Br J Surg 2004;91(3):362–7.
2. Bittner R, Schwarz J. Inguinal hernia repair: current surgical techniques. Langenbecks Arch Surg 2012;397(2):271–82.
3. Macrae WA, Davies HT. Chronic postsurgical pain. In: Crombie IK, LS, Croft P, et al, editors. Epidemiology of pain. Seattle (WA): IASP Press; 1999. p. 125–42.
4. Nienhuijs S, Staal E, Strobbe L, et al. Chronic pain after mesh repair of inguinal hernia: a systematic review. Am J Surg 2007;194(3):394–400.
5. Aasvang E, Kehlet H. Chronic postoperative pain: the case of inguinal herniorrhaphy. Br J Anaesth 2005;95(1):69–76.
6. Alfieri S, Amid PK, Campanelli G, et al. International guidelines for prevention and management of post-operative chronic pain following inguinal hernia surgery. Hernia 2011;15(3):239–49.
7. Poobalan AS, Bruce J, Smith WC, et al. A review of chronic pain after inguinal herniorrhaphy. Clin J Pain 2003;19(1):48–54.
8. Cunningham J, Temple WJ, Mitchell P, et al. Cooperative hernia study. Pain in the postrepair patient. Ann Surg 1996;224(5):598–602.
9. Hakeem A, Shanmugam V. Current trends in the diagnosis and management of post-herniorraphy chronic groin pain. World J Gastrointest Surg 2011;3(6):73–81.
10. Kehlet H, Jensen TS, Woolf CJ. Persistent postsurgical pain: risk factors and prevention. Lancet 2006;367(9522):1618–25.
11. Kalliomaki ML, Meyerson J, Gunnarsson U, et al. Long-term pain after inguinal hernia repair in a population-based cohort; risk factors and interference with daily activities. Eur J Pain 2008;12(2):214–25.
12. Werner MU, Mjobo HN, Nielsen PR, et al. Prediction of postoperative pain: a systematic review of predictive experimental pain studies. Anesthesiology 2010; 112(6):1494–502.
13. Hinrichs-Rocker A, Schulz K, Jarvinen I, et al. Psychosocial predictors and correlates for chronic post-surgical pain (CPSP) - a systematic review. Eur J Pain 2009; 13(7):719–30.
14. Sajid MS, Kalra L, Parampalli U, et al. A systematic review and meta-analysis evaluating the effectiveness of lightweight mesh against heavyweight mesh in influencing the incidence of chronic groin pain following laparoscopic inguinal hernia repair. Am J Surg 2013;205(6):726–36.
15. de Goede B, Klitsie PJ, van Kempen BJ, et al. Meta-analysis of glue versus sutured mesh fixation for Lichtenstein inguinal hernia repair. Br J Surg 2013; 100(6):735–42.
16. Zhang C, Li F, Zhang H, et al. Self-gripping versus sutured mesh for inguinal hernia repair: a systematic review and meta-analysis of current literature. J Surg Res 2013;185(2):653–60.
17. Nordin P, Zetterstrom H, Gunnarsson U, et al. Local, regional, or general anaesthesia in groin hernia repair: multicentre randomised trial. Lancet 2003;362(9387):853–8.
18. Kehlet H, Aasvang E. Groin hernia repair: anesthesia. World J Surg 2005;29(8): 1058–61.
19. Franneby U, Sandblom G, Nordin P, et al. Risk factors for long-term pain after hernia surgery. Ann Surg 2006;244(2):212–9.
20. Rab M, Ebmer And J, Dellon AL. Anatomic variability of the ilioinguinal and genitofemoral nerve: implications for the treatment of groin pain. Plast Reconstr Surg 2001;108(6):1618–23.

21. Amid PK, Hiatt JR. New understanding of the causes and surgical treatment of postherniorrhaphy inguinodynia and orchalgia. J Am Coll Surg 2007;205(2): 381–5.
22. Harms BA, DeHaas DR Jr, Starling JR. Diagnosis and management of genitofemoral neuralgia. Arch Surg 1984;119(3):339–41.
23. Starling JR, Harms BA. Diagnosis and treatment of genitofemoral and ilioinguinal neuralgia. World J Surg 1989;13(5):586–91.
24. Bradley M, Morgan D, Pentlow B, et al. The groin hernia - an ultrasound diagnosis? Ann R Coll Surg Engl 2003;85(3):178–80.
25. Ferzli GS, Edwards ED, Khoury GE. Chronic pain after inguinal herniorrhaphy. J Am Coll Surg 2007;205(2):333–41.
26. Aasvang EK, Jensen KE, Fiirgaard B, et al. MRI and pathology in persistent postherniotomy pain. J Am Coll Surg 2009;208(6):1023–8 [discussion: 1028–9].
27. Knockaert DC, Boonen AL, Bruyninckx FL, et al. Electromyographic findings in ilioinguinal-iliohypogastric nerve entrapment syndrome. Acta Clin Belg 1996; 51(3):156–60.
28. Ellis RB, Ceisse H, Holub BA, et al. Ilioinguinal nerve conduction. Muscle Nerve 1992;(15):1195.
29. Filler A. Magnetic resonance neurography and diffusion tensor imaging: origins, history, and clinical impact of the first 50,000 cases with an assessment of efficacy and utility in a prospective 5000-patient study group. Neurosurgery 2009; 65(4 Suppl):A29–43.
30. Bushnell MC, Ceko M, Low LA. Cognitive and emotional control of pain and its disruption in chronic pain. Nat Rev Neurosci 2013;14(7):502–11.
31. Garnock-Jones KP, Keating GM. Lidocaine 5% medicated plaster: a review of its use in postherpetic neuralgia. Drugs 2009;69(15):2149–65.
32. Bischoff JM, Petersen M, Uceyler N, et al. Lidocaine patch (5%) in treatment of persistent inguinal postherniorrhaphy pain: a randomized, double-blind, placebo-controlled, crossover trial. Anesthesiology 2013;119(6):1444–52.
33. Derry S, Sven-Rice A, Cole P, et al. Topical capsaicin (high concentration) for chronic neuropathic pain in adults. Cochrane Database Syst Rev 2013;(2):CD007393.
34. Mick G, Correa-Illanes G. Topical pain management with the 5% lidocaine medicated plaster–a review. Curr Med Res Opin 2012;28(6):937–51.
35. Bjurstrom MF, Nicol AL, Amid PK, et al. Pain control following inguinal herniorrhaphy: current perspectives. J Pain Res 2014;7:277–90.
36. Aasvang E, Kehlet H. Surgical management of chronic pain after inguinal hernia repair. Br J Surg 2005;92(7):795–801.

Moving?

Make sure your subscription moves with you!

To notify us of your new address, find your **Clinics Account Number** (located on your mailing label above your name), and contact customer service at:

Email: journalscustomerservice-usa@elsevier.com

800-654-2452 (subscribers in the U.S. & Canada)
314-447-8871 (subscribers outside of the U.S. & Canada)

Fax number: 314-447-8029

Elsevier Health Sciences Division
Subscription Customer Service
3251 Riverport Lane
Maryland Heights, MO 63043

*To ensure uninterrupted delivery of your subscription, please notify us at least 4 weeks in advance of move.

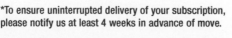

Printed and bound by CPI Group (UK) Ltd, Croydon, CR0 4YY

07/10/2024

01040502-0009